Mastering

₹ole

ators

RN, BC

 F. A. DAVIS COMPANY • Philadelphia

F.A. Davis Company
1915 Arch Street
Philadelphia, PA 19103
www.fadavis.com

Printed in the United States of America

Last digit indicates print number: 10 9 8 7 6 5 4 3 2 1

Publisher: Joanne Patzek DaCunha, RN, MSN
Developmental Editor: Kristin L. Kern
Manager of Art and Design: Carolyn O'Brien

As new scientific information becomes available through basic and clinical research, recommended treatments and drug therapies undergo changes. The author(s) and publisher have done everything possible to make this book accurate, up to date, and in accord with accepted standards at the time of publication. The author(s), editors, and publisher are not responsible for errors or omissions or for consequences from application of the book, and make no warranty, expressed or implied, in regard to the contents of the book. Any practice described in this book should be applied by the reader in accordance with professional standards of care used in regard to the unique circumstances that may apply in each situation. The reader is advised always to check product information (package inserts) for changes and new information regarding dose and contraindications before administering any drug. Caution is especially urged when using new or infrequently ordered drugs.

Library of Congress Cataloging-in-Publication Data

Mastering the teaching role : a guide for nurse educators / [edited by] Barbara K. Penn.
    p. ; cm.
  Includes bibliographical references and index.
  ISBN 978-0-8036-1823-7 (pbk. : alk. paper)
  1. Nursing—Study and teaching. I. Penn, Barbara K.
  [DNLM: 1. Education, Nursing—methods. 2. Educational Measurement—methods. 3. Faculty—standards. 4. Planning Techniques. 5. Students, Nursing—psychology. 6. Teaching—methods. WY 18 M4233 2009]
  RT71.M35 2009
  610.73071'1—dc22
                                                                    2007039734

Foreword

Becoming an effective teacher, like becoming an effective parent, is not necessarily an innate skill in everyone. Granted, some people have stronger instincts toward teaching, but most of us benefit from learning, being mentored, and practicing the teaching role. Education for students is far more than merely learning information. It is learning how to think, act, problem-solve, and develop team-working skills and knowing one's own skills and areas for improvements.

For faculty to be useful guides, mentors, and role models, they, like their students, benefit from learning about how people learn, the skills and techniques of contemporary instruction, including both classroom and clinical, and the important tools of evaluating learner attainment of the instructional goals.

In 1987, Chickering and Gamson[1] outlined seven principles for good teaching in undergraduate education. These principles state that good teaching:

1. encourages contact between students and faculty;
2. develops reciprocity and cooperation among students;
3. encourages active learning;
4. gives prompt feedback;
5. emphasizes time on task;
6. communicates high expectations; and
7. respects diverse talents and ways of learning (p. 121).

Now, more than two decades later, these principles remain a useful framework when considering teaching for nurse educators because they acknowledge the roles played by both students and faculty in the learning exchange. It is the responsibility of the faculty member to provide content for the

---

[1] http://www.mnsu.edu/cetl/teachingresources/frg-2005-06.pdf#page=120; Chickering, A. and Gamson, Z. (1987, March). Seven principles for good practice in undergraduate education. *AAHE Bull.*

student, but these principles acknowledge that more should be done in order to provide a classroom environment conducive for learning; for example, communicating high expectations. That is not to say that students do not have any responsibility in the exchange; they are much more than a vessel to be filled with knowledge. Students must also recognize their duties as active learners and be open to interacting with faculty as well as their peers in order to have a rich learning experience.

Effective teaching in nursing is critical to the field for many reasons. The first, and most obvious, reason is that teaching is the avenue used to prepare future nurses. Through classroom and clinical instruction, students learn the skills and nuances of nursing practice and apply what they have learned directly to their work with patients. Effective teaching does more than transfer information. It teaches students how to think critically and creatively in order to handle a situation, which in some cases is the most valuable lesson a student can learn.

Another reason that teaching is important to nursing is the fact that it is a precious commodity. The faculty shortage has illuminated the number one challenge faced by nursing schools, and some are surprised to learn that it is not a lack of students who want to be taught—it is a lack of professionals to teach them. Through their effective teaching and contributing, faculty members model the life of an academic for students and make it an attractive possibility for those who love to teach. In this sense, teachers beget teachers, which is the single best way to address the faculty shortage.

A final reason that teaching in nursing is significant is that it affects patient care. The lessons taught in the classroom about best practices in nursing become a reality when implemented in a health-care setting. Through effective teaching, nurses learn how to use technology that can save lives, communication techniques essential to the interpersonal work of teams, and an ethic of care that is at the heart of the profession. Patients benefit from the teaching done in today's classrooms, and those benefits will be felt for years to come.

Further, essential to mastering the role of teacher is understanding the scope of what may be called "academic citizenship."

That is, what are the expectations of a faculty person to understand the norms, values, and goals of the unique institution in which he or she works? We think these are key expectations and often not taught or role modeled. This text brings to faculty the tools for effective role implementation. Chapters are written by those considered as good at what they do and who willingly share with others what they have learned. We hope using this text will help you grow in your teaching role.

JEANETTE LANCASTER, PhD, RN, FAAN
PRESIDENT, AMERICAN ASSOCIATION OF
COLLEGES OF NURSING

FAY RAINES, PhD, RN
PRESIDENT-ELECT, AMERICAN ASSOCIATION OF
COLLEGES OF NURSING

GERALDINE (POLLY) BEDNASH, PhD, RN, FAAN
EXECUTIVE DIRECTOR, AMERICAN ASSOCIATION OF
COLLEGES OF NURSING

Contents

SECTION III

Clinical Teaching 177

SECTION IV

SECTION V

SECTION VI

Introduction

I'm so glad you are considering or recently made the important career choice to be a nurse educator, or maybe you have been teaching for some time and want to improve your educational practice. Regardless of your length or degree of experience, the nursing profession needs strong educators. I welcome you as faculty colleagues and applaud your desire to master this important role. You are probably aware that our country's nursing programs must prepare hundreds of thousands more nurses to meet the shortage in the next decade or so, and qualified faculty members are central to this important task. Thousands of teachers in hundreds of schools of nursing across the country are currently engaged in the important business of educating nurses, and many more faculty members will be needed in the next few years as current ones retire. If you have been teaching a while, you may want more information about a particular aspect of the faculty role, but your colleagues may assume that, because you're experienced, you "know it all." If you're new to the faculty role, your colleagues will welcome you, but they simply may not be able to give you as detailed or individualized an orientation to the role that they and you would prefer.

That's why this book was written—to offer you some guidance as you refine your established educational practice or move into a new role. If you are an experienced nurse educator, you may have mastered the basics and now want to shake up what you've been doing, be more effective, consider some new approaches, investigate an unfamiliar aspect of the faculty role, or become more active in planning your academic career. If you're a new faculty member, this whole transition may seem a bit daunting. As experienced teachers can confirm, beginning in the nursing faculty role can be intimidating. It's not just about presenting a class or supervising students in clinical (which can be anxiety-producing enough). New faculty members will find that there are several distinct aspects to the faculty role: many unfamiliar educational concepts, issues, and tasks to learn; a new higher education setting and culture to understand; and a great deal of nuance to grasp—insights and "lore" that can't always be passed on by experienced people to new teachers in the fast-paced educational environment. You are probably an expert clinician—the first criterion for good teaching—and you may be a natural teacher. However, the full faculty role, like any other, must be learned. But be patient with yourself. It takes *years* to become an expert teacher, to be a catalyst for active learning, to demonstrate intuitive grasp of higher education issues and teaching-learning of adults, and to become expert in one or more aspects of teaching nursing.

It is my hope that this book will offer a comprehensive look at the breadth of issues you'll need to consider as part of the faculty role. However, the book is not exhaustive. Each chapter is intended to be a primer on a topic, to get you started in understanding the ideas and applying them to your educational practice. Most chapters offer references and resources that will help you explore the topic further as you progress in the faculty role. The book is intended for nursing faculty in higher education settings but will be a useful guide for educators in any type of nursing education program.

I have been very fortunate throughout my educational career to have had exceptional colleagues and supervisors who have contributed to my professional development. Over the years, I have benefited from conversations with educators across the country who answered important, timely questions that enabled me to proceed with my immediate work. Or they offered different ways to think about an issue or approach that stayed with me, crystallized over time, and became part of who I am as an educator. In a sense, I'm hoping to capture these types of conversations for your benefit; thus the question-and-answer format of this book. Chapters are meant to mimic conversations you might have with an expert on any number of topics important to nursing faculty. So, enjoy your dialogues with these experienced faculty colleagues from around the country. They offer excellent ideas that will help you formulate or improve your approach to the nursing faculty role. Thank you for choosing to teach nursing. You will literally shape the future of our profession.

BARBARA PENN, PhD, RN, BC
JANUARY 2008

PERSPECTIVES ON ADULTS AS LEARNERS

1

How Adults Learn

Barbara K. Penn, PhD, RN, BC

---

1 Why is it such a big deal to think about adults learning differently than children?

Think of children sitting in neat rows in a classroom, with the teacher at the front of the room serving as the primary source of information. These students, who generally have limited experience with the subject, rely on the teacher to provide content, set the pace, and direct all learning activities. In contrast, adults come to learning with a wealth of life experiences, some knowledge about the topic, and expectations that their specific learning needs will be met so they can apply their learning immediately in practical ways to solve real-life problems. In a real sense, they are consumers, looking to you to provide a service (teaching) and a product (information), and they want to have input to what they are getting.

---

2 What are adults seeking in an educational experience?

Most adults have very definite ideas about what and how they learn, and they seek practical applications. But they are not completely independent learners; they need your expert guidance—to understand the importance of what they are learning, to learn the norms of the profession, and to navigate the educational experience successfully. And underneath it all, they need to know the learning experience is relevant and helping them achieve what they have set out to do.

---

3   Is there a particular theorist who is associated with adult learning?

Over 50 years ago, Malcolm Knowles was one of the first educators to devote significant time and energy to describing this unique population of learners and recommending specific strategies to teachers of adults. He popularized the concept of "andragogy," the study of teaching adults, and differentiated it from "pedagogy," which literally means the art and science of teaching children (although the term pedagogy is used to describe the study of teaching, even to adults). Although some might argue that Knowles' notion of andragogy is not strictly a theory, Knowles undeniably contributed to an understanding of adults as learners. Many other adult learning thinkers and theorists have continued in this distinct educational specialty area, and the professional literature on adult learning has exploded in recent decades.

Nursing education needs faculty members who are prepared at the graduate level in nursing and who are experts in specialty or advanced nursing knowledge and practice. These skilled clinicians also need to have insight into the characteristics of adult learners, which is pivotal to being able to create positive and rich learning experiences. I urge you to become more familiar with the current thinkers in adult learning to strengthen your teaching practice in nursing.

---

4   What should an adult learner look like?

Although the age range and characteristics of students in higher education are wide, for practical purposes we can consider them all adults. The ideal adult learner is goal-directed and able to manage his or her time and other resources to meet the demands of class and clinical. The student is self-directed, utilizing the instructor as a resource and role model, while taking responsibility for learning and being accountable for behavior. This motivated student is prepared for class or clinical, interested in learning, and actively contributes to discussions and other activities. We see these behaviors fairly consistently in graduate students and more frequently in undergraduate students, who are increasingly older. These students may have their own families and jobs and so are juggling many roles and responsibilities. These aspects of their lives help them be more mature and responsible, but the many demands on their time also may make some students impatient if they do not see practical applications to what they are learning.

---

5   Are adults as open to learning as children?

Yes and no. Adults may be more eager to learn than children if they have an immediate need for the information they are learning. They stay motivated to learn as long as they are mentally stimulated, get useful and frequent feedback from faculty, make progress, gain practical knowledge and skills, and enjoy the process. Conversely, adults tend to be less receptive to learning if their classes or clinical experiences duplicate what they already know or if they believe their time is being wasted. Adults are less willing than children to take risks in the classroom, because they do not want to appear stupid in front of classmates. In my experience, dignity is of paramount importance to adults, and if they feel discounted, disrespected, or embarrassed in the learning environment, they often stop participating.

---

6   I thought I was teaching adults, but I do not always see adult behavior in my students. Why?

We can expect learners to be accountable for their own learning and growth, but we also need to provide guidance to those who do not know how to make this transition to a higher level of behavior. Unfortunately, many adults are products of teacher-directed learning in their K–12 experiences, and they remain passive learners, even in higher education. They may not have been encouraged to develop strong reasoning or problem-solving skills. They may need to take more responsibility for their behavior.

Consequently, it is important that nursing instructors make expectations explicit that students will be prepared for (and attend) class, participate actively, take advantage of various opportunities to learn the required material, and further explore topics of personal interest. Younger students (and even older, less self-confident students) need frequent feedback, specific guidance on how to be a successful learner, and clear deadlines and performance expectations. We may need to encourage them to be more active, but I have found that most adult learners welcome this challenge, even if the approach is unfamiliar or uncomfortable at first.

---

7   How can I increase the self-directedness of my students?

You can gradually give more responsibility to students over the time you work with them. For example, try being very explicit with grading criteria for an early assignment in the course and then less directive in each subsequent assignment, allowing for increasing learner creativity and preferences. Or you can assign research topics or activities early in the course and, as the semester progresses, give learners more choices about what they study or how they demonstrate mastery of the content. You may want to work with faculty colleagues so that as learners progress through the year or the total educational program, there is a planned evolution of student performance expectations requiring gradually less specific faculty guidance. With faculty support, most learners ultimately become less reliant on the teacher for detailed directions, but throughout their educational experience, they will look to you and other faculty members to set the standard and provide expectations.

---

8   Are there certain conditions under which adults learn best?

Absolutely. Teachers of adults need to be aware of these conditions in order to be successful. Adult learners need:

- **Physical comfort.** For example, let students have food or beverages in class if possible. Provide reasonable breaks that allow them to meet personal needs. Rearrange the furniture to encourage face-to-face inter-action and prevent strained necks. Adjust the lighting and temperature if you can.

- **Emotional safety.** Engage students on a personal level so they feel included. Create an environment that makes them feel safe enough to engage in discussion, express opinions, and disagree with classmates and even you. Guide learners how to engage in profession-al dialogue with each other to maximize interaction and minimize hurt feelings. Offer encouragement. Give positive feedback. Be friendly and engaging. These approaches do not diminish you as a respected leader.

- **Active involvement** in what they are learning. Passive receipt of endless lectures is not the best way to keep modern students involved! Several other chapters sug-gest active strategies to keep students mentally stimulat-ed and physically active.

---

9   Should I tell learners what they need to know?

To a certain extent, yes, because you are the expert. You must guide learners to a fuller understanding of any topic you teach. But adults want practical answers to their questions and content that relates to their own lives. They want to be involved with what they are learning, not having you always tell them about it. I use the abbrevia-tion TNT: *Telling is Not Teaching* (Fig. 1–1). Blow up your ideas about telling learners in traditional lectures. Rather, ask thoughtful discussion questions. Draw on experiences students already have with the topic. Emphasize the practical aspects of the content. Involve students in real-life clinical scenarios or case studies. Have them analyze symptoms, laboratory results, pictures, or video clips. Create assignments that allow learners to seek information actively. Encourage animated discus-sion in class. Teaching adults by merely "telling" is rarely successful.

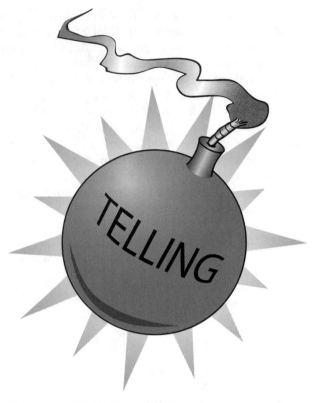

Figure 1–1. TNT: Telling is Not Teaching.

10 If adults are in class to learn about a topic, how can they contribute to discussion?

It is hard to know what experiences students bring to class unless we ask. I almost always have learners in my classes who have very relevant experiences to share, and they enjoy doing so. For example, in a class about responding to emergencies you might ask, "Who has seen or participated in a medical emergency?" You may find that a number of students have assisted at a car accident, been with a relative who had a heart attack, witnessed a near-drowning during a vacation, or have sophisticated experience in resuscitation as an emergency medical technician, firefighter, or nurse. When I solicit the real-life experiences of the learners, it validates their contributions, offers inexperienced students some peer resources, and makes class discussion more powerful and relevant to the group.

---

11 How does learning actually occur, and are there things I can do to facilitate the process?

As a guide, I have included a model of how adults learn (Fig. 1–2). It depicts a relatively linear process based on the cognitive theory of learning. Cognitivism describes learning in terms of mental processes like thinking and remembering and gives teachers good ideas about how to enhance or impede those processes to maximize learning.

---

12 How does the model work?

The left side of the model shows several important early aspects of learning:

- **Environment.** This includes the various stimuli that are available from the environment. Some of these, including some types of light and sound, are not available for humans and so are screened out.

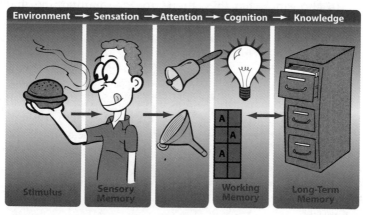

Figure 1–2. How adults learn.

- **Sensation.** What we can see, hear, smell, and feel stays in our consciousness for only seconds and must be processed further in order to be remembered or used. These are subjective events, and most of us can remember what a hamburger feels, smells, and tastes like and may be able to hear it sizzling in our memory. To maximize sensory information, we need to ensure that students *can* see and hear well in our classrooms by closing the door, brightening the lights, reducing glare, or whatever is required.

- **Attention.** The point at which we can begin to affect the learning process is at the funnel in the model. This represents the finite capacity of attention and the individual's need to filter out extraneous distractions (such as the hum of the air conditioner or traffic noise) in order to focus on learning. It also depicts how we as teachers need to minimize distractions. For example, discourage personal conversations, prohibit the use of cell phones, and deliberately direct student attention to the learning activity.

---

13 Why is gaining students' attention so important?

"Attention" refers to a level of psychological and physical arousal and addresses the energy students have to devote to choosing what they attend to and maintaining that attention. This is not just asking the group to settle down before you launch into your lecture or doing a fun "icebreaker." This is using a strategy that gets students *focused on the new content* that will be introduced. This is particularly important in large classes where students may be less active and therefore less attentive. We have all been tired or distracted, so we can identify with students who may not be as efficient at focusing on learning activities at a particular time. But we can still engage these students if we encourage interaction or activity related to the lesson early in the class. If we do not gain students' attention, we probably will not be able to teach them very much.

14 What techniques can I use to gain students' attention?

Remember, this is not just clearing your throat or rapping on the podium. It means actually focusing learners toward the lesson *content*. For example, at the beginning of the class or whenever you introduce a major new subject:

- **Invite students to define a term** or solve a small problem in groups. This is not intended to cover content (that comes later) as much as to introduce a concept and get them involved and more curious about the content to follow.

- **Share a dramatic fact** concerning the topic. You can find something spectacular in almost any subject you are teaching. For example, if you are teaching about a particular disease, give the percentage of the population affected and/or the total dollars spent in the United States on it each year. If you are teaching about a certain drug, give a vivid example of its *mis*use or a life-threatening side effect.

- **Tell a related story** from your professional experience that evokes a vivid mental picture and that learners can imagine as the class progresses. For example, I had a memorable hyperthyroid patient over 30 years ago who refused to stay dressed, tore down window blinds, and complained to the hospital hierarchy. These behaviors were explained by his disease, and when he was treated they all disappeared. Whenever I taught about hyperthyroidism in subsequent years, I told students about this patient's erratic behaviors to get them "hooked" and wanting to know more.

- **Solicit examples** from students who have had direct experience with the pending content, and ask for their impressions of that experience. Do they have experience with a disease or procedure? Do they have stories of their own about the topic? This strategy not only introduces content but also respects student experiences, an important way to increase their participation and provide learners insights about the topic other than yours.

- **Ask questions about the content** that you are fairly sure the students do not yet know but will at the end of the class. This is not a formal pretest, which is stressful and counterproductive, but more like a game, maybe even with small prizes. The purpose is to make them aware of the gap between what they know and what they need to know.

All these techniques give the subject some "wow" factor so that students want to learn more. Using one or more of these techniques does not have to take any more than a few minutes and will focus learner attention on what is to come—an excellent investment of your time.

---

15 What is working memory?

In the model, working memory is depicted by a light bulb because this is where all thinking (cognition) occurs, where the conscious brain processes information. But working memory has limitations. It:

- **Lasts only a few seconds,** so people have to work at keeping thoughts processing in the working memory. You do this when you repeat something again and again that you need to remember until you are able to act on it or write it down (a phone number or an item for the grocery list).
- **Has a finite capacity.** Only five to nine unrelated bits of information can be accommodated in the working memory at any one time, shown by the eight compartments. For example, have you ever been driving in traffic and needed to turn off the radio or asked the kids to stop talking so you can concentrate? This shows that consciousness can only handle so many things at one time.
- **Is disrupted by anxiety,** shown as several *A*s taking up room and preventing use of the full capacity of cognition. This is an important concept for teaching nursing, in which the seriousness of the tasks can fluster students and adversely affect their performance. Can you remember a time when you were so nervous or anxious that your performance suffered? Learners who are anxious

tend to focus more on their anxiety than learning; clearly not a good thing.

---

16 Should we get students used to stress and anxiety so they are able to function better in the real clinical setting?

A certain amount of anxiety actually drives us to think clearly and function well, but too much is too much! Some teachers believe we need to replicate reality, including stress, in our educational activities, but I disagree strongly. If students are anxious, they *cannot* learn, and learning is our goal. Nursing education can seem daunting to learners simply because of the seriousness of patient care, the volume of important content, and the rapid pace of the educational experience. Even teachers who do not mean to be personally intimidating may appear that way to beginning students, causing them anxiety.

To reduce students' anxiety, I urge teachers to remain approachable. Be open to student ideas. Give encouragement. Tell a joke, or relate a personal story or example. Reassure learners they *can* master the new content or skills, that you will do all you can to help them succeed. Break down complex new content or tasks into small, sequential steps, and help learners get comfortable with each small segment before expecting them to put it all together. Allow lots of practice, and give plenty of constructive feedback. Acknowledge what students do *correctly* as they are learning complex new material. Sometimes, our expectations are just too high for the level of our students. Remember, you are an expert teaching novices, and adjust your expectations accordingly. There will be time in later classes to help learners put it all together under more realistic circumstances, but they have to master requisite content and skills before this is possible.

---

17 How is long-term memory different from working memory?

Basically, working memory (WM) is cognition or the act of thinking, and long-term memory (LTM) is what we know, depicted by a file cabinet. Learning results from transferring information from the LTM to the WM for processing and then back again to LTM for storage. Although a real file cabinet ultimately becomes full, LTM has an almost infinite capacity, representing total knowledge gained from learning. The information stored in LTM is not immediately conscious and may be voluminous and sloppily organized. Just like a real file cabinet, the correct mental "folder" has to be located, retrieved, and brought to the conscious WM, where it is utilized and augmented. In successful learning, the contents of the file are well organized and understood, and the information can be processed efficiently in the WM and then returned to LTM for relatively permanent storage and easy retrieval next time it is needed.

18 How does understanding WM and LTM help me design instruction for adult learners?

For learning to occur, learners must remember important features of what they already know, actively think about linking the new content with their prior knowledge in meaningful ways, and use the new information in different contexts before moving on to another topic. To facilitate this, help learners recall important prior knowledge. This does not mean remedial work or comprehensive review. It simply means helping students find the right file in their LTM to add to as they learn new content. To make lessons memorable, use rich clinical examples. Devise simple but clever ways to help students remember complex information such as short acronyms, simple diagrams, and funny sayings. Ask learners to consider hypothetical situations in which they use the new information. Require learners to explain aspects of the new information based on their current understanding. This allows you to assess their mastery and make adjustments as necessary. These techniques ensure that the new information is truly learned, that it is stored well in the LTM and available for future use. Information that is heard but not *learned* is filed superficially, if at all, and is soon lost.

19 I have so little time to get the content covered. Should I just remind students of a few facts we covered in the last class, and move on to the new content?

This is a common problem in nursing education, but it speaks more about teaching and content to be delivered than learning. For learning to occur, there is an important distinction between recognition and recall that is helpful.

- **Recognition** is quick but does not necessarily indicate accuracy or depth of thinking. Recognition is involved when you remind students of a fact and they nod, indicating that they remember; when a student selects a simple answer on a multiple-choice test; or when you are struggling to remember a word or a name, someone says it, and you think, "Of course!" These are examples of recognition, which may be insufficient to support new knowledge because active thinking is not occurring.
- **Recall** is an intense process that takes a few minutes and requires some cuing (usually from you) to help the student find the right mental file. For example, when you ask students to define a term or relate pathophysiology to a certain diagnosis, you are asking them to remember and use what they already know. It is a deliberate process that takes time, but it forces them to do important, active thinking. Prior knowledge is the scaffold that supports the addition of new knowledge. If we help learners recall and use prior knowledge as they are learning, it will make them link old and new information, remember it better, and be able to retrieve and use it in the future.

20 Are there different kinds of learning, and should I be concerned about including them all in what and how I teach?

Yes. You have probably heard of three "domains" in learning: cognitive, psychomotor, and affective. Considering all three in everything you teach is important. Developing familiarity with the three domains will help you develop useful objectives and evaluation strategies:

- **Cognitive Domain.** The cognitive domain is primarily associated with Benjamin Bloom (1956) and refers to mental skills or thinking processes. The domain includes increasing levels of sophistication, from knowledge of basic facts to comprehension, application, analysis, synthesis, and evaluation. Although facts are important, nursing especially values the more complex learning represented in the higher levels of this domain. We want nurses who can apply knowledge, analyze clinical situations, explain complex phenomena they see, and justify their decisions using intellectual criteria.
- **Psychomotor Domain.** This domain addresses skills that require physical action and neuromuscular coordination. Of course, all skills have a cognitive component, but it is not enough to just think or talk about them. If you want learners to do something, you need to create an environment in which they *do* the skill, with enough repetition and guided practice so that they increase their proficiency over time. There are a number of psychomotor taxonomies available representing different disciplines, but Dave (1970) is most commonly associated with this domain in nursing education. However, although his domain is widely used by nursing, his work is hard to find in the professional literature. Dave's five-level taxonomy progresses from low-quality imitation of a procedure, through doing procedures with increasing speed and accuracy, to high-level habituation that requires little thought.
- **Affective Domain.** This domain addresses feelings, attitudes, values and beliefs: subjective perspectives that are often hard for people to change but that are so important in nursing. Krathwohl (1964) is the name most commonly associated with this domain, although he had help from colleagues. The affective domain describes progression through five levels, from simply being aware of differing perspectives to consistently acting on one's own firmly held value system.

21 Should I be concerned about matching my teaching style to students' learning styles?

First of all, it is important to recognize that learners have preferred styles of learning. You have probably seen a wide variation of learning styles in your classes. Some students prefer to read, whereas others prefer to listen. Some want to learn by working in groups, and others simply want to be left alone. Some like to role-play, and others favor a methodical lecture. Most people keep using learning strategies that have brought success and discard those that are uncomfortable or were not as useful. There are dozens of learning style instruments available and any number of ways to conceptualize learning "style."

These tools are helpful for learners to understand themselves better, but they are not meant to pigeonhole learners into categories or suggest that only the preferred styles will yield positive results. Learners actually should expand their repertoire of approaches, including those that stretch their skills and comfort, in order to be broadly prepared to learn in a variety of situations.

It seems intuitive that if we match our teaching style with the learners' style, then outcomes will be more favorable. However, I do not recommend using commercial tools to assess students' learning styles so we can adapt our teaching accordingly. The bulk of research does not support this approach. Most scholars in this area recommend that teachers offer as wide a variety of teaching-learning strategies as possible so that learners can use their favored styles and expand their skills to include methods they do not prefer but that will strengthen their learning. This allows you to teach in ways that are most genuine and comfortable for you and offer your students choices in how they learn, a hallmark of adult learning.

References

Bloom, B.S. (Ed.) (1956). Taxonomy of educational objectives: The classification of educational goals. Handbook I: Cognitive domain. White Plains, N.Y.: Longman.

Dave, R.H. (1970). Psychomotor levels. In R.J. Armstrong (Ed.) Developing and writing behavioral objectives. Tucson, Ariz.: Educational Innovators.

Krathwohl, D., Bloom, B., & Masia, B. (1964). Taxonomy of educational objectives, Handbook II: Affective domain. New York: Longman.

Resources

Graetz, K.A. (2006). The psychology of learning environments. Educause Review 41(6), 60–74.

Knowles, M.S. III, Holton, E.F., & Swanson, R.A. (2005) The adult learner, 6th ed. San Diego: Elsevier.

LeFrancois, G.R. (1999). Psychology for teaching, 10th ed. London: Wadsworth Publishing.

Merriam, S., Caffarella, R., & Baumgartner, L. (2006). Learning in adulthood: A comprehensive guide, 3rd ed. San Francisco: Jossey-Bass.

2

Traditional Nursing Students

Heidi Taylor, PhD, RN

---

1 Who are traditional students?

When college faculties and staff use the term "traditional students," they are usually referring to a set of characteristics that many now consider antiquated notions of who the traditional college student is. In the academy, traditional college students are those who have come to college within a few months of their graduation from high school, are typically 17 to 19 years of age when they enter college, live on campus, and may rely on parental support to attend college. Despite our tendency to classify traditional students as a group sharing these characteristics, students usually come from diverse backgrounds, making generalizations about this group difficult at best.

Because generational differences among students are well discussed in another chapter, I want to focus on the unique needs, challenges, and opportunities surrounding teaching students who enter college directly after graduation from high school. These students are sometimes referred to as "Generation Y students," "Millennial students," or "Generation NeXter's" (Taylor, 2006).

2   What proportion of students is considered traditional?

Traditional students may constitute a small minority of the students you will be teaching, with some reports indicating that traditional students comprise as little as 16% of the total university enrollment. It is fair to say that the percentage of students in any university or college that meets the general characteristics of traditional students will vary. It is helpful, then, for all faculty members to assess the generational makeup of the students in their classes.

3   What cultural milestones have shaped the experiences of traditional students?

The cultural milestones experienced by students are interesting to consider when discussing students of any generation. Beloit College publishes a useful set of cultural characteristics that shape student experiences called the Mindset List. This list generalizes about the cultural realities of students entering college each year. For example, Beloit College's Nief and McBride (2007) report that the mindset of students who will graduate in 2010 has been shaped by the following:

- The Soviet Union has never existed.
- Smoking has never been permitted on U.S airlines.
- DNA fingerprinting has always been admissible as evidence in U.S. courts.
- Text messaging is their e-mail.
- Reality shows have always been on television.
- They have always preferred going out in groups as opposed to dating in couples.

4   Why is it important to understand younger students' cultural milestones?

While such observations may seem trite at first, understanding the student's unique cultural perspective is as important to effective teaching as the cultural perspective of a patient is to effective nursing. Making a reference to Nurse Ratched from *One Flew Over the Cuckoo's Nest* (Ken Kesey, 1967) will probably not be effective when illustrating how *not* be a nurse, unless, of course, you have required the reading or you have used the film. Cultural competence applies to teachers, and being effective with this group of students will require some study on your part to become culturally competent.

---

5   What do you think is a major distinguishing characteristic of traditional students?

A major consideration for this population of students is the extent to which technology has become a major part of the culture and these students' lives. Technology as a collection of tools to make life easier has become an extension of the students themselves. Information that was once something "out there" to be retrieved is now only as far away as the student's own fingertips. This immediate access to information, which is now so internalized by students that many are able to text-message and access information while tending to other multiple tasks, changes the teaching role in profound ways.

---

6   How do I best prepare to teach this type of student?

Your classroom will be filled with multiple generations of students who have multiple learning styles and abilities. No single strategy will meet the unique needs of all of your students, nor will it make you a good teacher. The challenge, then, is to create a learning experience in the classroom that will actively engage as many students as possible. Teaching is a personal and collective experience in which you, as the teacher, are also a learner. Likewise, the learners can be teachers. There are several approaches to prepare for your multiple roles in the learning experience of your students.

Know who you are: Parker Palmer writes in his book, *The Courage to Teach* (1998): "Teaching, like any truly human activity, emerges from one's inwardness, for better or worse. As I teach, I project the condition of my soul onto my students, my subject and our way of being together. The entanglements I experience in the classroom are often no more or less than the evolutions of my inner life. Viewed from this angle, teaching holds a mirror to the soul. If I am willing to look in that mirror and not run from what I see, I have a chance to gain self-knowledge—and *knowing myself is as crucial to good teaching as knowing my students and my subject*" (p. 2, emphasis added).

Palmer calls for deep self-examination and self-understanding among teachers and informs us of the importance of knowing the best and the worst of what lies in the hearts of those who teach. He argues that it is, indeed, the human heart that is the source of good teaching (p. 3). He further posits that "...good teaching cannot be reduced to technique; good teaching comes from the identity and the integrity of the teacher" (p. 10). In his eloquent descriptions and from his own study of good and bad teaching over the years, Palmer explains that all good teachers do not use similar techniques. Some good teachers use only lecture, some use very different techniques, but the characteristic that they all share is a passion for their work and the subject. Students can quickly identify bad teaching when teachers distance themselves from the subject, and "(t)heir words float somewhere in front of their faces, like the balloon speech in cartoons" (p. 11).

To prepare our students for the world in which they will work and live, the ability of the teacher to weave complex connections between and among the students and the subject is key to teaching and learning. Therefore, recognizing your own strengths and weakness, understanding your own heart as it guides your teaching, and allowing yourself to be vulnerable to your failures and your weaknesses are all important in developing yourself as a person who teaches from the "heart."

On a more pragmatic note, seek teaching assignments for which you can be genuinely excited. It is hard to be authentic when you are assigned to a course for which you have little enthusiasm. If you cannot demonstrate enthusiasm for teaching, do not expect your students to generate enthusiasm for learning.

Generation NeXters, born between 1980 and 2000, will quickly disengage when they sense that you are acting toward them in a way that is not true to who you are. For example, adopting the slang of the youth culture of the time may make you feel more connected to students (or may give you a false sense of connecting), but it is likely to make you appear disingenuous in the eyes of the students. They have a general idea of how old you are, and nothing can make you appear more foolish in their eyes than adopting the language and the style of their generation. If they cannot trust you to be true to yourself, how can they trust you to be true to them? They really do not want teachers who act and talk like them, they just want you to understand them.

Develop knowledge of the "best practices" in teaching: An important and humbling principle to remember is that you are not the master of all knowledge. You may be an expert clinician in your area of nursing practice, but teaching is about more than just telling students what you know.

Persons new to the faculty role often make the mistake of teaching the way they were taught, teaching according to their own learning style, or simply allowing their egos about their own clinical expertise to get in the way of good, student- and subject-centered teaching. There are significant resources available to guide nurses in pedagogical theory and strategies that engage students and improve learning.

---

7 How can I find out more about teaching traditional and other students?

Just as we insist on evidence-based practice in nursing, nurse educators should develop evidence-based teaching. The best preparation for teaching is to develop a consistent practice of reading the theoretical and research literature for best practices. There are fine professional journals dedicated to the teaching of nursing and teaching in general.

These should now become part of your regular professional reading, in addition to the professional clinical journals that keep you abreast of the latest research in your clinical area of interest.

There are often many resources on your campus to the person new to teaching. Do not be reluctant to ask for access to them. Your university may have a center for teaching excellence, a mentoring program, or other resources available to you. Find out who the best teachers are on your campus, and do not limit yourself to those teachers in your own discipline. Do not hesitate to ask to visit their classrooms or to meet with them over lunch. These experts can provide great ideas and strategies you might never have considered, and they are usually quite willing to share their knowledge and skills.

Finally, do not be shy about asking the students themselves how you are doing. Younger, more traditional students have good insights to share into their own learning and opinions about the learning environment. It is quite helpful periodically to ask the students how their learning experience is going. This requires that you be comfortable being vulnerable, because you may not hear what you want to hear. Nothing can be more disappointing than to discover that an activity you planned for weeks is not really meaningful to the students. But if you are committed to make learning meaningful, you must be prepared in earnest to ask for feedback.

---

8 What are some questions I can ask students to gauge how the class is going?

Here are some ideas:

- At the end of each class (or at periodic times during the term), allow some time for discussion about what is working and what is not working. Ask, "How did we do today?" "Did you find the [group activity, discussion, open book quiz, paired test, etc.] useful in helping you understand the concepts better?" "What can I do differently for you next time that will be more helpful?"

- At the beginning of the term, ask the students to think about the courses they have enjoyed the most, and ask them why they think they enjoyed it. Was it because of the subject, convenience of the schedule, use of technology, style of the teacher, types of assignments, and so on. Let their answers guide your instructional design.

9   How should I design instruction to engage traditional students effectively?

The first key is to *design* the instruction. Persons new to the faculty role often take too much time organizing *what* they will teach and too little time thinking about *how* they will teach what needs to be learned. For older students, the traditional lecture *may* work best. The traditional lecture may also work well when the faculty member is uniquely talented to enliven the content for the student. But for most Generation NeXters, most teachers need to employ a variety of strategies in a single teaching-learning episode to effectively engage students in the classroom.

10   Do lesson plans work well with traditional students?

I prefer to call these "learning plans." Designing instruction means carefully planning each class or learning session with the student. Class sessions can be as short as 50 minutes to as long as 3 to 4 hours. Clinical sessions are usually longer. Planning the use of the time is essential work for the teacher. Learning or lesson plans are common in primary and secondary schools and can be highly useful in the collegiate environment.

When planning a learning session with students, it is important to remember that Generation NeXt students can generally focus on something for about 15 to 20 minutes (some research indicates as briefly as 10 minutes) at a time. Therefore, learning activities need to be scheduled for some change about every 15 to 20 minutes.

Consider using the process described in Table 2–1 when creating the learning or lesson plan for a class period.

Table 2–1

The Learning/ Lesson Plan

LEARNING PLAN FOR FUNDAMENTALS OF NURSING ON 2/4/08 FROM 10:00 AM TO 10:50 AM

By the end of today's learning session, I want students to:
- Understand fully the concept of blood pressure

  - Systolic
  - Diastolic
  - Pulse pressure

- Recognize blood pressure findings that are not expected in several specific case studies
- Develop a beginning level of knowledge about the nursing implications when assessing expected and unexpected blood pressure findings

This learning session is important because:
- This knowledge is essential to assessment of the patient's condition
- This knowledge is necessary before students can adequately understand the effects of antihypertensives, which will be discussed next week
- Students will be expected to learn how to measure blood pressure using a sphygmomanometer this week in clinical practice

The necessary antecedent knowledge for this session is:
- Anatomy and physiology of the circulatory system
- Basic knowledge of blood pressure, based on reading and assignment prior to class session

Students are expected to come to class with the following completed before class:
- Pages 35–39 in their textbook
- Guided reading assignment for these pages completed

Audiovisual and other materials needed for class: [fill in as needed]

TIME	ACTIVITY
10:00–10:05	Take attendance, settle in, set the tone for the day
10:05–10:15	Small group work
	Students discuss their answers to the guided reading assignment
10:15–10:25	Large group discussion of guided reading assignment and clarification of any erroneous information
10:25-10:35	Small groups analyze case studies including nursing implications (each case study different)
10:35–10:45	Small groups report on findings to large group
10:45–10:50	Answer questions

11 Table 2–1 refers to a guided reading assignment. What is that?

This strategy is very useful in helping students make their way through voluminous material in the textbook. Nursing textbooks are filled with a tremendous amount of information and provide tremendous resources for students. The Generation NeXter is often confounded and frustrated by the amount of information in the book, especially when teachers assign large chunks at a time of material to be read.

Nursing instructors often complain that students do not read the assigned readings and come to class unprepared for meaningful discussion. (We can argue whether reading before or after class is most effective. In some situations, it may be better for students to hear your discussion before they attempt to read the material in the text.) Unless the student is guided to the important information and how to make sense of it, teachers cannot expect the student to know how to prepare through reading alone. It is simply not fair to say that everything they read is important. It is not humanly possible to master every factoid and idea in a nursing textbook. Keeping them guessing about what you want from them is no way to ensure good learning. Guiding students through the volumes of information and assisting them in learning what is truly important are major tasks for the teacher.

The purpose of the guided reading assignment is to break the content of a chapter into manageable pieces. It helps the student focus on what you believe is most important in the chapter rather than spend time memorizing facts that may have little relevance to your intended purpose. Guided reading assignments are particularly useful in assisting the Generation NeXter in staying focused for shorter periods of time.

The creation of a guided reading assignment requires significant work on the front side of your teaching (Table 2–2). However, once the assignments are completed, they can serve as a powerful method for guiding class discussions and identifying areas that are well or poorly understood. They can also help you organize your thoughts. This approach is useful not just in guiding students through textbooks; it can be used to guide students through any information source.

Table 2–2

Guided Reading Assignment

GUIDED READING ASSIGNMENT FICTIONAL CHAPTER 1

After you read this chapter, I want for you have a better understanding of:

a. _____

b. _____

c. _____

d. _____

Before you read anything, write what you know about hypertension (the major concept in the first piece of reading). It is OK if you do not know much about it.

Do you know anyone with hypertension? How have you noticed this condition affects her/his life?

Read pages 35–37 in this chapter, and answer the following questions before you move on to the next piece of reading. (In this section, ask questions about the major concepts and ideas present in these pages. These questions should guide students to the pieces of information you think are important.)

1. *In your own words, what is the definition of _____?*

2. *Explain what you think is meant by _____?*

Read pages 37–39, and answer the following questions before you move on to the next piece of reading.

3. *What is happening in the heart and the circulatory system when you hear the systolic sound?*

4. *What is the nurse's role in (choose an intervention)_____*

Continue to break the chapter into smaller sections, and ask the types of questions that are consistent with your objectives for the learning session and for the course. This should provide an excellent resource for the student to prepare for examinations, quizzes, and other evaluation activities.

At the end of the guided reading assignment, ask something like:

What were the most interesting things you learned as a result of completing this assignment?

What [surprised, frustrated, saddened, excited, etc.] you the most about what you read?

12 What is "engagement," and why is it important to traditional students?

Student engagement is characterized by active learning. Engaged students are excited about learning, enjoy attending classes and being involved in the learning process. Engaged students are more successful than disengaged students, and they are certainly more fun to teach! They become engaged students because of engaged teachers. Generation NeXters need to be challenged by a learning culture in which they are fundamentally changed by the learning experience. It is no longer effective to share knowledge-level information in the classroom through lecture or even through lecture complemented by discussion.

According to Taylor (2006), Generation NeXters have little patience for educational methods they see as outdated. Dyads, triads, and small group activities, even in large classes, should become the norm in most classes. These students are not engaged when the memorization/regurgitation process is used as the primary mode of teaching. They want to interact with the content and information, incorporate knowledge into theory, apply theory to real life, and understand the inherent value of what they are learning.

13 How do I prepare young students for the difficult and emotional nursing work ahead?

Despite growing up in a culture with more openness about sexuality, violence, and graphic realism in the media, many of these young students have never personally witnessed death and dying; the naked, traumatized bodies of others; or the intense emotions of human suffering. They may be unwilling to share their fears related to clinical experiences or about potentially harming someone through their own acts. It is helpful for these students to have an opportunity to discuss their private concerns about such issues with you in confidence.

If you are teaching beginning students or even students in a later course who are just now dealing with trauma or death, a writing exercise can be helpful to identify students who need extra support. Even more mundane aspects of nursing may require the student to grapple with unfamiliar emotions or reactions. For example, ask students to reflect in writing on their experience with helping people who were, for example, bleeding or vomiting, and allow them to privately express any fears or concerns they had about their own reaction to these kinds of situations. Although they may appear quite confident about the intimate nature of the work ahead of them, particularly around their peers, they may be quite anxious about their experiences with another person's blood, emesis, sputum, stool, and urine. This anxiety may cause significant performance issues on examinations and in clinical experiences. Hone your own assessment skills for student anxiety about such things, and be prepared to offer compassionate support for students experiencing the sights, sounds, and smells of nursing for the first time.

---

14 How do I help younger students who are accustomed to communicating in abbreviations and slang to communicate in the professional world?

This generation may lack the civil and social interaction skills that are expected of them from patients, particularly those in an older generation. Although they care deeply about patients and want to participate meaningfully in their healing experience, they will need specific guidance in recognizing the difference between a social interaction and a professional, therapeutic relationship.

There has probably never been a time when teaching therapeutic communication skills and professional language has been more important. These students need assignments that help them develop a strong professional vocabulary, and they need their teachers to model these behaviors consistently. Although it is easy to slip into the jargon of the day when discussing nursing work (and these moments can be quite amusing and provide a nice moment of humor during class), it is important that the teacher use this as a teachable moment and to model professional communication for the students. By that I mean, if jargon or slang is being used in the course of the discussion, take a moment to say something like, "Well, that's an interesting way to describe this, but let's think about how we might talk about this when we are talking to or in the presence of a patient.") Students need specific examples of how to talk about nursing work in a professional way.

---

15 I am a teacher, not an entertainer. How can I teach to this generation of students who expect to be entertained?

It is true that this generation of students, which grew up with educational entertainment on television and computers, expects learning to be fast, easy, and fun. But it is not true that a teacher necessarily has to be an entertainer. Remember that to engage a student effectively in anything, teachers have to be engaged themselves. If you are truly passionate about what you teach, your energy will be contagious.

Think back to professional workshops you have attended. The ones you truly enjoyed and from which you learned the most were probably not the ones where you sat for hours listening to a talking head drone on about a topic. You probably liked the ones where the facilitator mixed things up a bit. The instructor might have presented some new information, had you break up into small groups to work together on something, brought you back together to discuss things with a larger group, and then may have played a game. He or she used media in interesting ways throughout the workshop and probably employed a variety of techniques to get the participants talking more.

As you think about your teaching with Generation NeXters, consider yourself a facilitator and a guide. The students have access to high-quality information in many sources, including their textbooks and the Internet. Your role, then, is to guide the students through the maze of information to what is truly important, to facilitate their learning, and to help them become resourceful nurses.

They will be routinely disappointed and probably unsuccessful if your class is nothing more than a repetition of information they can get elsewhere. You have to make the information relevant, role-model the critical thinking and civility you expect from them, and engage your own passion for nursing.

References

Palmer, P. (1998). The courage to teach. San Francisco: John Wiley and Sons.

Nief, R., & McBride, T. Beloit College Mindset List. Retrieved April 26, 2007, from http://www.beloit.edu/~pubaff/mindset/

Taylor, M. (2006). Generation NeXt comes to college: 2006 updates and emerging issues, a collection of papers on self-study and institutional improvement. Retrieved March 30, 2007, from http://taylorprograms.org/images/Gen_NeXt_article_HLC_06.pdf

Resource

Upcraft, M.L., Gardner, J.N., Barefoot, B.O. (2005). Challenging and supporting the first-year student. San Francisco: Jossey-Bass.

3

RN-to-BSN Students

Diane Graham Webb, MSN, RN, CNE, and
Ann Deshotels, MSN, RN, CNE

---

1 Why do RNs return to school to earn their BSN?

Although nurses have their individual reasons for returning to school, most say they return to:

- Advance their knowledge or professional growth or increase their salary.
- Increase their career and promotion opportunities, i.e., for management positions.
- Meet entrance requirements for graduate programs.
- Meet current position requirements.

---

2 What is the difference between a student who is already an RN and the generic baccalaureate student?

We typically use the term "generic" baccalaureate student to refer to young people straight from high school who usually do not have any clinical nursing, hospital, or patient care experiences. They often do not work so they can attend school full time, whereas the typical RN student is licensed, works in a health-care setting, and often takes care of a family. The RN student is fulfilling two roles simultaneously: the role of expert clinician at work and the role of student at school. The RN student has been educated in an associate degree (AD) or diploma program and returns to school with a basic understanding and knowledge of nursing and can draw on experiences from health-care backgrounds. The RN student is used to working in the "real" world and wants immediate application of what is learned in the classroom.

---

3   What barriers, educational conflicts, and stressors do RN-to-BSN students encounter?

Because many RN students typically occupy multiple roles (spouse, parent, employee), several factors are perceived as hindrances to continuing their education that may include:

- Time management issues: limited time must be balanced among home, work, and school.
- Work schedules: work schedules often conflict with class schedules.
- Financial strain: tuition, books, and time off from work can deplete resources.
- Role conflict: the "expert" at work becomes the student at school.
- Fear and anxiety related to academic performance.
- Resistance from coworkers who question their decision to return to school.

---

4   How can I encourage RNs to return to school?

One of the best ways to encourage nurses to return to school is to talk with them *before* they graduate from their AD or diploma programs. You will probably meet these students and nurses in the clinical setting and will have the opportunity to plant the "continuing education" seed early and encourage them to take courses that will apply to their BSN degree. Schools may have articulation agreements with schools that facilitate transfer of credits between programs and make academic progression smoother. The receiving school may have mechanisms for awarding academic credit for previous knowledge and experience. These mechanisms may include credit by examinations, blanket credit, or portfolio review. It is important to keep repetition of previously learned skills/knowledge to a minimum. Flexibility of class scheduling for the working RN is very important as is collaboration with health-care facilities in regard to tuition reimbursement, educational pay differential, and employer support.

---

5   Where is the best place to recruit RNs into baccalaureate programs?

Recruiting RNs to advance their degrees is best done in the health-care settings where they work. Recruitment days at local colleges that have associate degree and diploma programs are successful as well. Other potential recruiting sites include your school's Web site and state and specialty nursing organization newsletters, magazines, and conferences. (The authors' school has a nursing continuing education department, so RN-to-BSN program brochures are included in all CE packets. "Word of mouth" has also been one of our most successful tools. We always say that our graduates are our "best recruitment tools.")

---

6   What can I offer in the way of support and advice for the RN student?

Helping the RN student assess his/her reason for returning to school and discussing the demands that will be placed on his/her personal and professional life are the first steps. In our experience, RN students want to graduate in the shortest time possible and therefore often overload themselves in academic credit hours per semester. We advise determining how quickly a student wants to graduate, plan a schedule for this time frame, and discuss the feasibility of such a schedule. Having the student set realistic goals cannot be overemphasized. No matter what time frame a student decides on, an entire proposed schedule, from the first course to graduation, should be planned and discussed. Support for RNs include:

- Offering orientation programs
- Arranging mentors (students currently in the program or recent graduates)
- Giving prompt, constructive feedback from instructors
- Making the student an active participant in the learning process
- Emphasizing critical thinking, not memorization

- Making application assignments
- Providing a syllabus that includes a course calendar with assignments and due dates
- Providing explicit guidelines and evaluation tools for all assignments
- Offering a "friendly ear" to listen to feelings and frustrations

Because of work schedules, RNs may not be able to access resources such as the library during regular school hours; therefore, remote access to such resources should be made electronically on a 24-hour, 7-days-a-week basis.

---

7 Is teaching RN students really different from teaching traditional baccalaureate students?

Yes. As mentioned, RN students can relate to health-care scenarios in more depth and with more expertise than can traditional students. RN students have health-care work experience that can result in critical thinking at clinical and management levels.

---

8 Do course requirements differ between the RN-to-BSN program and the generic BSN program?

The answer depends on your BSN program and how well you think that program meets the needs of your RN-to-BSN student population. For example, in our school's program, several courses such as pharmacology, critical care nursing, and skills labs are not a part of our RN-to-BSN program. Other courses such as health assessment, leadership and management, research, and nursing informatics are the same between the RN-to-BSN program and the generic BSN program.

---

9 Does the teaching format and style differ between RN-to-BSN and generic BSN programs?

It is important that faculty members adjust adult learning principles according to the experiences the RN students have had in their clinical settings as well as introduce critical thinking and reasoning methods of decision making. The generic student often needs the "ideal" situation presented in order not to be confused by the many problems of reality. Active learning, in which the RN learns through taking part in determining content of courses, is also important. Teachers act as facilitators, often utilizing and building on the clinical expertise of RNs in learning experiences.

10 How should classroom assignments differ for RN students and generic BSN students?

Classroom assignments for RN students are aimed at developing their professional roles; mastery of technical skills is assumed. Assignments that are applicable to the RN workplace are preferred and serve a twofold purpose: a learning experience for the student and an improvement in nursing care for clients. RN students often collaborate with faculty members and preceptors to identify areas of real concern in their clinical settings. Generic students need more foundational assignments that develop their basic understanding of health-care scenarios.

11 How do clinical assignments differ for RNs compared with generic students?

RN students are usually employed in a health-care setting, working under their own state license. Their technical skills were accomplished in the basic RN program; therefore, clinical assignments are geared toward individual learning needs that have been identified by the students and their preceptors. Their assignments are designed to build on their current knowledge base; it is important that they not spend time on what they have already mastered. Generic BSN students require clinical supervision related to technical nursing skills as well as decision-making and critical thinking assignments.

12 Can RN students function independently under their own license as students in clinicals?

Yes. This ability is one reason to require a minimum of 1 year's experience as an RN before enrolling in clinical nursing courses. In a clinical setting related to school assignments, the RN student works with a mentor who collaborates with the student and faculty. In our school, we require RN students to purchase professional liability insurance.

13 What are some of the challenges in finding/selecting meaningful clinical settings for RN students?

Clinical settings are shared by many nursing students in each community. RN students have the distinct advantage of being able to fulfill many assignments in their clinical setting. If an RN student needs to complete an assignment that is not possible to do in a present work setting, then faculty, supervisors, mentors, or the student can make contact with another facility to complete the assignment.

14 Should I prepare clinical preceptors/mentors to evaluate RNs differently than other students?

Fortunately, many health-care agencies have preceptor programs in order to orient newly hired nurses, so preceptorship is not a novel idea. At our school, we orient preceptors to the purpose and objectives of each clinical experience, emphasizing the focus of that particular experience. Collaboration between faculty and each preceptor aids in troubleshooting or problem-solving individual situations. The RN student usually does not require direct supervision by the clinical preceptor.

15 How can I validate basic nursing knowledge as well as clinical skills for the RN student?

Basic, safe nursing knowledge is validated by the RN's graduation from a basic nursing program and successful completion of the NCLEX-RN examination. Clinical preceptors can be utilized in specialty areas for additional knowledge required for safe, competent practice in those areas.

Other validation methods include:

- Self-assessment
- Checklists completed by supervisors
- Credentialing documentation
- Portfolio review

16 Because the RN student is already licensed to practice, should I use different evaluation methods?

Traditional objective testing is usually not part of the evaluation of RN students. Assignments related to development of critical thinking and clinical reasoning skills may be done with the use of clinical projects. Application of knowledge is emphasized. Traditional objective testing can be a portion of evaluation in specific courses such as health assessment and pathophysiology.

17 How can I promote professional socialization of RN students?

Classroom discussion about professional behavior is very helpful in students' socialization. Encouraging students to belong to professional organizations or volunteer for committee or community work is emphasized. Faculty members acting as role models and introducing students to others who embody professional socialization are important. Collegial relationships between faculty and students in which students are recognized for their areas of expertise facilitate socialization.

18 What challenges are encountered in teaching RN students who are highly specialized in an area of nursing in which the faculty may not have experience?

Nursing faculty members are facilitators of acquiring new knowledge, not experts in all areas of nursing. Initially, you may find yourself intimidated by such students, but this is a wonderful opportunity to identify and utilize students' strengths and utilize their expertise. Let them fulfill a teaching project in class or with their colleagues. Such an assignment lets students realize that we all have individual strengths and can learn from one another.

19 Can any nursing program instructor teach in an RN-to-BSN program?

The most effective teachers are those who:

- Philosophically believe in RN-to-BSN education and who recognize AD and diploma graduates as adult learners who want to build on their previous education and experience.
- Believe the roles of the teacher are facilitator, collaborator, consultant, and coach in the educational process.
- Can form warm, caring relationships.
- Act as role models for professional socialization.
- Respond constructively to student frustration and anger.
- Are flexible and have a good sense of humor.

20 How can I prepare myself to teach in an RN-to-BSN program?

Review the principles and techniques of adult learning and active teaching. Examine your philosophy of education, teaching, and nursing. Stay abreast of current nursing knowledge. Be an active participant in the nursing community; volunteer for community services. Make nursing informatics a priority. Be a role model for professional socialization.

21 What do you see as a model for RN-to-BSN education?

RN-to-BSN education involves an active, collaborative learning process between students and teachers who bring their own sets of variables to the equation. Learning occurs

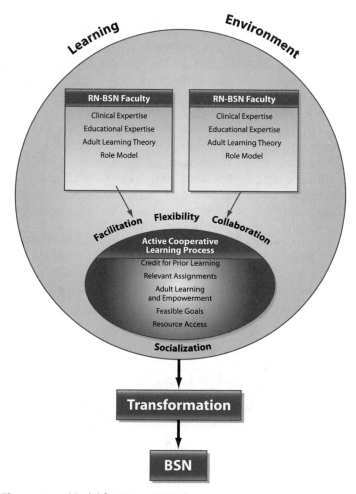

Figure 3-1. Model for RN-to-BSN education. (Copyright 2007 Diane Webb and Ann Deshotels.)

in an interactive relationship, with focus on the "real" world and in such a manner that fosters socialization and transformation. Figure 3–1 depicts such a framework.

The model for RN-to-BSN education involves two sets of variables. The student enters the learning environment with prior education and current educational needs, clinical experience and expertise, and a professional identity, an identity in which he or she is the "expert." As a result, when the "expert" becomes the student, the person often experiences role conflict and role strain. Teachers bring their own clinical and educational expertise, their knowledge of adult learning theory, and their ability to act as role models to the scenario.

These two sets of variables meet in an active learning environment that involves flexibility, collaboration, socialization, and facilitation. Students are given credit for prior learning assignments relevant to their clinical practice and access to necessary resources. Teachers apply active learning techniques, and students are empowered to set and achieve feasible goals.

Within the context of this active cooperative learning process, a transformation occurs, and the student emerges with a different perspective on professional nursing and the role of the nurse. The student is transformed into a baccalaureate-prepared nurse.

Resources

Billings, D.M., & Halstead, J.A. (2005). Teaching in nursing: A guide for faculty, 2nd ed. St. Louis: Elsevier Saunders.

Cangelosi, P.R. (2006). RN-to-BSN education: Creating a context that uncovers new possibilities. Journal of Nursing Education 45(5), 177–81.

Delaney, C., & Piscopo, B. (2004). RN-BSN programs: Associate degree and diploma nurses' perceptions of the benefits and barriers to returning to school. Journal for Nurses in Staff Development 20(4), 157–63.

Eckhartdt, J.A., & Froelich, H. (2004). An education in service partnership: Helping RNs obtain baccalaureate degrees in nursing at their practice sites. Journal of Nursing Education 43(12), 558–61.

Jacobs, P.M. (2006). Streamlining an RN-BSN program. Nursing Education Perspectives 27(3), 144–47.

Lillibridge, J., & Fox, S.D. (2005). RN to BSN education: What do RNs think? Nurse Educator 30(1), 12–16.

4

Second-Degree Master's Students

Melanie Dreher, PhD, RN, FAAN

A half century ago, professional nursing leaders, in considering the future of health care and the preparation necessary for nurses to address these challenges, boldly launched the movement to locate nursing education in collegiate rather than hospital settings. That action has probably been the single most influential factor in advancing the profession during the twentieth century. The action was controversial, disrupted the status quo, and required nursing leaders to move beyond their own backgrounds, experience, and work settings to pioneer a new educational approach for future nurses. We are now facing a similar decision point for the profession. Increasingly, we see the development of programs that prepare entry-level nursing professionals with graduate degrees (e.g., the nursing doctorate and the generic master's program). These programs are able to build on a broad base of education already acquired by students and the focus on several years of professional nursing education. These innovative models provide us with a variety of graduate education approaches for professional entry, and they need to be carefully examined and evaluated. (American Association of Colleges of Nursing, 1998, p. 20)

---

1 What was the thinking behind this statement?

This caveat to be mindful of the future when the requirements of professional nursing practice outstrip the capacity of baccalaureate education is rapidly becoming a reality.

The need to teach the expanding body of nursing knowledge is already eroding the liberal arts foundation for which our nursing leaders fought so hard. At the same time, the health-care system is demanding an expanded skill set from nurses. In addition to being excellent clinicians, professional nurses, including new graduates, are now expected to be clinician leaders. As patient advocates, they are expected to communicate effectively with other health professions; build clinical teams at the bedside; monitor patient safety; improve quality; incorporate evidence into practice; and understand how to collect, store, mine, and interpret data that will improve clinical outcomes for patient populations (Institute of Medicine, 2003).

---

2   Are master's entry programs successful?

These new programs have demonstrated success in attracting extraordinary college graduates, generating highly qualified and highly diverse applicant pools, and preparing excellent graduates actively sought by employers. Yet such programs remain controversial and somewhat challenging for the faculty members who teach in them. Part of the challenge has to do with the students themselves, and part has to do with the reaction of nursing colleagues to these programs. The following questions are those most commonly asked about master's entry generalist programs and their particular challenges. They should help the reader not only to better understand the programs and the students but also to participate in an informed manner in the debate and dialogue that surround these programs.

---

3   Why has postgraduate nursing education not been explored before?

Postgraduate entry into nursing is not new. In the early 1900s, even before the first baccalaureate program had opened at the University of Minnesota, Radcliffe College in Massachusetts collaborated with Massachusetts General Hospital to offer a nursing education program for college graduates, many of whom became distinguished nurses in World War I. The number of postgraduate programs offering a *second bachelor's degree*, sometimes referred to as an *accelerated bachelor's degree*, has since proliferated significantly. In 1990, 31 colleges or universities in the United States offered such degrees. By 2002, there were 168, with 46 more in the planning stages. Such programs usually offer a compressed bachelor's degree in nursing, typically awarded after 12 to 18 months. But even before the second bachelor's degree programs began to flourish, a few schools began to experiment with graduate nursing education for applicants with degrees in other fields.

---

4   Where were the first graduate nursing programs for people with degrees in other fields?

Perhaps the most well-known and controversial of these was the ND (Doctor of Nursing), originally developed at Case Western Reserve University and then adopted at University of Colorado, Rush University, and the Medical University of South Carolina. Unfortunately, the ND was an idea ahead its time; although it did not proliferate broadly, the four schools in which it was adopted produced excellent graduates who went on to successful careers in nursing. Ultimately, these four programs took different trajectories, ranging from comprehensive generalist practice to advanced specialty practice to clinical leadership and management.

In 1974 Yale was the first university to accept individuals with degrees in other fields into the School of Nursing's Graduate Entry Pre-specialty in Nursing (GEPN); these students then went on to the advanced practice phase of the program to receive a master's degree. Although not as widely adopted as the second bachelor's degree, these *direct-entry master's* programs preparing advanced practice nurses caught on, and by 2002 there were more than 50 programs in the United States, most of which were about 3 years in duration and required that students sit for the RN licensure examination during the course of study.

5 Are graduates from these programs all prepared for advanced practice?

Relatively recently, schools and colleges have offered a new kind of postgraduate master's entry program in which students are prepared, not for advanced or specialist practice, but rather as clinician leader generalists. While similar to bachelor's programs, in that they prepare graduates for generalist practice, these direct-entry master's programs include the comprehensive clinical leadership content that most bachelor's programs are unable to include: delegation and clinical team building, interprofessional communication, evidence-based practice, informatics, fiscal accountability and quality improvement, and clinical outcomes management. As a result, such programs are typically longer than second bachelor's degree programs, ranging from 18 months to 2 years and ordinarily requiring an immersion residency at the conclusion of course work.

6 How many direct-entry master's programs are there in the United States?

From data available in early 2007 (American Association of Colleges of Nursing, 2006–2007), there were 60 master's entry programs nationally, only 7 of which had direct-entry master's students enrolled in the generalist option. But programs are emerging rapidly in response to the need for leadership at the point of care, particularly hospitals, where the shortage of qualified nurses is the greatest. DePaul University in Chicago was the first to offer a generalist master's program in 2000, and it continues to be their only prelicensure program. The University of Iowa followed the next year, and in early 2007, 15 colleges and universities throughout the United States offered programs that awarded generalist master's degrees, although not all are direct-entry programs (American Association of Colleges of Nursing, 2006–2007).

7 What is the benefit of master's-prepared generalists for health care?

Contemporary nursing practice is very complex and sophisticated and becomes increasingly so each day. The intellectual challenges professional nurses and students encounter in providing high-quality, safe care for patients require extensive education to guide clinical judgment. In its series on the broken health-care system in the United States, the Institute of Medicine called for the education of all health professionals to include patient-centered care, evidence-based practice, information technology, interprofessional communication, and quality improvement. In professional nursing education, with the already mushrooming undergraduate curricula, it is highly unlikely that the knowledge deemed essential for nurses, physicians, physical therapists, dentists, pharmacists, and so on, can be taught without extending the length of the programs. And when an undergraduate program moves from 4 years to 5, it begins to look a lot like graduate professional education.

The value added by these programs is the opportunity to focus on clinical leadership as well as clinical scholarship. In our current baccalaureate programs, it is all we can do to provide the clinical knowledge and skill required by our students. Leadership is usually relegated to one course in the last semester. Consequently, students never learn how to delegate and build the clinical teams required for patient safety at point of care. We expect our graduates to be patient advocates, but we are unable to give them sufficient practice in interprofessional communication. We want them to be fiscally responsible, but we do not give them the tools to create economical approaches to high-cost, high-volume clinical activity. We want their practices to be evidence-based, but we do not introduce them to the organizational strategies needed to incorporate research findings into practice. We want the graduates to improve clinical outcomes for their population of patients, but we do not teach them how to collect, store, organize, and analyze data. The nursing shortage is not just a quantity problem. The need for well-qualified nurses who are better educated is plain.

8   Why not just stick with the popular master's entry programs that prepare advanced practice nurses?

Since Yale first opened its direct-entry master's programs, it has educated the college graduate for careers in advanced practice specialty programs, including nurse-midwives, clinical specialists, and nurse practitioners. Although such programs are superb courses of study, their graduates often do not provide direct care in hospitals, the single greatest employer of nurses and where the nursing shortage is greatest. Although acute care nurse practitioners and clinical specialists may practice in hospitals, they are less likely to provide direct patient care and more frequently function in a consultative or managerial role for the entire hospital.

An equally important consideration is the shift of specialty and advanced practice nursing education from a master's to a doctoral degree. The groundswell of support for the Doctor of Nursing Practice (DNP) degree is good indication that by the year 2015, the majority of specialty practice education will occur in DNP rather than master's programs (American Association of Colleges of Nursing, 2007a). With the exception of specialty knowledge and practice, the core content of the DNP curriculum can be offered in a master's generalist program. Graduate-level epidemiology, biostatistics, informatics, fiscal management, evidence-based practice, health-care policy and economics, pathophysiology, pharmacology, and health assessment, which comprise the generalist master's course work, also constitute the foundation course work for DNP programs. The simultaneous emergence and integration of these two new graduate programs provide a great opportunity to put nursing on a parity with other health professions.

9   Why would we use our faculty resources to educate more master's students when we need more nurses to provide direct patient care?

This question and its sequitur "Who will be at the bedside for the patient?" assume that direct patient care is less challenging and therefore less appealing for the college graduate thinking of a career in nursing. I am disturbed when I hear faculty members tell students that "there is more to nursing than care at the bedside." What could be more interesting, challenging, and rewarding than caring for people and their families during the most critical times of their lives? The Institute of Medicine (2007) report on quality and safety speaks to the need for astute, critical thinking and multifaceted clinical intervention, requiring more, rather than less, education for those managing the care of clients and patients.

Reference to the "bedside nurse" does not take into consideration that safe, effective, and comprehensive management of a patient requires the organization and coordination of a team of providers, educated at many levels. One of the factors leading to the development of the clinical nurse leader role is the acknowledgement from hospital nursing leaders, in particular, that patients and families are not well served by the existing system; that there is a need for nurses who will take charge of the clinical management of a patient, delegating those aspects of care that can be accomplished by nursing staff with less education, coordinating care with other health professionals, and being supported by continuous communication among the care team. Effective patient advocacy requires leadership as well as clinical expertise. We know that nurses who demur from requesting a "time out" to assure the safety of the patient before the surgeon begins or who are fearful to request that the physician put on gloves before examining the patient are not successful advocates.

Finally, the experience of those schools that have developed master's generalist programs suggests that many of these students left seemingly lucrative and prestigious careers to engage in meaningful, emotionally satisfying and intellectually stimulating work. They are eager to practice clinically and provide direct patient care. Physicians do not believe that direct care of patients is boring or less intellectual or less demanding or less rewarding.

10 How does the curriculum of the direct-entry master's generalist program differ from the curriculum for second bachelor's degree programs?

Unlike the second bachelor's degree programs, in which bachelor's level content is compressed and taught in an accelerated format, the master's generalist courses are taught on the graduate level. These students take many of the same courses that are typically offered as core for master's specialty programs, i.e., graduate-level nursing theory, evidence-based practice, pharmacology, physical assessment, pathophysiology, informatics, epidemiology, and biostatistics. There are other differences as well. As in medical education, most direct-entry master's generalist programs include a full-time residency in the last phase of the program, which may include several clinical rotations. There are opportunities for clinical practice prior to the residency, but they are not often organized around the specialty designations that traditional prelicensure programs follow. Although they must have the clinical *theory* that pertains to the care of elders, the care of persons with a behavioral disorder, or the care of communities, they do not need to have clinical practice in each of these areas. Rather, faculty members need to take some time to determine what are the *general* elements of clinical practice that *transcend* all specialties, e.g., observation and assessment; communication (in person, telephone, electronic, and public presentation); consultation and guidance, and synthesis and adaptation of clinical knowledge to meet the needs of specific clients, whether they are individuals, families, or whole communities.

11 What are the concerns of faculty teaching in direct-entry master's programs?

Stepping out of teaching within a specialty and into a generalist orientation is often a great hurdle for faculty members who are used to teaching solely within their specialty, whose research is specialty-oriented, and who resonate most with their specialty organization. But revisiting and articulating the essential aspects of nursing, i.e., those components of education that *must* be included to claim membership in the profession of nursing, is a good exercise for the entire faculty. Like medicine, nursing has become so specialty-focused that we often forget our common concepts such as wellness, patient advocacy, family centeredness, community focus, and so forth. It is also important for the faculty to come to terms with the reality that each one of these students will have a different educational experience and that they do not have to be taught *everything*. These students are aggressive learners, and with our *guidance,* they will find ways to learn. Our responsibility, as a faculty, is to help them understand that continued learning is their professional responsibility as clinician leaders and to provide direction regarding how they can do that effectively.

---

12 I have heard that these students have an attitude problem and think they know more than the instructors.

Faculty members who have worked with these students in second bachelor's degree programs or in direct-entry master's programs soon discover these students are truly adult learners who bring knowledge and practice of other fields. We need to respect their rich backgrounds and life experience, build on it, and think of these people as junior colleagues rather than as acolytes. It is also a good idea to think of ourselves as "coaches" rather than "instructors."

So the real question is whether faculty members are intellectually and experientially equipped to guide the education of these more educated and mature students. Most faculty members who have worked with this population of students cite the comparative ease with which they are able to provide instruction. Comments such as "highly motivated," "mature," "independent learners," "committed," "strong performers," and "high academic expectations" pepper the conversations about these students. Indeed, most educators find that they are a joy to teach. As one faculty member observed when questioned whether she could make a nurse out of a drama major, "if they don't know something, they look it up....What a concept!"

At the same time, one is equally likely to hear about students "with an attitude," who "don't know their place," "challenge their preceptors," or "debate the faculty member." Such observations beg the question whether the problem really rests with the students or the faculty or perhaps with our whole profession. We coach students on how to debate issues and present a different point of view, as long as they do not disagree with us. We must remember that our profession has been plagued by an overabundance of timid, deferential, risk-averse nurses. We can benefit greatly from these assertive, well-informed, mature college graduates who will not back away from constructive dialogue and debate. We need as many aggressive nurses as we can get to transform health care.

Fundamentally, these master's generalists and even the second bachelor's students cannot be taught the same way high school graduates are taught. Therefore, they cannot be taught *with* high school graduates. They need to have specially designed courses and clinical experiences that move at a pace that is ordinarily too fast for traditional bachelor's students; otherwise they become impatient. In nursing, we are not used to teaching classes in which there may be an oboist, a firefighter, an accountant, an advertising executive, an applied anthropologist, and a retired space engineer in the same room or clinical practice setting. While this can be a bit daunting at first, we have to remember that each of them chose this journey and is vitally interested in our guidance along the way. Such students respond well to clinical problem solving and learning how to learn.

Even with these advanced students, we cannot teach them everything they need to know for every patient encounter they may have. Rather, we must teach them the skills and strategies they need to be creative problem solvers, which includes being excellent observers, communicators, and synthesizers of knowledge. Today, teaching any nursing student how to care for a person with a myocardial infarction (MI) does not add value to their education. Protocols for the care of patients with an MI are available everywhere for students. Our job is to assist the student to adapt that protocol to meet the needs of a particular patient so the care delivered is patient-centered and culturally appropriate.

13 How do we teach these students to be effective clinician leaders when there are so few role models in practice?

This may be the greatest challenge that we have in educating direct-entry master's generalists. Because most hospitals have put the least prepared nurses at the bedside, it is difficult to identify appropriate preceptors. This was the same problem that faculty members faced in the early days of preparing nurse practitioners. Yet somehow we made do and muddled through until we had graduated sufficient numbers of nurse practitioners to provide the expert preceptors that we needed. Yes, for a while it will be a trial for faculty members to prepare students for roles that may not exist in many places. But this is always the case as nursing practice and education evolve. Indeed, our greatest challenge as educators is to prepare graduates for a health-care system that does not yet exist but for which we will give them the tools to create. The lack of role models in practice is commonplace in nursing education. Faculty members must engage students in envisioning what the clinical management of the patient *could* be and prepare them for the reality that they will create.

14 How can we strengthen the residency?

Because the residency is ordinarily a very important part of the direct-entry master's generalist program, it is essential that faculty members work closely with the *leadership* of the clinical practice partner to fully explain the program goals and intentions. This program cannot be taught without full cooperation from the affiliated practice sites. This, by the way, has not been difficult. Hospital nurse executives are quick to acknowledge the importance of both the education and the clinician leader role, and many have already constructed positions that activate the role. When the negotiations reach the unit level, however, it becomes problematic. Many existing staff members are skeptical about the master's degree and whether it is really needed for direct care. They have also heard these students might feel "superior" and not follow their direction. With regard to the residency component, most units have never had a full-time (40 hours a week) student on the staff, who will rotate to evening and night shifts along with the preceptors.

The faculty members must acknowledge staff concerns (most of which disappear after hosting these students for a week or two). They must work with the associate directors and unit managers to present the program to the entire staff but carefully select those nurses (who must be at least bachelor's level) who can work most effectively with these students.

The presentation to the whole staff must include the intent of the program and the clinical goals for students. It is critically important that staff members know that the students' goals and objectives are not procedural; rather they are focused on critical thinking, patient care management, and clinical leadership. This is not to say that it is not useful for a master's generalist student to learn how to perform nursing procedures, but the real goal of the clinical practice component (particularly the residency) is to learn how to develop, oversee, and implement the care of patients; to make good clinical decisions; to delegate within and to build well-functioning clinical teams; to incorporate new evidence and protocol reviews into practice, to use information to assess performance and set performance goals for a population of patients (e.g., persons with diabetes, neurosurgical patients, newborns, hospice patients, etc.); and to engage in interprofessional teamwork and communication. It is equally important for staff members to know these students will be mature; they have set high academic expectations for themselves and are not hesitant to question and even debate the care plan and implementation.

15 What prerequisites are necessary for admission to the program?

The answer to this question varies from school to school. Most postgraduate programs in nursing, whether they are bachelor's or master's programs, have found that students from diverse professions and backgrounds all performed exceedingly well. The obvious prerequisites include anatomy and physiology, microbiology, psychology, and statistics. Some schools require chemistry; some a foreign language; some require epidemiology while others make it part of the curriculum. I believe all nursing students should have a course in cultural anthropology before they come into nursing because the discipline of anthropology and the profession of nursing are so aligned.

16 Is requiring a college degree for entry into master's nursing education programs viewed as elitist, and does it exclude persons from underrepresented populations?

It is critically important that nursing educators everywhere commit to building a diverse workforce as a primary strategic objective. This workforce should include gender diversity as well as ethnic diversity. Colleges and universities offering these innovative second degree master's programs are reporting applicant pools, acceptance rates and, most important, graduation rates in which there is a much higher proportion of both men and underrepresented ethnic groups than in the traditional and even second bachelor's degree programs. In my experience, African American, Latino, and American Indian students have an even greater appreciation of and need for an excellent education and strong credentials. This may be the reason that the proportion of master's nurses among the African American nursing population is higher than among the white population. Faculty members teaching these students have observed anecdotally that successful completion of a college education as well as maturity and life experience generate a high level of self-confidence in these students, making them competitive in these rigorous programs.

17 Will there be jobs available for graduates of master's generalist programs?

It is difficult to imagine a scenario in which employers refuse to hire new graduates because they are too well educated and too well credentialed to practice nursing. It is also hard to imagine that quality health-care employers would not want the best-educated clinician they can find to provide leadership at the point of care, where the impact on quality and safety is felt most keenly. Prelicensure master's programs report a high demand for these graduates, who are prepared for high-level clinical practice. Although graduates are qualified for a variety of practice settings, the majority have their first employment in hospitals, where they have been reported to be leaders comparatively early in their careers. Employers indicate they are superior patient advocates, excellent problem solvers, and committed to high-quality care at the bedside.

Employers have also reported better retention of these graduates. The reason for this is still unclear, and there may be several explanations. One may be the maturity these graduates bring to their careers and the associated problem-solving skills. Another may be their ability to move more quickly through the clinical ladders in their employment. Still another may be that, unlike younger students, most of whom are women, they are not leaving to follow a spouse or begin families. Given the cost of turnover, commonly estimated to be between $80,000 and $120,000 per nurse, retention is an important issue economically and in terms of continuity, safety, and quality of care.

18 Should students taking their first job expect to be paid more because they have a master's degree?

In many ways, this question reflects a lack of understanding of the health-care marketplace and the illogic that governs nursing compensation. On the one hand, professional nurses believe, and rightly so, they deserve higher compensation for the enormous responsibility they undertake. On the other hand, there is not another occupation in which someone with 2 years of education can command the wages that many registered nurses earn. Some enlightened hospitals and health agencies are making an effort to adjust compensation for nurses with more education so as to attract and retain the very best talent. For other hospitals, this is not a priority. As long as there is a nursing shortage, graduates will be in an optimal position to work in an organization that invests in its employees rather than just hires workers.

Will a master's degree ultimately result in more money? Yes. Employers of these graduates quickly assess the value they add to patient care, particularly with regard to quality and patient safety, and find ways to foster their commitment to the organization.

A more critical problem than the illogical compensation practices is that most nurses employed in hospitals are not salaried professionals but hourly workers. In the best of all possible worlds, master's-prepared clinician leaders, with their firm grounding in other disciplines and political skills, will be better positioned to advocate for a more professional orientation to recruitment and retention of nurses. This includes, for example, salaried positions, incentive plans, differentiated roles based on education, and so on. Finally, many college graduates who come into nursing find the standard compensation quite attractive in comparison with their current earnings with a bachelor's degree in psychology, music, biology, or anthropology.

19 With master's degrees, what will prevent graduates of these programs from trying to take leadership roles that exceed their capability?

It is highly unlikely that employers would consider placing new graduates into leadership positions with no prior experience. It is equally unlikely that master's graduates would seek such positions without sufficient experience. Graduates of these program feel the same sense of anticipation combined with hesitancy as all new nurses. On the other hand, because they typically bring greater maturity to their new work, they may feel ready and be encouraged to take leadership roles fairly early in their work life. The limited experience of master's generalist programs thus far is that graduates view themselves as beginning nurses but quickly distinguish themselves as clinical leaders. The challenge for the faculty members who work with these students is to help them understand that they are beginners in nursing while at the same time assisting them to leverage their rich backgrounds and life experience and assure them they will have the knowledge and skill to become clinician leaders quickly.

---

20 My colleagues say that these programs contribute to the alphabet soup that will make the public even more confused. What's your perspective?

The public understands very well that a doctoral degree signifies a more learned and accomplished professional than a master's degree and that a master's degree signifies a more learned and accomplished professional than a bachelor's degree. If anyone is confused, it seems to be our own profession. Early graduates of these programs encountered this confusion when they applied for their first positions and were told that they were not qualified because they did not have a bachelor's degree in nursing. It is important for faculty members to warn students that this could happen and that it is easily resolved by a letter from the school or just a phone call. Military scholarships for bachelor's preparation in nursing also had to be renegotiated to support these students. Nursing may be the only profession in which we have to prove that there is a relationship between education and performance. The registered nurse licensure designation for all levels of education does create some confusion, but a simple explanation that the RN degree signifies that all nurses have passed an examination to assure minimal safe practice usually suffices to end misunderstanding.

I view this point in the history of nursing as an opportunity to simplify and standardize our education and credentials. We may very soon come to the time when the bachelor's degree is the minimum education required for professional nursing practice, the master's will signify clinical leadership, the doctor of nursing practice (DNP) will designate advanced and specialty practice, and the PhD, like all other disciplines, will be solely for preparing nursing scientists and researchers. What a happy ending that would be to a century and a half of experimentation.

21 Will this program drain the already depleted faculty resources?

Another very important reason for moving to a post-bachelor's program in nursing is that more students can be taught with fewer resources. Many of the courses that we feel compelled to offer our typical undergraduate students are unnecessary. Other content should be advanced instead. Graduate-level pathophysiology can be managed by these students, many of whom have science backgrounds and life experience that facilitate their rapid progress. Furthermore, such students are the equivalent of other health sciences students entering with a college degree and could take interprofessional courses offered by other health science schools. Teaching 80 post-bachelor's students in an 18-month program simply requires less time and fewer faculty members than teaching 80 undergraduate students in a 2-year program.

Another advantage is that postgraduate courses of study are easier to administer. Essentially all the courses taken by such students are taken within nursing; no one has to worry about fitting in pharmacology with liberal arts requirements or scheduling clinical practice so that it does not interfere with the class schedules of another departments. This is very liberating and can open up enormous possibilities for creative clinical practice. Electives are accounted for by their undergraduate majors, bringing a rich and diverse set of knowledge and experience into the nursing profession with music, geography, business, biology, and psychology, to name just a few.

22 How are these programs related to the clinical nurse leader movement?

The proliferation of master's generalist preparation (sometimes referred to as a "generic master's") has been accelerated by the development of the clinical nurse leader (CNL) role. See the American Association of Colleges of Nursing Working Paper (2007) on this innovative role. The CNL requires a master's degree and completion of a national certification examination. The CNL curriculum is nursing education's response to the Institute of Medicine's series on quality and patient safety. Although the majority of master's programs educating students for CNL certification require a bachelor's degree in nursing for admission, a smaller but growing cohort of colleges and universities have designed direct-entry master's generalist programs that admit students who have a college degree in another field.

Although the CNL role has accelerated the development of master's generalist programs, such programs should not be role-specific. Opportunities abound for clinician leaders who are needed everywhere in health care. It would be possible, but not very prudent, to launch a prelicensure generalist master's curriculum that is not consistent with the essential curriculum content for CNL certification. Fundamentally, the proposed CNL curriculum prepares graduates to be leaders at point of care in any context (AACN 2007), and all generalist master's programs would be wise to assure that their graduates are eligible to sit for the CNL certification examination. The combination of systems knowledge with a comprehensive clinical orientation will produce nurses who have the potential to be high performers in any position they choose to take.

23 Many nursing education programs are located in smaller liberal arts colleges that typically do not grant master's degrees. What will happen to their nursing programs?

There are many undergraduate college programs that offer master's degrees in business education, education, and social work. A strong financial argument could be made to presidents and provosts that if nursing departments included both pre-professional and professional curricula, the departments could extend the number of years that students were on campus and attract students from other campuses. It is interesting that the economics of such programs has escaped the attention of presidents and provosts of colleges and universities. If faculty members have the potential to graduate twice as many students in the same period, simply by requiring different admission criteria and streamlining the curriculum, why do they continue to support a more expensive, labor-intensive, time-intensive program, particularly during a nursing shortage?

---

24   How will this degree add value to the nursing profession?

All postgraduate students in nursing add value to the profession. They bring maturity and motivation along with a wide array of life experience and preparation in other fields that have the capacity to enrich nursing and affect the quality of care. A graduate degree has even greater potential to attract career-oriented, ambitious men and women into nursing who are seeking the same opportunities for leadership and status that exist in other professions. As the last health-care profession to adopt graduate entry, nursing has been on an unequal playing field in the competition for the best and brightest college graduates. The experience of the doctor of pharmacy (PharmD), initiated just a little over a decade ago, is instructive. Recently, I attended a graduation ceremony for a PharmD program. I was struck by the larger proportion of women in the graduating class (approximately 75%) and thought that 10 years ago, these same women would have been nursing students. In my opinion, these PharmD graduates discounted the opportunity for a career in nursing to pursue a more highly regarded credential and greater opportunity for leadership and career advancement. Direct entry into *graduate*-level nursing practice is a huge draw. It is useful to imagine a college senior seriously considering a career in health care: the choices include a doctor of medicine, pharmacy, dentistry, physical therapy, audiology, optometry, and podiatry and a second bachelor's in nursing. During the admissions interviews for the University of Iowa master's generalist program, one applicant told the committee she was aware of how competitive this program was and therefore applied to the College of Dentistry as a backup. *This* is the kind of student we want and need in order to advance our profession.

Arguably, there are successful, well-enrolled second bachelor's programs all over the country that produce graduates in 12 months. In my mind, the question is not why offer a master's degree, it is why *not* offer a master's degree? Nursing is the only health-care profession that has not moved universally to an entry-level graduate degree. What is it about the nursing paradigm that makes us gravitate to lower-degree options? Why do we make our students work harder than any students on campus and then award them the lowest degree available? Sometimes I think there is some form of self-denunciation operating and a disregard for our own profession, which is seen as not worthy to warrant a degree that is consonant with the education required. When we opened the prelicensure generalist master's program at Iowa, we debated for months whether the degree should be a second bachelor's or a master's. Interestingly, it was the Dean of Medicine who ultimately created the tipping point when he said, "Melanie, you have been telling me for the past 4 years how sophisticated and complex contemporary nursing practice is. Why would you *not* offer a master's degree?"

References

American Association of Colleges of Nursing. (1998). The essentials of baccalaureate education for professional nursing practice. Washington, DC: Author. Available at http://www.aacn.nche.edu/education/bacessn.htm

American Association of Colleges of Nursing, Institutional Data Systems, Research and Data Center, 2006–2007.

American Association of Colleges of Nursing. (2007a). Doctor of nursing practice. Available at http://www.aacn.nche.edu/DNP/index.htm

American Association of Colleges of Nursing. (2007b). Working paper on the role of the clinical nurse leader. Washington, DC: Author. Available at http://www.aacn.nche.edu/Publications/WhitePapers/Clinical NurseLeader.htm

Institute of Medicine of the National Academies. (2003). Health professions education: A bridge to quality. Washington, DC: Author.

Institute of Medicine of the National Academies. (2007). Keeping patients safe: Transforming the work environment of nurses. Washington, DC: Author.

5

Intergenerational Perspectives

Lydia R. Zager, MSN, RN, CNAA-BC

1 Why are the multigenerations a challenge for faculty and our students?

We are facing four generations in the workplace. and this includes the academic setting. All four generations have many differences in their characteristics and values. The majority of faculty members are Baby Boomers, with a few Traditionalists and Generation Xs. The majority of students are Generation X and Y, also known as the Millennial Generation. Generation X and Y student characteristics, values, and learning styles are a challenge for faculty members as they realize old methods may not work for these new technology-savvy students. Generation X and Y students are ethnically diverse, are socially aware, value family and their time off, and believe being smart is "in."

2 Why is it important for our students to understand the differences in the generations?

Just as faculties need to understand their students, students need to know about the different generations they will be caring for when they graduate. The differences can be as simple as addressing Traditionalists formally with Mr. or Ms. and being able to relate informally with Generation

X patients. This knowledge for the students will make a significant difference in students' ability to establish rapport with patients and the health-care team with which they will be working. In the questions below, the characteristics of the different generations are addressed.

---

3 Who is the Traditionalist/Silent/Veteran Generation?

Who are they?
Born 1900–1945
Major world events: World Wars I and II and the Depression
What do they need?
Leave a legacy and share their work and life experiences
What are their values?
Believe in the "tried and true"
Believe that "no news is good news"
Want to be respected for their experience and knowledge
Challenges for faculty who are Traditionalist
Learning new technology
Accepting that the tried and true ways do not always work
Adapting to "less is more" in communicating with Generations X and Y. What do they *need to know* versus *nice to know, with regard to information?*
Being asked by students about how they are doing

---

4 Who is the Baby Boomer Generation?

Who are they?
Born 1946–1964
Comprise 45% of the workforce; 76 million persons
Shaped world policies and politics
Question authority and "stand up" for what they believe in
Changing the way aging is viewed as they enter retirement
Service-driven and will "go the extra mile"
What do they need?
Want to find personal meaning in their work
Need recognition for their work
Like to share their opinions, talk (brag) about themselves and their families
Can be critical but do not like criticism; need praise

5   Who is Generation X?

Who are they?
Born 1965–1980
Approximately 46 million persons in the workforce
Highly independent and good problem solvers
Creative; get things done smarter, better, safer
Parallel thinkers, able to multitask
Responsive and focused
Technology-literate
High moral and ethical standards
Believe in marriage and family
Tremendous loyalty to peer groups
Optimistic about quality of life
What do they need?
Want to know why they need to learn "this"
Desire personal interaction with the faculty
Want constant feedback
Prefer specific information
Want the instructor to be a partner
Like informality and to have fun
Want balance now, not when they are 65 years old

6   Who is Generation Y?

Who are they?
Born 1979–1994
Largest group since the Boomers: 71–80 million persons
Culturally diverse:

- 36% non-white, or Latino
- 20% have at least one immigrant parent

Family characteristics:

- Single-parent families
- Children of late Boomers or early Generation X

(continued)

- Increased parental attention and involvement
- Trophy children: high expectations

Realistic view of the world
Risk-tolerant
Cultural influences:

- Advancing technology
- DVDs, CDs, cell phones, computers
- Internet
- Violence: Columbine, Oklahoma City bombings, 9/11
- Mass media and consumerism: MTV, music (rap, hip-hop, pop)

What do they need?
Very reliant on the group
Respond to humor, irony
Upgrade use of technology
Needs similar to Gen X

---

7 What important teaching strategies do faculties need in developing partnerships for learning with Generations X and Y?

The word COACH can help faculty members work successfully with Generations X and Y. See Figure 5–1.

- **C: Collaborate and create partnerships**

Generations X and Y neither consider instructors as the only ones with information nor see them in a power position. They respect the teacher as an expert, but they want the faculty to partner with them in the learning process.

COACH THE STUDENT

- **C:** Collaborate and create partnerships
- **O:** Off with the toggle switch
- **A:** Acquire the knowledge
- **C:** Connections and communication
- **H:** Have to give frequent feedback

Herman J., Manning L., & Zager, L. (in press). Publishing, leading learning: The eight-step approach to teaching clinical nursing. Bosier City, La.; I Can Publishing.

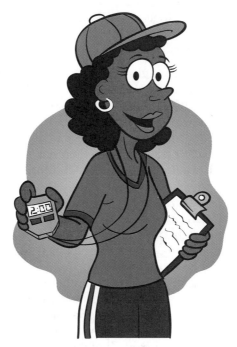

Figure 5-1. Picture of coach.

This requires the faculty to establish a relationship with students and use multiple methods to help them learn based on their different learning styles. Generations X and Y see learning as a social activity and believe it should be fun. Technology such as blogs and wikis can be very effective, whether it is in the classroom or in clinical. Clinical faculty members can post reflection questions and allow the students to reflect on their clinical day through the blog with interaction between members of their clinical group.

Clinical provides an optimal opportunity to capitalize on teamwork. Working in pairs is a very effective way to help novice clinical students gain confidence as they rely on each other's strengths and knowledge. Faculty members can encourage student clinical groups to use wikis to solve problems when they are faced with newly learned information or skills. Students learn how to build cohesive teams by working together and relying on peer support, a major variable in positive job satisfaction (Herman, Manning, and Zager, in press).

- **O: Off with the toggle switch**

The ability of Generations X and Y members to talk on the cell phone, do instant messaging and surf the Internet, all while they are writing a paper is impressive. However, the more we learn about the way we think, we realize it is impossible to think about more than one thing at a time. In fact, what we do is toggle back and forth between the subjects. Generation X and Y's ability to access large amounts of information is a great skill but can lead to superficial learning. There is danger in never spending enough time with any one subject to learn it in depth. In addition, it is difficult for novice learners to discern relevant from irrelevant information.

Considering the size the of the textbooks and the amount of reading that is required, students do not know what is important to learn relative to the vast amount of information contained in the textbook. As faculty we can no longer feel obligated to lecture on all of the content. According to Arhin and Johnson-Mallard (2003), students read only the highlights and scan the rest of the chapter. Generations X and Y are looking for guidance and direction from their faculty to help them prioritize their learning. By doing this, instructors help the students turn off the toggle switch (Herman, Manning, and Zager, in press). It is important that students be able to think critically and to make good decisions. This requires more than superficial learning, which results from assignments of large volumes of reading material without guidance from the faculty.

- **A: Acquire the knowledge**

It is as important today to know how to access information as it was to know and memorize information in the past. This becomes a challenge for faculty members as they struggle to integrate new technology into classrooms and learning experiences. As faculty, we know the importance of trying to keep students engaged while learning and experiencing clinical, where in-depth knowledge is critical.

The use of wireless laptops is very effective in the classroom for accessing knowledge students do not understand. Skiba and Barton (2006) state that because Generation X and Y seek information and knowledge by connecting to the Internet, not reading their textbooks, faculty members must introduce and encourage students to use discipline-specific databases like CINAHL or MEDLINE versus just seeking information randomly from the Internet. In the same way, databases like CINAHL and personal digital assistants (PDAs) in clinical are excellent tools students can use to access information about their patients' conditions, diagnostic tests or procedures, or a medication they do not know.

The use of wireless laptops, PDAs, and iPods is more than a fad; it is here to stay and is changing education at all levels. Prensky (2001) describes the difference between Generations X and Y compared with Baby Boomers and Traditionalists by the way they view technology. Prensky states, "digital immigrants" (the latter) reach for the Yellow Pages to find a bookstore, and "digital natives" "Google" the information on the Internet. Which are you? Faculties are going to have to continue to be creative in how they engage students in the learning process (Herman, Manning, and Zager, in press).

• C: Connections and communication
Generations X and Y have grown up in a multicultural, multiethnic, and global world. They live in neighborhoods with families that may be biracial and come from many different cultures. These students have been experiencing the customs, dress, and food of many cultures since they were in elementary school. They have traveled extensively with their families and are very open-minded and accepting of different races, cultures, and individual differences. They have been e-mailing and instant messaging all of their lives and may interact with people from different countries through the Internet.

This open-mindedness, acceptance, and appreciation for cultural differences is a valuable asset; however, because of the lack of personal interaction and the cryptic nature of their communication, faculty may find it is imperative to help the students with the interpersonal skills of face-to-face communication, unlike students of the past. Courses in "therapeutic communication" become very important and need to include interactive role playing and practice for students to learn. Interpretation of nonverbal communication, such as body language and facial expressions, may need to be taught and practiced, whereas in the past it may have been sufficient just to read about it. Even more essential will be their ability to detect the nonverbal cues of patients with critical medical or psychosocial needs. Clinical instructors will need to give feedback and model effective caregiver and patient interactions. Simulation laboratories are an excellent addition to clinical resources, but sessions must include relationship-building if students are to be successful in their face-to-face interactions with their patients. Their often short answers or boredom with tedious conversations will present a barrier to effective interactions with Traditionalist and Baby Boomer patients (Herman, Manning, and Zager, in press).

- **H: Have to give frequent feedback**

Generations X and Y want it now! Instant messaging is in, e-mail is out. Even with cell phones, text messaging is used as much as the phone. These generations grew up with interactive games such as Nintendo and expect immediate feedback about how they are doing. Unlike Traditionalists and Baby Boomers, Generations X and Y expect feedback on a daily basis. As with the games, they use this feedback to adjust and learn what works and what does not work. If there is no feedback, they are unable to proceed in the learning process, or like any of us, they will assume they are correct. It is very important for faculty members to communicate to students when they can expect to receive feedback.

Teachers have to set expectations and communicate when they will be available. It is important that teachers also communicate the limits about when they will not be available: 24 hours a day, 7 days a week is not an option! Skiba and Barton (2006) suggest faculty members should post office hours when they are available for instant messaging or for chat rooms. Regardless what faculty members choose, using only midsemester and final evaluations is inadequate to meet the needs of two generations for whom instant messaging is the norm (Herman, Manning, and Zager, in press).

---

8   Why is it important for faculty to continue to evaluate teaching strategies?

The evaluation process cannot be ignored in an attempt to create new and innovative learning environments for students. Teachers must still remember to assess their students' learning styles and preferences, not merely make assumptions because the students are Generations X and Y. The information that needs to be learned must be analyzed and compared with the needs of the students. Skiba and Barton (2006) indicate that the content that needs to be learned needs to be matched with technology that will best support and enhance it. They pose six questions for faculty members to ask themselves in planning their learning experiences for their students:

1. Do you know your students and their preferences?
2. Once you know their preferences, how will you adapt or accommodate?
3. What balance between the physical (classroom) and virtual worlds of learning is appropriate for your student population?
4. Are there renovations to your physical space that need to be targeted for your learners?
5. What is the balance between faculty and student perspectives?
6. How do you engage your learners and what are the best methods for incorporating IT into your teaching? (p. 8).

The optimal goal for today's higher education institutions is for faculty to offer options in creating interactive learning environments that can meet a vast array of learning styles and preferences that keep pace with the needs of the learners.

References

Arhin, A.O., & Johnson-Mallard, V. (2003). Encouraging alternative forms of self-expression in the Generation Y student: A strategy for effective learning in the classroom. The ABNF Journal, Nov/Dec, 121–122.

Herman, J., Manning, L., & Zager, L. (in press). Leading learning: The eight-step approach to clinical teaching. Bosier City, La.: I Can Publishing.

Prensky, M. (2001). Digital natives, digital immigrants. On the Horizon 9(5), NCB University Press. Available at www.marcprensky.com/writing/ Accessed February 16, 2007.

Skiba, D.J., & Barton, A.J. (2006). Adapting your teaching to accommodate the NET generation of learners. The Online Journal of Issues in Nursing, 11(2). Available at www.nursingworld.org/ojin/topic30/tpc30_4.htm. Accessed February 16, 2007.

Resources

Donley, R. (2005). Challenges for nursing in the 21st century. Nursing Economic$ 23(6), 312–318.

Hu, J., Herrick, C., & Hodgin, K.A. (2004). Managing the multigenerational nursing team. The Health Care Manager 23(4), 334–340.

Kupperschmidt, B.R. (2006). Addressing multigenerational conflict: Mutual respect and carefronting as strategy. Online Journal of Issues in Nursing 11(2), 1–14. Available at http://www.nursingworld.org/ojin/topic30/tpc30_3.htm Accessed October 4, 2007.

Martin, C.A. (2004). Bridging the generation gap(s). Nursing 2004, 34(12), 62–63.

Martin, C.A., & Tulgan, B. (2002). Managing the generation mix from collision to collaboration. Amherst, Mass.: HRD Press.

Martin, C.A., & Tulgan, B. (2001). Managing Generation Y. Amherst, Mass.: HRD Press.

Oblinger, D. (2003). Boomers, Gen-Xers, and millennials: Understanding the new students. Educause 38(4): 37–47.

Siela, D. (2006). Managing the multigenerational nursing staff. American Nurse Today 11(3), 47–49.

Tulgan, B. (1997). The manager's pocket guide to Generation X. Amherst, Mass.: HRD Press.

Weston, M. (2006). Integrating generational perspectives in nursing. Online Journal of Issues in Nursing 11(2). Available at

www.nursingworld.org/ojin/topic30/tpc30_1.ht Accessed
    November 10, 2006.
Zemke, R., Raines, C., & Filipczak, B. (2000). Generations at work.
    Managing the clash of veterans, Boomers, Xers, and Nexters in
    your workplace. New York: American Management
    Association.

6

Adults as Students: Special Considerations

Esther H. Condon, PhD, RN

1 Are there any simple rules that should be kept in mind when teaching adult learners?

Being helpful and respectful are two important aspects of what mature learners expect from their teachers. Knowing that each of us has something to learn from others is an important leveling factor in teaching-learning situations. Always being truthful with students is another important rule. Adult learners especially enjoy humor and will participate in making the classroom a fun place to be when given the chance.

2 How do I deal with the fact that I am younger than some of my students?

Sometimes it is uncomfortable to realize that there are adult learners who have knowledge and experience beyond our own. But it *is* comforting to know that most adult learners recognize that we cannot be expected to know everything. Generally, they expect that we, as faculty, are qualified and know our subject matter regardless of our age. By encouraging students to share their knowledge, observations, and experience, the classroom becomes a learning community that values diversity of opinion and abilities.

3 Will I feel less intimidated by mature learners as time goes by?

That depends on you. Having "confident humility" can help
you overcome feelings of insecurity in teaching-learning situations. Developing true partnerships with mature learners
can win you their confidence and diminish feelings of anxiety for all. Often, feelings of insecurity or intimidation can
lead to a desire to control, and this is likely to upset the egalitarian relationship that mature learners prefer in teaching-
learning situations. Showing consideration and respect for
mature learners will earn the same for the teacher.

4 Are there theoretical approaches that work best for mature learners?

Any approach that empowers adult learners is helpful.
Acknowledging that the learner is an adult is very important. Participatory course and assignment development,
teaching strategies, and evaluation strategies that place
responsibility on students work well for mature learners.
Adult learners bring a wealth of knowledge and experience to the classroom if they are encouraged to do so.
Remembering that teaching and learning require a partnership between teacher and students that, among peers,
sets the stage for a positive teaching and learning experience. Being flexible is greatly appreciated by mature learners. However, adult learners do not appreciate having their
time wasted by trivial assignments or being in a classroom
where learning is not taking place.

5 Suppose my students do not like me?

The first obligation that we as teachers have toward our
students is to be effective in teaching. This does not mean
that we should not be likeable or liked by students, but
students tend to prefer teachers who are effective rather
than simply likeable. Not being liked by students may
give you reason to reflect on the effectiveness of your
teaching ability. Consider whether this is situational
(giving challenging but fair examinations) or because of
your methods or style of teaching. Students may not prefer some personality traits in teachers, so modifying one's

behavior may be required to increase student satisfaction with the teaching-learning process. Universally, students abhor feeling intimidated by their teachers. Threatening remarks, even in jest, can quickly lead to feelings of dislike and distrust between students and faculty. Earning the respect of students is a worthy goal of all teachers, and this can be achieved through being effective in the classroom and being available to students to discuss their concerns.

6   Why do some adults in class appear highly motivated, and others seem not to want to be there at all?

Remember that adult learners arrive with prior knowledge that has served them well. Education is about change, and adults need to be sure that new knowledge, values, and beliefs will serve them at least as well as those with which they arrive. Equally important, and maybe more so, are the experiences they have had in other educational settings. These experiences strongly influence how the current situation is perceived and interpreted and the responses that adult learners have in the new learning situation. It is important to be supportive of adult learners who are in the process of changing their perspectives through learning. They are taking a leap of faith that the new learning will be helpful to them.

7   How can I affect the apparently unshakable values and belief systems that are in opposition to what I am trying to teach in class?

Often as teachers we forget that adults have developed values and beliefs over time that are second nature to them. It is not until values and belief systems are challenged or critiqued that their strength and the learner's reliance on them become clear. It is not reasonable to expect that values and beliefs formed over a long period will be changed easily or quickly. Helping adult learners become aware of their own and others' values and beliefs allows them to examine their values and beliefs in the light of new learning and to change them in ways that make them congruent with changes that have taken place as a result of learning.

8 How can I best support the adult learner who is often in class with students who are much younger?

There are times when being the oldest member of the class is not negative. Adult students can often bring a different perspective to their less experienced classmates and demonstrate a work ethic that comes with maturity. Such students are often good role models for their younger counterparts who are struggling with adopting the professional role of nurse. Giving recognition to these students can be a boost and can lead to a mentoring relationship that enhances the adult learner's career. Younger students also gain the opportunity to learn from the more mature student's perceptions of classroom and clinical experiences in a nonthreatening way. Having a mix of younger and older students in a class can be very enriching for all concerned.

9 What do I do when adult and younger learners display conflicting values in class?

Conflicting values are equally likely to appear in classrooms with students who are similar in age. However, the conflict that may appear between adult and younger learners may be generational rather than ideological. Fortunately, conflicting values offer opportunities for dialogue and discussion among diverse students. You need to be skillful in conducting these discussions to allow the expression of all points of view. This is an excellent opportunity to show that conflict has a growth-promoting function and that it can be managed to enhance learners' understanding and tolerance of diverse values. Values clarification exercises can be very rewarding to learners when conducted in an open and supportive forum.

10 What should I know about cultural aspects of teaching adults?

Remember that all cultures define and interpret who and what a teacher is, and this establishes expectations that cannot be ignored. Look at your own cultural values and beliefs about teachers and teaching. This may help you be more sensitive to what students are experiencing. Observing student responses is important. For example, what might seem to be appropriate to a teacher from a majority population might be perceived differently by a student from a minority population. When unexpected responses occur, try to learn what the student has experienced, and respond in a way that clarifies intent and promotes understanding. Some students may feel uncomfortable about raising sensitive topics such as the impact of race, class, gender, age, sexual preference, and disability on life experience and health. Incorporate these topics in the classroom where they can be discussed openly. International student and faculty exchanges are increasingly common, and these, too, provide opportunities for developing understanding of cultural context and meaning.

11 What is the best way to approach the mature learner who is not succeeding in class?

Generally speaking, a considerate and straightforward approach works best. Adult learners need practical advice about how to improve performance. Often they know what is holding them back and will share this, but being an adult is not necessarily sufficient preparation to identify and resolve academic challenges. Adult learners appreciate the time and effort you give them helping them to understand class material, and they are willing to make considerable efforts to reach the required standard. Be flexible if you can with the adult learner who has work and family obligations to provide support and motivation to encourage him or her to persevere and be successful.

12 What are some not-so-optimal scenarios regarding adult students?

Fortunately, teaching adults usually is professionally rewarding and personally satisfying, but there are some unique situations that may occur simply because the students *are* adults. These include the student who:

- Dominates or takes over the class.
- Makes personal advances.

- Brings a child to class.
- Threatens you.
- Is impaired by alcohol or drugs.
- Complains about another faculty member.

---

13 How should I respond to the adult learner who wants to take over the class?

Novice teachers are particularly likely to feel threatened by a perceived loss of control in class. Time and experience in the classroom will alleviate those feelings. Knowing that adults expect to be heard in class and are eager to demonstrate knowledge and competence with peers makes it imperative for us to be willing to share control of the teaching-learning process. There will be times when students have knowledge and experience that surpass yours. In those circumstances, acknowledge the expertise of the student by asking the student to lead discussions on the topic or to give real-life examples that make the theory easier to understand. On the other hand, there will be times that students will want to talk as much as possible even if it deprives others of the opportunity to speak. When this occurs, set a time limit for speaking, and actively call on students who are less inclined to participate. Sometimes asking eager students to "hold that thought" and returning to them after others have had the chance to speak can help to alleviate the problem.

---

14 How do I handle adult learners who are personally attracted?

As a reflective teacher, one should consider how this affects the relationship of trust that must exist between students and teachers. This relationship must take precedence over other kinds of relationships with students. A student may feel admiration for and even be attracted to the teacher, but this should not become the focus of the relationship for a least two reasons. First, the teacher is in a position of power over the student, regardless of how egalitarian the relationship might appear. Teachers make important decisions that affect the lives and the futures of students that could be compromised by romantic involvement. Students become vulnerable when they become romantically involved with teachers, and teachers open themselves to real or perceived conflicts of interest. Second, in the classroom, teachers and students are not peers; teachers are expected to make prudent decisions regardless of decisions that a student might make. Does this mean that the teacher should take action that would hurt the student's feelings? No. Gently reinforcing the appropriate relationship and behavior is the most appropriate action. By taking an even-handed approach toward all students, the teacher can avoid being perceived as "available" in a romantic way.

15 What do I do when an adult learner brings a child to class?

First, knowing the institutional policy about bringing children to class is important. There are possible liability issues should the child be injured as a result of being in the classroom. Second, consider the effect on other learners. When there is a clear policy about children in class, it must be communicated to the entire class at the outset. If it is at the discretion of the teacher, then the entire class must be involved in making the decision. Adult learners appreciate involvement in structuring teaching-learning situations.

16 What should I do if I feel threatened by a student?

Do not ignore these feelings. Assessing the level of threat is an important action to take, and then communicate with the appropriate authority. Often, feelings of anxiety and hostility can be tempered by having another person present, such as a colleague or an advocate for the student, when conferencing with students. There are times when teacher and student feel that the relationship has become adversarial because of a particular issue. There are even times when the student may not behave rationally. The teacher must take all precautions to protect him- or herself and the student from harm.

17 What should I do if I suspect that a student is under the influence of alcohol or drugs in class or clinical?

The abuse of alcohol, street drugs, and prescription drugs has become prevalent among health-care providers. If you suspect a student is abusing alcohol and/or drugs, you must consider the effect on the individual, peers, the teaching-learning environment, and the safety of patients. The safety of patients takes the highest priority if a student's judgment and performance are impaired. There can be no tolerance of drugs or alcohol-related impairment in clinical settings. By the same token, a student will be unable to participate effectively in classroom or other teaching-learning environments when drugs or alcohol-related impairment exists. You must make clear that no student abusing drugs or alcohol will be allowed to participate in teaching-learning situations because of the potential for endangerment to self and others. If impairment is suspected, take steps to protect patients, and bring the situation to the attention of appropriate others. You will need to implement school policy concerning counseling the student. The issue of substance abuse by professionals and options for treatment should be included in student professional leadership courses.

18 What should I do if students come to me with complaints about a faculty colleague?

This is a difficult problem, especially when you have a good relationship with the complaining student and you want to listen. However, students must understand that solutions to complaints about other teachers must be the result of responsible action. Generally, there are procedures in place to address problem resolution, and those should be followed. Often, a student just needs to process a situation and values an opportunity to express a heartfelt opinion about the problem, but this must not take precedence over following the established procedures designed to ensure a fair hearing for all concerned. However, we are obliged to take appropriate action if students are being abused or intimidated by a colleague who refuses to respond to student concerns. Confidentiality should be maintained, and rumor and speculation should not be entertained.

19 What do I do if I believe a colleague is behaving in an arbitrary manner with students?

True colleagues will tell each other the truth about a situation. It is important to have colleagues who can be trusted to do this. There are times when teachers lose perspective, especially when they feel threatened by a situation. It is at these times that a trusted colleague can provide a sounding board and some balancing advice. Teachers and nurses have the same obligation to treat those with whom they interact with respect.

20 What must I know to be successful in teaching adult learners?

Teaching adult learners brings its own challenges and opportunities. Adults often prefer to know the relevance of knowledge to their lives and tend to evaluate it using this criterion. Knowing that adult learners bring a capacity for thoughtful appraisal and often insightful critique of what is being taught gives the teacher an opportunity to think about why and how the content is important and how to convey that importance to learners. Adult learners flourish when their past and current knowledge is valued, when open-mindedness is encouraged, and when learning leads to understanding that produces professional and personal satisfaction. To teach is to change a life, forever.

Resources

Buresh, B., & Gordon, S. (2000). From silence to voice. Ithaca, New York: Cornell University Press.

Clark, C. M., & Springer, P.J. (2007). Incivility in nursing education: A descriptive study of definitions and prevalence. Journal of Nursing Education 46(1), 7–14.

Collins, P. (1993). Black feminist thought. New York: Routledge.

Conro, J.L. (2006) The faculty parking lot is not for planning:

Becoming an effective first-year teacher. Blue Ridge Summit, Pa.: Rowman & Littlefield Education.

Frangenberg, R. (1995). The social construction of whiteness. Minnesota: University of Minnesota Press.

Freire, P. (1970). Pedagogy of the oppressed. New York: Seabury.

Freire, P., & Freire, A. (1997). Pedagogy of the heart. New York: Continuum.

Luparell, S. (2007) The effects of student incivility on nursing faculty. Journal of Nursing Education 46(1), 15–19.

Roach, M.S. (2002). Caring, the human mode of being, 2nd ed. Ottawa, Ontario, Canada: CHA Press.

TEACHING ADULTS

Planning a Course

Patsy Maloney, EdD, RN, BC, CNAA, CEN

1 **What is the difference between planning a course and writing the syllabus?**

Planning a course is analogous to planning patient care and uses similar steps—assessment, planning outcomes (objectives), planning interventions (activities/assignments), implementation (structuring the activities and assignments), and evaluation. The course-planning process begins with an assessment of context, subject, students, environment, and teacher. After the assessment, the planner decides on learner-centered objectives. In other words, what skills and knowledge should the students have by the end of the course? Then the faculty member plans the interventions or activities and assignments that facilitate achievement of the objectives. The next question is how best to structure or implement these activities. The final question is how to evaluate achievement of the objectives. The syllabus is the tool that documents the plan and communicates the course plan to the students. It is analogous to the written nursing care plan that communicates the care.

2   How do I get started planning a course?

The first thing a course planner does is to assess the context, subject, environment, students, and the teacher. These are the specific context of the course or the course environment, the general context of the course, the nature of the subject, the characteristics of the learners or the students, and the characteristics of the teacher.

3   How do I assess the general context of the course?

Answer the following questions: What is the purpose of this course? How does this course fit into the larger picture? It is not just the teacher who determines the purpose of the course. The university, the college, school or department of nursing, the profession, and society as a whole have expectations of nursing courses. The course is part of a larger curriculum that addresses the larger context. The faculty member needs to know at what level the course will be offered—at the beginning of the program, in the middle, or near graduation. What courses are prerequisites? What courses come after this course? What knowledge and skills do the teachers of the course expect from the students?

4   How do I assess the nature of the subject or content?

Ask if the subject is practical, theoretical, or a combination. Nursing students are usually more motivated to learn practical courses, such as medical-surgical nursing and pharmacology. Theoretical courses, such as research and history, are often not considered as useful by students. What is essential information to be covered? Are there controversies or important changes in the field that need to be addressed?

5   How do I assess environment?

The environment of a course is more than the physical space in which it will be delivered, such as a laboratory, clinical agency, or technologically advanced classroom. It consists of the number of students, the length and frequency of class meetings, and whether the course will be delivered live or online, or a combination of both.

6 How do I assess the students?

When planning a course, it is important to assess the students who will be taking it. Are they primarily working students with families, or traditional college students? What prior knowledge and experiences do they bring that relate to the subject? In nursing it is not unusual to have 50-year-old working students and 20-year-old traditional students in the same classroom. Many students come with previous health-care experiences, such as those of an emergency medical technician, renal dialysis technician, or phlebotomist. Many come with college degrees in fields other than health care. All students come with different learning goals, expectations, and preferred learning styles.

7 How do I assess the teacher?

Finally, if you are the course planner, you must assess yourself as a teacher. What are your beliefs about teaching and learning? What are your attitudes about the students and about the subject? What is your level of content knowledge? What are your strengths and challenges as a teacher?

8 How do I know what the objectives should be?

Start with the end in mind. What skills and abilities should the students have at the end of the course? What should they retain for 2 to 3 years after the course is over? Should they value lifelong learning? These become the learning-centered objectives. In general, faculty planners use Bloom's Taxonomy: cognitive, affective, and psychomotor domains for writing content objectives. The outcomes—objectives—for significant learning should include subject knowledge beyond simple memorization and basic understanding. This includes the higher levels of Bloom's cognitive domain: application, analysis, synthesis, and evaluation as well as what Fink terms the human dimensions, which he describes as interactive and reflective skills, caring (he describes it as valuing), and finally learning how to learn, which is practicing skills and abilities and valuing learning. Learning outcomes can fit under these objectives categories for universities and schools of nursing. For example, at Pacific Lutheran University our categories are subject knowledge and methodology, critical reflection, interaction with others, expression, valuing, and using multiple frameworks. One course is not expected to have objectives addressing all areas, but it should reflect more than basic understanding of the subject. Really think about what the student should know and the skills and abilities that each student should have by the time he or she has completed the course.

---

9 How do I determine progress toward the course objectives?

Progress is determined by assessment of the student's work and feedback to the student. Fink recommends "forward-looking assessment." Wiggins terms this "authentic assessment." Forward assessment is looking ahead to real-life situations in which the student will need to use these skills. Forward assessment creates a real-life problem for the student to solve. It is best if this problem is unstructured and open-ended. For example, assign a student in a health assessment class to evaluate an individual or family and develop a health promotion plan to include a health teaching plan. This assignment requires the student to use subject matter, critical thinking, and interpersonal skills.

Traditional assessment is differentiated from authentic assessment, and both are necessary. Traditional assessment requires a student to respond, whether in multiple choice, essay, or fill-in-the-blank. It is teacher-contrived and -structured and offers indirect evidence of the ability of a student to perform. Authentic assessment is a real-life task performance structured by the student and provides direct rather than indirect evidence of skills and abilities. An example is the state driver's license examination: a multiple-choice examination and a driving performance test, a combination of traditional assessment and authentic assessment. Student self-assessment should be part of the course plan as well as frequent feedback. Feedback should be provided frequently at least weekly, if not daily. It should discriminate poor from adequate from excellent work, and it should be offered with care and concern.

10 How do I choose the learning activities and/or assignments for the course?

Include experiential and reflective activities as well as the more traditional lecture and textbook reading activities. When a student accesses information and ideas from primary sources, it increases learning over merely reading about it or having the teacher lecture. Experiencing is a powerful way of learning. This is the true value of nursing clinical experiences. In-class experiences include debates, simulations, role playing, and dramatizations. Outside of class, students may be involved in authentic projects, situational observations, and service learning. But the experiences are not enough. Students must reflect on what they are learning and how they are achieving their objectives. Each student should consider what still needs to be learned. The reflective dialogue can take place with self in the form of a journal and/or portfolio or with others in a group setting or on a Web site discussion board. The instructor should facilitate and monitor these activities to make sure students are progressing well.

11 How do I know if my course components—objectives, assessment, teaching and learning activities—are integrated?

Review the assessment plan to see if it addresses all course objectives, allows for adequate feedback to students on all objectives, and allows for student self-assessment. Ask the following questions:

- Are the teaching/learning activities appropriate for outcome achievement?

- Are there extraneous assignments that do not address an objective?
- Do the teaching/learning activities and feedback on the activities prepare the student for the final course assessments?

---

12 Once I have planned the outcomes, the assessment, and the activities, how do I organize the course into a whole?

The first step is to divide the quarter or semester into four to seven sections that focus on the major topics of the course. Arrange the topics in the best manner for introducing them to students, and decide on how many class sessions to devote to each topic. Take advantage of the organizational scheme to create progressively challenging assignments working toward a capstone assignment at the end of the course.

---

13 How do I grade the assignments and activities?

The grading system should reflect your objectives and teaching/learning activities. A teacher is not required to grade everything. Early assignments may be given strictly for feedback. For example, allow students to present several times for feedback before grading a presentation. The grading weight assigned to an activity or assessment should reflect the importance of the activity. Decide on the components of the course that you will grade. Grading should not be overwhelming; weigh each assignment. Students can often give valuable input into what should be graded and the value of any particular assignment. You can build the request for student input into your course plan.

---

14 How do I decide upon how many out-of-class assignments are necessary and beneficial?

Build a template that includes every class meeting. On the template, include in-class and out-of-class teaching/learning activities. The out-of-class activities need to prepare the students for in-class work, keep them connected to the subject, and allow them to practice skills between classes. A good rule is to expect 2 hours of outside classwork for every hour of in-class work. In other words, for a three-credit class, 6 hours of out-of-class work per week is a reasonable expectation. Any assignment, whether in-class or out-of-class, should be directly related to a course objective.

---

15 How do I choose the course resources?

Course resources include the textbook or collection of articles, videos, or any other material necessary to facilitate the students' achievement of course objectives. Textbooks are designed to cover the subject matter and often have accompanying instructor resources with suggested teaching and learning activities as well as a test bank. It is important for a new faculty member to realize that far more attention goes into the writing of the content as opposed to the instructor resources to facilitate achievement of objectives. Therefore, do not count on instructor resources. To select the text, get copies of different publishers' texts covering your subject. Get input from students and other faculty on the text. You are not just looking for subject coverage but a resource to facilitate the achievement of course objectives. If new material becomes available after you choose a text or a topic is not covered in the text, choose articles to supplement. In addition to written material, films allow students to experience something that they would otherwise miss. For example, the film *Wit* shows the diagnosis and treatment of advanced ovarian cancer and then death. It is a powerful resource for end-of-life care or informed consent.

---

16 How do I evaluate the entire course, not just assess student learning?

The simplest way to evaluate the course is to use a survey and ask students a variety of questions concerning the course. Most universities have a system for doing this and then give the feedback from these surveys to the course faculty. The students' performance on the assignments, particularly the final capstone assignment, is helpful information. Many universities have faculty teaching consultants available that can meet with the class and get anonymous feedback for the course instructor.

---

17 If this is the best way to plan a course, why is it so rarely used?

Course design and planning is a complicated and time consuming process. Often, new teachers are given a course to teach with a syllabus used by the previous teacher. The new teacher has anywhere from a couple of weeks to a whole semester to prepare, but in any case this course is one of many responsibilities. Excellent courses require time, knowledge, application, and reflection on the latest evidence on learning. Without the time and dedication involved in creating a course, the previous syllabus, which is meant only to communicate a course design to students, becomes the plan. The topics for the syllabus, often coming from the table of contents of the textbook, become the driving force for the course rather than learning outcomes that include skills and abilities. Should your course be purpose- and objectives-driven or content-driven by a textbook? What should drive the teaching and learning process—the students' learning needs or the textbook manufacturer?

Resources

Fink, L.D. (2003). A self-directed guide to designing courses for significant learning. Accessed March 31, 2007, at http://www.ysu.edu/catalyst/PastEvents/2005/FinkIDGuide.htm

Grady, G. (2001) Designing and planning a successful course: Bridging the gap between common practice and best practice. Accessed March 31, 2007, at http://www.cdtl.nus.edu.sg/brief/v4n6/default.htm

Mueller, J. (2006). Authentic assessment toolbox. Accessed April 8, 2007, at http://jonathan.mueller.faculty.noctrl.edu/toolbox/whatisit.htm

Wiggins, G.P. (1993). Assessing student performance. San Francisco: Jossey-Bass Publishers.

Wiggins, G., & McTighe, J. (1998). Understanding by design. Alexandria, Va.: Association for Supervision and Curriculum Development.

8

Developing a Course Syllabus

Debra P. Shelton, EdD, APRN-CS, CNA, OCN, CNE

---

1 What is a syllabus?

The syllabus is a written communication tool that provides an overview of the course and what will be taught during the course. When a faculty member is interested in teaching a new course, he or she develops the syllabus. Typically, the syllabus is submitted to the curriculum committee before a course can be taught within the college or department to ensure that the content is not taught in other courses and is either a required or an elective course. If the course has been taught before, a syllabus will be on file in the department.

---

2 Why do I need a syllabus?

All courses require a syllabus. The syllabus conveys important information about the course to the students. Like going to a foreign country, you need a map to know how to navigate the place; students and faculty need the syllabus to navigate through the course.

---

3 What is the purpose of the syllabus?

A syllabus defines the instructor's role and the student's responsibilities in the course. The syllabus will identify the course content, convey the course requirements, and detail the student's involvement in the course. The focus should be on student learning.

---

4 I am teaching a course for the first time, but I do not like the existing syllabus. What do I do?

Certain components of the syllabus cannot be altered. Once the curriculum committees have approved the course, the course must stay essentially the same: the course number, description, pre- and co-requisites. But the faculty member can incorporate current concepts and content related to the course and can identify new forms of evaluation and learning activities.

---

5 Is there a format for the syllabus?

The format is generally standardized for the entire college or university. In some instances, all departments use a template. The syllabus should be succinct and not overload the student with information. Too much detail is a detriment to learning. On the other hand, there must be enough guidance that learners know what is expected of them. Decide what the student needs to know in the beginning to start the course and progress through the course content successfully.

---

6 What is included in the syllabus?

A general rule for syllabus content is:

- Course number, course description
- Pre- and co-requisites
- Course and unit objectives
- Required textbooks, materials, and supplies
- Course content/outline
- Grading system
- Learning activities
- Evaluation process
- Policies regarding attendance, late work, and makeup work

More information can be added that defines the student responsibilities for course work. Grading criteria for assignments, handouts, course calendar, and other learning resources can be included. Some departments include policies with which students should be familiar.

---

7   If I do not like the grading standards, can I change them?

Generally, grading standards are developed by the entire department. If a faculty member wants to change the grading scale for a course, often such a request must be taken to the curriculum committee for approval. In addition, the accrediting agencies will want to know the rationale for the proposed change.

---

8   Can I change the assignments?

Assignments can be changed as needed by the instructor and/or the department. When changing an assignment, consider how the assignment fits into the course and how it will be evaluated. Make sure you have identified the critical elements and grading criteria for the new assignment before making changes, because assignments that are not well thought out may not accomplish what you intend.

---

9   How do I select and convey reading assignments to learners?

Required textbooks and readings should be included in the syllabus. Review a number of textbooks well in advance of the course before selecting one or more. Textbook decisions are made at least a semester before the course is taught to ensure that the bookstore can obtain the books. When selecting textbooks, focus on the currency of the content and difficulty level. The required readings help the student understand the course content and supplement the lectures and the learning activities. Recommended readings are usually optional for students, but they should also supplement the course content. Other learning resources can be included in the syllabus—Web sites, videos, CDs, and so on. Consider the cost of the books as well as the cost of copying or obtaining the required and recommended readings.

---

10 Do I need to include a schedule that describes each class?

A course schedule or calendar should be available to the students. This does not necessarily have to be included in the syllabus. The schedule helps students prepare for each class and also know when assignments are due or tests are scheduled. Students can plan their semester and know what to expect during the course. List class holidays and important dates on the schedule.

---

11 How detailed does the content outline need to be?

The course content can be in a number of formats. Generally, the course content is in outline form. The course content should build from the basic concepts to the more advanced concepts. The outline can be as detailed as you want it. A very detailed outline does take up a lot of space. The course schedule, content, and required/recommended readings can all be placed in the syllabus.

---

12 How do I select learning experiences for the content?

The learning experiences should reflect the course content and should encourage critical thinking and application of the course concepts. The learning experiences should promote students' engagement in the course and promote active learning. Assignments, papers, projects, and case studies are just a few of the various learning experiences that can be incorporated into the course. Offer a variety of activities, and be sure to analyze how the learning experiences develop the students' skills and application of knowledge and enhance learning.

---

13 Do the learning experiences need to be identified in the syllabus?

The learning experiences should be outlined in the course syllabus so that students are aware of the various activities that comprise the course and what will be expected of them. Descriptions of learning experiences can be brief or detailed. If brief descriptions are included, spend class time reviewing the learning activities in more detail. Students are eager to discover what and how they will be learning in the course, so this is important to get right.

---

14 Can I put articles in the syllabus?

Placing articles in the syllabus presents a whole new issue. If you are the author of the article and you have the copyrights to the article, then you can include the articles. Most of the time, faculty will provide citations for articles, and students are expected to obtain their own copy, or the article can be placed in the library on reserve. If the article is not available to the students, you can obtain permission from the publisher to duplicate copies for students. Because obtaining permission can be a lengthy process, you will need to allow ample time, and you may also be required to pay a fee.

---

15 Why does the university want to copyright my syllabus?

Copyrighting is a form of protection provided by U.S. law for intellectual works. Copyrights are provided for unpublished and published works. A syllabus can be considered a "work for hire," which is a work developed by the author within the scope of a position. In this case, the employer is considered the author of the syllabus. The faculty member and the university need to agree in writing that the syllabus is considered a work made for hire. The copyright of the material is secured automatically when the work is created, according to the 1976 Copyright Act. For more information on copyright law, see the government Web site http://www.copyright.gov

---

16 How do I go about revising a syllabus?

Time and thought need to go into the revision process. Consider the purpose of the syllabus and what needs to be conveyed to the learner. If other faculty members have taught the course, you might want to get input from them on changes that need to be made to the syllabus. At the completion of the course, faculty should review the course evaluations and revise the syllabus at that time. If you wait until the next time the course is taught, you may forget the changes that need to be made. Bear in mind the logistics of providing the syllabus to the students. Getting the syllabus copied may take weeks to ensure sufficient copies are available.

17 How can I make my syllabus user-friendly?

The syllabus should be organized and easy to read. Avoid elaborate fonts. Highlight or bold important information that you want to stand out to the students. One good way to make it student-friendly is to provide faculty contact information, office number, and office hours. A letter to the student or comments about the instructor's philosophy can set the tone of the course and can help the students understand how the class will be conducted. The syllabus can communicate your openness to questions as well as the direction of the course.

18 How can I make my syllabus learner-oriented?

The focus of syllabus development has changed from being a brief two-page handout to a learner-centered work. The learning-centered syllabus promotes student engagement in the course and becomes a learning tool that promotes active, purposeful, and effective learning. A learning-centered syllabus requires that the faculty member develop a positive learning environment using creative teaching and learning strategies to engage the student.

19 How is the syllabus shared with students?

Handing out copies during the first class is one option for providing the syllabus to the students. Other means include having copies available in the bookstore. In the current technology-oriented environment, posting online has become a means of providing the syllabus to students. The syllabus can be placed on a local server, a Web home page, or through courseware such as Blackboard and WebCT. When placing the syllabus online, consider your own computer skills and those of the students. Faculty members should still require that students have a hard copy of the syllabus and refer to it frequently during the course.

Resources

Davis, B.G. Creating a syllabus. Accessed April 27, 2007, at http://teaching.berkeley.edu/bgd/syllabus.html

Davis, B.G. Preparing or revising a syllabus. Accessed April 27, 2007, at http://teaching.berkeley.edu/bgd/prepare.html

Grunert, J. (1997). The course syllabus: A learning-centered approach. Bolton, Mass.: Anker Publishing.

Singham M. (2005). Moving away from the authoritarian classroom. Change 37(3), 50–57.

Numerous other Web sites are available on writing and developing a course syllabus.

9

Learner-Centered Teaching

Jean E. Bartels, PhD, RN

---

1 What do the experts say about the nature of learning and knowing?

Most experts believe that learning and knowing are very individualistic activities. Individuals approach learning based on acquired cognitive styles and learning approaches that are used and developed over time. What one knows is grounded in perceptions gleaned from interaction with the world and learning environments. Eventually, individuals build personal knowledge bases and trend toward preferred ways of gathering, interpreting, analyzing, and storing information, all the while establishing ways to use that knowledge across applied contexts.

2 What is the process by which individuals actually learn?

Learning occurs most effectively when it is integrative and experiential, self-aware and reflective, active and interactive, developmental and transferable. Marilla D. Svinicki (1994) states the following about learning theories:

- Information is learned only after it is recognized.
- Learners use information in ways that make it meaningful to themselves.

- Learners store learned information in their long-term memory, organizing it in a way that is consistent with their understanding of the world.
- Learners return to their understandings, test them in new contexts, and then refine and revise what they have learned.
- Learners do not automatically transfer learning to new contexts but rather apply learning only after exposure to multiple situations.
- Learning as a process is most effective when learners become aware of their learning style and actively decide on the best approaches to use in a given situation.

3   Are there really differences in how individuals learn?

Research has shown that people do learn in different ways, often returning to learning approaches that are comfortable for them. Some individuals learn best from very specific, hands-on, and involved experiences; others learn best when they can observe others. Some learn by imaging or conceptualizing their experiences, creating mental explanations for what they observe. Others like to experiment with new information and experiences, using abstract theories to solve problems and make decisions. The most effective learners, however, develop a full range of learning styles in order to accommodate the wide variety of learning situations they are likely to encounter. They understand how to use multiple learning approaches depending on the context in which they find themselves.

4   Are these differences important in nursing education?

Traditionally, nurses have learned through what has been identified as four fundamental ways of knowing. Kolb's (1984) experiential learning theory also provides a useful theoretical framework and terminology for each, in parentheses:

- Scientific reasoning (abstract conceptualization)
- Ethical or moral obligation (reflective observation)

- Personal involvement (concrete experience)
- Aesthetic appreciation (active experimentation)

Significant to nurse educators, these distinct yet interdependent ways of knowing require a holistic approach to the educative process preparing nurses for the full scope of their practice. Attending to each ensures that learners experience and reflect on the full scope of the practice discipline. The educational experience must help learners understand what they need to know and why, appreciate the rights and responsibilities of their practice, develop an appreciation of their lived experiences, and attribute significance and meaning to their work.

---

5   What are the characteristics of a successful learner?

Successful learners develop characteristics that prepare them for a lifetime of learning. They understand how to integrate and build their learning to maximize their personal effectiveness. They are independent and creative, consistently aware of their own capabilities. They are committed to demonstrating their best, and they are habitual in doing so. Successful learners participate as active and independently aware learners, adapt effectively to the learning environment, adopt the perspectives and practices of the discipline they are attempting to learn, develop intellectual habits that make connections between prior and present learning, and understand the importance of self-assessing their own strengths and challenges.

---

6   Are some approaches to the teaching-learning process better than others?

The most critical learning that an educator must do is to understand that learning goes beyond knowing to doing something with what one knows. Educators are responsible for making learning available to students by clearly articulating outcome expectations, identifying the criteria for successful performance, and making those expectations public. In order to do that, teaching and learning processes must be flexible and adaptive to the context and desired outcome of the learning experience and individualized to the variety of learning styles and learning needs of students. Approaching the teaching-learning process from this perspective allows for learning to be integrated, self-aware, active, developmental, and transferable.

7   What is the real goal of learning?

The real goal of learning is to foster independence in learners, preparing them for a lifetime of personal and professional development. Ultimately, learners must independently seek their personal learning goals, and those goals must be understood as a lifelong pursuit. Independent learners possess the critical thinking skills that will ensure their ongoing growth. They understand how to evaluate evidence; identify assumptions that influence behavior; bring multiple perspectives to their interpretation of situations and problems; evaluate an argument; consistently assess the quality of their own thinking; employ increasingly complex, nuance-sensitive thinking to each context in which they find themselves; and communicate their understandings to others.

8   What are the assumptions and principles that underpin learning?

Learning is an interactive and dynamic process that requires both the learner and the educator to engage in outcome-directed activity. Borrowing from Alverno College (Mentkowski & Associates, 2000), the following educational assumptions should form the foundation of learning:

- Learning goes beyond knowing to being able to do something with what one knows.
- Learning becomes available to learners when educators articulate clear expectations/outcomes along with the criteria for successful learning.
- Learners should have multiple opportunities to develop and analyze their learning in varied ways and contexts.

- Learners vary widely in their learning style, motivation for learning, and development as learners.
- Expectation/outcomes must be carefully identified and compared with what contemporary life requires.
- Learning involves making actions out of knowledge—using knowledge actively to think, judge, make decisions, discover, interact, create.
- Active learning involves the clarification of information, determined (purposeful) practice in using information, assessment of one's progress toward meeting learning expectations, and feedback on successes and areas yet to be developed.

---

9 How might those assumptions and principles affect my approach/attitude toward teaching?

Active learning approaches require that educators take responsibility for making learning more available to learners. We do this by clearly articulating our expectations and making them public to the learner. We become, then, more responsible for developing new ways to teach the growing amount of knowledge and skills required of new graduates. Using active learning strategies and real-life experiences, along with an integrated approach to teaching across the curriculum, educators create the context and structure that places learners clearly in the center of the learning experience.

---

10 What is the difference between developing competence and developing abilities in the learning process?

Abilities are learned dispositions to perform in ways that reflect specialized knowledge, attitudes, skills, motivations, and self-perceptions. For example, one develops an ability to communicate that reflects one's level of education or development, knowledge, experience, and self-understanding. Developing competence with an ability requires that the learner can habitually use that ability effectively in a variety of contexts, consistently attentive and adaptive to the nuances each context presents.

11 What are the abilities learners need to develop to be successful in the current nursing practice environment?

Nurses practice in environments that are extremely complex and nuance-sensitive. This requires a well-honed ability set that can be adapted to multiple demands, audiences, and contexts. Minimally, nurses need to develop competence with the ability to:

- Communicate effectively with a variety of audiences in a variety of modes (e.g., writing, speaking, using technology, critically listening and reading, mathematically).
- Critically and creatively analyze and solve problems.
- Interact effectively with colleagues as well as clients.
- Work collaboratively in groups to accomplish tasks.
- Use values and ethics in making moral judgments.
- Act responsibly professionally and as a culturally sensitive global citizen.

These abilities have been highlighted in the AACN *Essentials of Baccalaureate Education for Professional Nursing Practice* (1998), a document that has been reaffirmed by nurse educators and practice partners studying contemporary and future educational needs for nurses.

12 How can abilities be leveled to ensure appropriate learning develops?

Abilities are best developed using incremental learning, determined practice, and multiple opportunities for performance in varied contexts. Picturing an ability at its expected endpoint is a good way to begin. What exactly should the learner be able to do with what he/she knows at the *end* of the learning experience? Put your vision of this end product into a full and detailed word description. From there, sequence how much and what type of development is needed, as the learner progresses from novice to experienced, in his or her use of the ability. What will the learner need to learn and practice at each stage of development? What increasingly complex context will provoke the ability? To master an ability, the learner and teacher must engage in an exchange of observations related to the development and assessment of the ability. What criteria will be used to measure success at each developmental level? How will the learner reflect on his or her progress toward development and comfort with the ability? How will feedback to the learner be arranged regarding progress toward the endpoint of the ability?

13 Can you provide an example of how an ability might be developed in a learning situation?

An ability essential to professional nursing practice is the ability to communicate effectively in multiple modes and contexts. By the end of a program of studies in nursing, the learner should be able to speak and write effectively for diverse audiences by establishing and maintaining context, developing ideas logically and congruent with theoretical perspectives, supporting ideas with evidence, using appropriate conventions, and addressing content appropriate to the context and audience. Initially, the learner should be given opportunities to perform the technical skills of speaking and writing with a consciousness of each element of the process. Support and feedback from the faculty are important and necessary as the learner begins to understand the elements of effective writing and speaking as well as how to evaluate his/her own effectiveness. As the learner develops, he/she should be able to write and speak with confidence, integrating all expectations for effective communication into a comfortable approach to speaking and writing that has become habitual. He/she should be given learning experiences that refine skills in multiple and diverse contexts. The learner self-assesses each performance, accepting responsibility for overcoming challenges to his/her own work. The advanced student independently demonstrates end-of-program expectations, integrating communication skills within the framework and context of the discipline. No longer dependent on faculty feedback, the learner creates and implements his/her own benchmarks for the ability.

14 How does developing an ability relate to program outcomes?

Program outcomes are sets of statements that describe the abilities that a learner will be able to demonstrate at the end of a set of learning experiences. These statements indicate the abilities expected of an individual who has progressed successfully through a program of studies. Taken collectively, the program outcomes should paint a comprehensive picture of what the graduate is able to do with the learning he/she has acquired. Outcomes should include the integration of knowledge, abilities, attitudes, and performance capabilities that the learner has been validated as achieving.

15 What is "experiential learning"?

Experiential learning is the activity of connecting what one knows with one's actions. It is active learning, purposefully constructed, and practiced so that the learner experiences a seamless connection between thinking and doing. Experiential learning involves making an action out of knowledge—using knowledge to think, judge, make decisions, discover, interact, and create. This active learning requires clear information regarding what is to be learned, determined (planned and guided) practice in using that information to achieve an outcome, regular assessment of progress being made toward mastery of the learning experience, and feedback on successes and areas needing development so that they too can be turned into successes.

16 Do students really learn better through performance?

Evidence suggests that performance-based learning endures because it encourages conscious connections between knowledge and action. Learners who put knowledge into actions tend to see the interrelatedness of their learning with both theoretical perspectives and the world of work. Through performance and active self-reflection, learners begin to take increasing responsibility for their own development as they are encouraged to bridge the conceptual and abstract with the reality of their experience. Such learning confirms the educational experience, gives meaning to the theoretical, and assists the learner in understanding and taking on a professional identity.

---

17 Can collaborative learning really work?

The old saying "two heads are better than one" could be replaced today with the understanding that "more than one head is needed for solving today's problems." Learning collaboratively places an individual in the situation of potentially experiencing both convergent and divergent opinions and thoughts, the very elements that are necessary for reflective and fully developed thinking. Learning in isolation reduces the learner's ability to challenge conventional thinking, learn from the divergent perspectives of others, and form cooperative bonds. Through collaboration, better solutions to complex problems are likely to be formed.

---

18 What is learning productivity?

Learning is productive when it results in growth and change for the learner as well as improved thinking and problem solving in the situation. Productive learning has occurred when learners are challenged to bring their best thinking to a learning situation, to apply their learning across multiple contexts, and to make their thinking public so that others can learn from and build on it. This means that learning must be active if it is to be productive. It must involve exploring relevant phenomena and making purposeful and well-considered judgments about courses of action to take. Learners who think productively think critically. Critical thinking requires learners to:

- Evaluate evidence.
- Identify the assumptions that influence behavior.
- Bring multiple perspectives into their interpretation of situations and problems.
- Evaluate all related arguments surrounding an issue.

- Assess the quality of their own thinking.
- Employ more complex, increasingly nuance-sensitive, contextual thinking in a situation.
- Communicate the results of their learning in context.

---

19 How can we help students learn better?

Educators have the responsibility for transforming teaching, learning, and assessment practices to focus on what students are able to do with what they know. Students should not be the last ones to know what is expected of them related to their learning. Educators must take the responsibility for making learning more available to learners by articulating outcomes and making them public. This means educators must develop new ways to teach the growing amount of knowledge and skills required of new graduates. They must create innovative ways to provide this knowledge and experience across multiple contexts. Successful students learn to connect their learning, bridging knowledge and experience. This requires educators to use an integrated, connected approach to teaching across the curriculum, being singularly focused on developing each student across all learning experiences.

---

20 What does it mean to create a community of learning?

A community of learning requires educators to not only have an interest in teaching but also be open to continuous improvement. We need to be willing to create the context and structures to support a system that makes students the center of the learning experience. We have to have an understanding of what the outcomes of student learning should be across the curriculum by having a public agreement on our educational expectations, assumptions, and values. We must explicitly incorporate those outcomes into our teaching. Last, we must enter partnerships with our learners, helping them to see that learning that is meaningful is learning that is collaborative, linked to shared experiences, developed over time, and continuously expanded.

21 How can we make learning last?

Learning that lasts is learning that transforms the individual, making him or her consciously aware of how what is known finds interpretation and meaning in the reality of one's life, career, and relationships. Learning lasts when it becomes a routine, effective way of approaching questions, problems, or new contexts. We make learning last when we give students opportunities to bridge didactic information with the realities of their chosen career. Successful learners are individuals who have developed the intellectual habits that connect prior learning with new experiences, making them able to connect relevant concepts and apply theories and abilities appropriate to the situation. We make learning available and lasting for students when we create places for this ability to be practiced, assessed, and modified until the learner experiences each ability as a habitual approach to exploring and addressing new, complex issues and situations.

22 Is it time for a new approach to learning?

It is clear that education must inevitably and powerfully change if we are to adequately prepare the next generation of nurses to participate as full partners in shaping the future of health care and the profession. The extraordinary amount of emerging information available today, coupled with the demands of the practice environment, requires that nurse educators find new ways to assist learners in developing the ability to locate, analyze, and apply knowledge. It is no longer adequate to just have information; one must now be able to use what one knows to create better solutions for increasingly complex practice challenges.

23 How do we change the undergraduate education paradigm from teaching to learning?

Changing the undergraduate education paradigm from teaching to learning requires a commitment by educators to place students at the center of the learning experience.

This requires that educators take full responsibility for making learning more available by articulating outcomes and related criteria for the successful achievement of outcomes. Educators must collaboratively determine what contemporary life requires, what these outcomes are as well as what abilities these outcomes require. They must develop these abilities, assisting learners to take action from their knowledge—using their knowledge to think, judge, decide, discover, interact, and create. Improving the quality of education in order to meet these demands, challenges, and opportunities of the future will require internal motivation, a collaborative culture, and the continuous cycle of using outcome assessment data to improve how we teach and learn. Becoming better will definitely require doing things differently.

References

American Association of Colleges of Nursing. (1998). The essentials of baccalaureate education for professional nursing practice. Washington, DC: Author.

Kolb, D.A. (1984). Experiential learning: Experience as the source of learning and development. Upper Saddle River, N.J.: Prentice Hall.

Mentkowski, M. (2000). Learning that lasts: Integrating learning, development, and performance in college and beyond. San Francisco: Jossey-Bass.

Svinicki, M.D. (1994). Practical implications of cognitive theories. In Feldman, K.A., & Paulsen, M.B., eds. Teaching and learning in the college classroom. Needham Heights, Mass.: Glenn Press, 274–281.

Resources

Association of American Colleges and Universities. (2002). Greater expectations: A new vision for learning as a nation goes to college. Washington, DC: Author.

Chinn, P., & Kramer, M. (2004). Integrated knowledge development in nursing. St. Louis: Mosby.

Hutchings, P. (2000). Opening lines: Approaches to the scholarship of teaching and learning. Menlo Park, Calif.: Carnegie Publications.

Lowenstein, A., & Bradshaw, M. (2001). Fuszard's innovative teaching strategies in nursing, 3rd ed. Gaithersburg, Md.: Aspen Publications.

Smith, B., et al. (2004). Learning communities: Reforming undergraduate education. San Francisco: Jossey-Bass.

10

The Power of the Classroom Climate

Patricia G. Coyle-Rogers, PhD, RN-BC

1 What do you mean by "classroom climate"?

The classroom climate is the relationship between you and your students as well as the relationship between each of the students. It depends on each individual in the group, the group dynamics, and the subject being studied. Classroom climate has two components: (1) physical environment and (2) psychological/emotional environment. These elements are always present; therefore, you must pay close attention to each, as a healthy classroom climate will enhance achievement and satisfaction in your teaching-learning process.

2 What elements of the classroom climate are particularly important for learners?

The physical environment and psychological/emotional environment are crucial to your classroom climate. The physical environment should be comfortable and encourage the learners to participate. The psychological/emotional climate, however, is the area over which you have greater control. Creating an environment that fosters mutual respect is key to establishing a positive classroom tone.

3 What is my role in establishing classroom climate?

Your role as faculty in creating a positive classroom climate is vital to the learning process. The first session of each class is pivotal for establishing a climate for learning that is respectful, supportive, challenging, friendly, informal, open, and spontaneous without being threatening and condescending. Mutual respect for individuals and their ideas are the most important principles you can foster. Creating a spirit of acceptance is important so students can feel confident to express their thoughts and feelings. To create this tone, you will need to role-model the desired behaviors.

Your role, therefore, is to "light the fire" for learning, help the student develop and use thinking skills, and provide an environment that nurtures motivation and active student involvement. In the classroom, teachers find this can be accomplished through strategies that:

- Utilize the learning processes and thinking skills inherent in the "learning loop."
- Engage participants in the learning process.
- Recognize the motivational potential both of nurses' inborn propensities and the design of the learning tasks.
- Provide a positive learning climate through supportive interaction.

You can most readily influence climate by focusing on two complementary aspects of classroom interaction: the rapport *between* you and the students and the rapport *among* the participants. In the first, you can promote a positive rapport by functioning as a facilitator of the learners' efforts, emphasizing supportive interaction and assuming the role of an ally who is working *with* them to *improve* their competency rather than a judge for whom they must *prove* their competency. This practice was called the "learning loop" above and is most successful when you and your students are engaged in tasks with a goal and purpose beyond the classroom.

By initiating and maintaining a supportive climate, you can promote a bond of trust, personal ownership of the learning, and a willingness of the students to take risks, be creative, and pursue learning independently In the second aspect, positive rapport *among* the learners promotes a sense of community that encourages creativity, a sense of security, an intrinsic desire to learn, and the risk-taking of self-initiated learning. You can nurture this rapport among learners by providing a noncompetitive, collaborative atmosphere and:

- Using teaching strategies that promote collaboration rather than competition such as small and large group work toward such shared goals as improving performance.
- Encouraging learners to use each other as resources.
- Setting up peer interviews, which help participants learn about and identify with each other.

Figure 10–1 illustrates the role of classroom climate and its impact. This concept is so vital for the process of learning to take place.

4   How do I create a positive physical environment?

You can adjust any of the following to provide a positive physical environment:

- Use tables and chairs rather than the standard classroom desk to encourage face-to-face interaction. Tables of four to six students work best.
- Use a nonlinear classroom setup, such as arranging seating in a circle or semicircle.

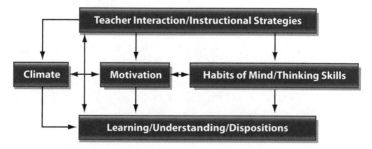

Figure 10–1. The role of classroom climate. (Pontious, M. [2005]. Classroom climate. Wisconsin School Musician 75[3], 10. Used with permission.)

- Make sure the room has good lighting and ventilation. Adjust lighting to reflect classroom activities (high for discussion, lower for video presentations).
- If possible, set classroom temperature between 68 and 72 degrees Fahrenheit, depending on the time of year.
- Identify designated break areas, and give appropriate breaks per institution policy.
- Close windows, blinds, or doors, if appropriate, to minimize outside distractions.
- Make sure you have functioning audiovisual equipment.

---

5   How do I create a supportive psychological/emotional learning environment?

- Be sensitive to the individual differences in each student by recognizing the multiple learning styles that exist in a single classroom setting.
- Learn students' names to signify a positive relationship between you and your students.
- Arrange seating to reflect your method of instruction for the session.
- Establish expectations on the first day of class by reviewing course syllabus, grading structure, and dates for tests/papers/projects.
- Establish rules that require listening while others speak, recognition of others' opinions, and prohibition of personal attacks.
- Create a safe environment for student participation through no ridicule of students' questions or remarks, confronting students who attack other students, and reinforcement of appropriate verbal and nonverbal communication.
- Make yourself available to the students by coming early before class or staying after class to build individual relationships with your students.

---

6   How important is developing a climate of mutual respect?

A dynamic relationship is created between you and your students when mutual respect is effective and honored.

This relationship fosters personal and intellectual development for all involved. This climate allows for collegiality, honesty, and fairness. When mutual respect is present in a classroom setting, the following expectations are fulfilled:

- Faculty members are:
  - Knowledgeable about their subject matter.
  - Prepared for class with materials and visuals designed for diverse student backgrounds.
  - Fostering an environment of collaborative learning and active participation.
  - Respectful of students as individuals, including their various styles of learning.
  - Setting high standards and communicating how to achieve the outcomes.
  - Responding to student inquiries in a timely fashion.
  - Honoring their office hours.
  - Refraining from using language, humor, or examples that may be insulting or insensitive.
  - A role model of self-respect and tolerance
- Students are:
  - Prepared for classroom and laboratory sessions.
  - Willing to be active learners.
  - Valuing diversity in the classroom.
  - Refraining from insulting and insensitive language.
  - Committing time and energy to the course.
  - Finishing assignments appropriately and in a timely fashion.
  - Communicating with faculty to prevent any issue from becoming an insurmountable problem.
  - Respectful of the learning environment by minimizing distractions.
  - Providing candid and truthful evaluations and recommendations for the faculty.

---

7 How can I create an environment that respects diversity?

Respect for diversity in your classroom can often prove very difficult for a novice faculty member. The difficulties you must overcome stem from several sources:

- Lack of knowledge about diverse peoples and lifestyles
- Inherited prejudices and stereotypes, many of which you may be unaware
- Guilt, anger, frustration, and anxiety that are stirred by discussing diversity issues

Creating the right environment starts with self-awareness, a desire to make all students feel respected and valued and your commitment to demonstrate that respect. Students are always observing a faculty member's behavior and rhetoric. Remember, too, that diversity is not just a racial/cultural perspective. It also focuses on gender perspectives (male, female, gay, lesbian) and multiple generations in the same classroom (new high-school graduates, returning students, second-degree students). Essentially, diversity is just major differences of opinion.

---

8 What are some effective teaching strategies for the increasingly diverse classroom?

Some teaching strategies that can be effective for you are:

- Use discussion and small-group work as elements of your teaching methodology.
- Allow your students to get to know one another.
- Establish classroom rules that celebrate everyone and denigrate no one.
- View all students as individuals rather than racial, ethnic or gender category. Make sure no one assumes the position of a particular *group.*
- Universalize the gender/ethnic experience whenever possible. Find examples from the nursing literature that illustrates how people of diverse identities share many common problems, issues, and solutions (e.g., *Sentimental Women Need Not Apply*, [PBS video]).
- Make your mantra "We are all the same in different ways."
- Establish respect for the values of diverse people by using specific examples from your field of study to show how culturally varied people have contributed to nursing.

- Use gender-neutral language.
- Use specific examples and ideas in nursing that exhibit stereotyping and its harm.

---

9 What can I do to create a classroom climate that fosters open communication?

Open communication is a combination of mutual respect and communication techniques. By following the steps in establishing mutual respect, the groundwork for a healthy environment for idea exchange in your classroom will be in place. Practice good verbal and nonverbal communication techniques. Good nonverbal communication techniques can include:

- Eye contact
- Open facial expressions
- Relaxed body posture
- Gestures that are congruent with your speech
- Appearing confident and knowledgeable of your topic

    Some ideas for good verbal communication techniques you can use are:

- Greeting the class at the beginning of each session
- Preview the topic for the day
- Review previous topics discussed through overview
- Allow for questions
- Make sure your transition from topic to topic is smooth and concise
- Never use media for media's sake, rather use them to enhance classroom presentation
- Know your materials so you do not have to read from your notes or overhead

---

10 What is anticipatory set, and why is it important?

Anticipatory set is a component of lesson planning. It is a brief activity at the beginning of the lesson that effectively engages all students' attention and focuses their thoughts on the learning objectives. You *hook* the students and make them anticipate the learning activity. The anticipatory set should relate to some previous learning. If successful, it should help the student get mentally ready for the lesson.

---

11 Can you provide some examples of anticipatory set?

Examples of anticipatory set may include:

- A handout given to students as they enter class
- A story or anecdote told at the beginning of class
- A prop set up in the classroom
- Discussing a pertinent news item
- Reviewing questions written on the board
- Be creative in planning your anticipatory sets

---

12 How does course "history" affect the classroom climate?

Students enroll in courses for a variety of reasons. Sometimes their course selection is based on what they have heard about a particular course and/or instructor. They have a perception that the course is easy or involves little effort or that the instructor is a hard grader. If students have a perception of the "history" of your course, that is what is awaiting you on your first day of class. Establishing a positive course history can be beneficial for you. Students enter your class understanding that you have high expectations, are knowledgeable in your field of nursing, are fair, and make class interesting for them.

---

13 How can I counteract negative course history?

By following the steps noted above in establishing a positive classroom climate and outlining course expectations, students will have a clear picture of your course. By establishing a clear picture of your classroom, you will help set aside any false perceptions that may have developed over time.

---

14 How will my class expectations affect the learning climate?

Research exploring how teachers' expectations can affect student performance began with *Pygmalion in the Classroom*

(Rosenthal & Jacobson, 1968). This study involved giving teachers false information about students' learning potential; by the end of the study, some of the targeted students exhibited the "expected" achievement. While it would be inaccurate to claim that a faculty member's expectations determine a student's achievement, the research clearly notes that teacher expectations have a major effect on student learning.

Your expectation may fall into two types: self-fulfilling prophecies or sustaining expectations. According to Good and Brophy (1984), self-fulfilling prophecies are the most dramatic type of teacher expectations because they involve preconceived ideas about potential changes in student behavior and achievement. Sustaining effects are those where you fail to recognize student potential, thus not allowing students to reach their potential.

While this evidence notes that low teacher expectations can have a negative effect, the reverse is also true. It has been documented that teachers who provide high expectations for their students see those students reach these high standards. By establishing high expectations for your students, you can set the stage for your students to excel. High and realistic expectations for your students are a key component in establishing your positive classroom climate.

---

15 What influence does my personality have on the classroom climate?

Your personality can be pivotal in the classroom. Your personal approach creates the classroom climate. Your mood affects each session. You have tremendous power to make a student's time with you miserable or joyous. Know yourself. Are you an introvert or extrovert? It matters. The introvert trying to be open, overly friendly, and vivacious will appear phony. The extrovert trying to be reserved will be miserable. Students know when you are "faking it." Just be yourself.

---

16 What impact does my physical appearance/demeanor have on the classroom climate?

Just as your personality matters, your personal appearance matters. Your appearance tells the students how much you value the interaction in the classroom with them. It sends a message of how you value yourself. A sloppy appearance sends the message that you are not organized and that more than likely your class presentation is dysfunctional. Be groomed neatly, and wear professional attire. While "business casual" may be appropriate for the clinical setting or office hours, professional attire like a dress or suit is an integral component of establishing a positive classroom climate. Research has shown that school administrators view faculty in business attire as "more professional" in their approaches as opposed to those in casual wear.

17 How does my enthusiasm for nursing affect the learning environment?

Just as your personality sets a tone in your classroom, so does your enthusiasm for nursing. Your enthusiasm is a synergy for all that happens in the classroom. Enthusiasm is contagious. Why would students want to enter a profession you are not enthused about? When this energy is missing in your classroom, a strained relationship can exist between you and your students. It sends a mixed message to them that while they need to know the classroom content, it is not worth your energy. Never tell students "We'll get through it" as it sends a message of nonimportance for course and content. Keep your passion for nursing alive through change, continuous improvement, and staying relevant. This should feed your zeal and enthusiasm.

18 How do my organizational skills affect the classroom climate?

Your organization of content and classroom activities is very important to the intended outcomes of your course. Your organization should be rational and based on program objectives, learner characteristics, and your own perspective and experience. Organization combines a twofold approach.

The first approach is to have an in-depth syllabus that shows your students the path your course will take for content acquisition. Nursing has traditionally had syllabi available for class work, and we are often cited in literature as a great example of class content organization. Be creative in your development of this syllabus. Include Web-based activities as appropriate. Many colleges place syllabi on the school Web site for the student to download.

The second approach is the classroom setting. Every class session should have an introduction, a body of content, a relevancy component, and a summary. Organizing your classroom content, similar to that of a written paper, helps clarify your content for students.

19 How do I encourage a participatory learning environment?

If you have established a classroom climate of mutual respect, you are well on your way to encouraging a participatory learning setting. Students must feel nonthreatened and free to participate openly in discussions and express their views. Once this climate has been established, the following activities will assist you in encouraging your students to participate actively:

- Pose open-ended questions.
- Allow all students to express their views.
- Explain incorrect answers.
- Use problem-solving exercises.
- Examine critical issues.

In a participatory learning setting, students are transformed when they encounter new ideas that challenge their prior assumptions. It is therefore important for the faculty member leading the participatory learning to push students to think critically about the issues or topics they address. Remember, when students are challenged to evaluate their beliefs, they are truly engaged in learning.

20 What are some additional strategies I can use in my classroom to enhance the learning environment?

Structure your classroom setting in such a way that multiple learning approaches are utilized. It is important that we move away from a strictly teacher-centered approach. Use techniques such as discussion; groups; demonstration/ simulation; forum, panel, or symposium; or computer or Web-based instruction. Enliven your classroom content by:

- Print (e.g., books, newspapers, programmed texts)
- Audio (e.g., tapes, audio books, computer streaming)
- Visual (e.g., slides, chart, flipcharts, PowerPoint, photographs, video clips)
- Stimulations (e.g., case studies, discussion guides)
- Examples (e.g., equipment demonstrations, mock-ups, practice stations)

As Malcolm Knowles wrote in 1984, "The typical classroom setup, with rows and a lecture in front, is probably the least conducive to learning that the fertile human mind could invent. It announces to anyone entering the room that the name of the game here is one-way transmission, that the proper role of the student is to sit and listen to transmission from the lecture" (p. 15).

We need to be a new generation of faculty using interactive methods and, once and for all, bury the old-fashioned lecture.

Reference

Good, T., & Brophy, J. (1984). Looking in classrooms, 3rd ed. London: Harper & Row.

Knowles, M. (1984). The modern practice of adult education. New York: Cambridge.

Rosenthal, R., & Jacobson, L. (1968). Pygmalion in the classroom. New York: Holt, Rinehart & Winston.

Resources

Avillion, A. (2001). Core curriculum for nursing staff development, 2nd ed. Pensacola, Fla.: National Nurses in Staff Development Organization.

Galbraith, M. (ed.). (1990). Adult learning methods. Malabar, Fla.: Kreiger Publishing.

Kiersey, D. Please understand me II. (1998). Accessed February 7, 2006, at www.keirsey.com

Ohio State University. (2001). The teacher's handbook. Accessed February 5, 2007, at http://www.ftad.ohiostate.edu/Publications/TeachingHandbook/contpdf.html

McIntyre, E., Rosebery A., & González, N. (2001). Classroom diversity: Connecting curriculum to students' lives. Portsmouth, N.H.: Heinemann.

Pontious, M. (2005) Classroom climate. Wisconsin School Musician 75(3), 10.

Russell, S. (2006). An overview of the adult learning process. Urologic Nursing 26(5), 349–370.

University of North Carolina at Chapel Hill. (1998). Diversity in the college classroom. A publication of The Center for Teaching and Learning. Accessed January 8, 2006, at http://ctl.unc.edu/tfitoc.html

11

Managing the Modern Classroom

Anita Wingate, PhD, RN

---

1 What do you mean by "managing the classroom"?

In addition to conveying content, you have several responsibilities for ensuring that class runs smoothly. These include making certain that you are prepared for class, learners feel comfortable participating, students interact positively with you and their classmates, content and discussions stay focused, there are clear policies regarding what occurs in class, and distractions to learning are minimized. Experienced teachers do these things with ease, but newer faculty members may not be aware of all the things that are involved in managing a class.

---

2 How can I calm the "before-lecture" nerves?

Before you even get to the classroom, you may find yourself the victim of anxiety bordering on panic. As coordinators of the teaching-learning environment, we all look forward to that moment of facing our classroom or auditorium of students with all the savoir-faire of the consummate teacher (or, increasingly, the entertainer that the technology-wise students have come to expect). The reality is that we also have those moments just as class is about to begin when our stomach hurts, our heart rate increases, and our voice threatens to give out entirely. Even if we are facilitating a participative class rather than strictly lecturing, anxiety can be an issue. What to do? That depends on your level of preparation. If your anxiety is at least partly related to a lack of confidence (read "lack of preparation"), then above all, getting prepared for class is key, so that your confidence in your ability to conduct the class is well placed. On the other hand, if you are prepared for class, then the best thing to do is pretend that you are calm. Visualize that effective, confident teacher you most admired in your student days, and then pretend to be that person. Because each class session is a new experience, remember that fear is part of the thrill of the unexpected and not all bad. It helps to practice the good habits of rest and nutrition so that you have the emotional and physical stamina to deal with the class. Also, if you focus on the students instead of yourself, you will find that your self-consciousness (and anxiety) will begin to diminish.

3 How do I prepare for each class?

Love your subject. Not every class we teach is necessarily our first choice of assignment, but if you are going to teach something, consciously try to work up enthusiasm for it. It is best to be educated in the content area. If that is not the case, think about taking formal coursework to increase your knowledge, or plan to spend extra time to become more proficient about the topic. This will build credibility as well as confidence in your teaching. And whenever possible, negotiate to teach content that is truly your area of expertise.

Months before the class starts, as you prepare the syllabus for the course, begin to think about class activities that you will want to incorporate into the course. Review the objectives that pertain to this class, organize and prioritize the actual content (being sure that you consider the syllabus for consistency and order), and review the material that you will need to present. If you use PowerPoint (or similar platforms), prepare early enough to allow you to review it several days prior to class, in case you need to revise it, or add Internet links for expansion or clarity. Do not embrace technology for the sake of the technology. The technology should be "transparent," letting the information shine through. On the other hand, be willing to explore new ways of promoting learning, and be willing to spend the time learning and incorporating new technology when it serves the students well.

---

4   What if I am not totally prepared for class?

"Totally prepared" gives the impression that learning experiences for each minute of the class time are thoughtfully and carefully planned for each class session. This is the ideal for which we all strive but rarely attain. Trust yourself to be able to facilitate good learning with a little spontaneity. Keep in mind what your general goals are for that class period, and use some creativity to meet those goals. Use a few questions to start a discussion, and the class may easily become more interesting than a well-structured lecture would be. Use some class time to give students an opportunity to give feedback about the course up to that point, or let students work in groups of two to formulate test questions about the content of recent class sessions. Remember with confidence that you are the expert on the topic, even when you are not as well prepared as you might be.

---

5   How do I get the students' attention so I can start class?

The larger the class, the more difficult it can be to get everyone to stop chattering. The days when any instructor could walk into a room and command a respectful silence are gone. At the beginning of the semester, you will need to suggest an agreement about a particular signal that will be used to indicate the start of class. This could be a raised hand, a cautious tap on the microphone, or stepping behind the podium. I use a cordless microphone in a large auditorium; turning that on usually silences the group as I begin to talk. If you use PowerPoint, starting the presentation by dimming the lights should be adequate warning that class is beginning. Starting each class period with a quotation or humorous saying begins a routine that has students anticipating the beginning of class. These strategies gain student attention so that the class can begin. Considering how adults learn, you also must use a technique to introduce the content in a novel way so that learning can begin.

---

6 How can I get to know all the students if I have a large class?

This is a challenge if you are teaching classes of more than 50 students, but there are strategies that can help. You can seek the permission of students to take their individual pictures and label them for your own review. If you already have pictures, spend time learning to link names with faces. To make this process easier, you can construct seating charts and request students to use the same seats during the semester, although many students prefer to choose their own seats. Large name tags or tents (folded paper with names in large type placed in front of each student) may be very helpful, especially during the first weeks of class. You can request that students introduce themselves by name each time they ask a question or make a comment during class for the early weeks of the semester.

---

7 Is it important that I recognize each student, especially in a large class?

Students, like all of us, enjoy being known, so they will appreciate the effort you make to get to know them. Even in a large class, you can make the effort to know many of the students. Unfortunately, sometimes you get to know those students best who are the least productive, as they are the ones requiring additional time with you. Not all instructors have the ability to accomplish the task of learning the names of all the students, but everyone can make the effort to learn at least some names each week. Spending time informally with students before and after class will help you remember them.

---

8 Should I ask students to sit in assigned seats?

If you need to keep attendance records, assigned seats will facilitate this immensely, but most courses do not require this at the college level. If you are trying to learn each student's name, having students sit in assigned seats is an excellent way to get to know them if you produce an alphabetical seating chart and use it daily. However, students may object to such a rigid protocol, so you need to decide which conflicting value (getting to know them versus their freedom to sit where they want each day) is more important. A variation of this idea is to give them their initial choice of seating and arrange the seating chart based on their preference.

---

9   How should I expect students to address me?

Be consistent with the university guidelines about this, if they exist, or take your lead from your peers. Some faculty members believe a formal title helps establish a respectful relationship with students and is a good model for students, especially those studying for professional careers. Others feel no loss of credibility if students use a familiar name rather than a formal title. In any case, be very clear about what you prefer so that students can follow your lead. If you really have no preference, leave it up to the students. If you state a preference, be prepared to have some students vary from your suggestion. If we expect students to use a title when addressing us, perhaps we should return that respect by using titles for them.

---

10   Should I give students any choices about class activities and, if so, which class activities might be open to student choice?

Imagine being in a situation in which you have no freedom to alter anything. Even if you respect the experts who have created the situation, you might find it downright annoying. Therefore, give students choices when possible. Obviously, the faculty member's judgment must prevail about issues such as how best to evaluate students (examinations, papers, projects, oral presentations, care plans), what the grading scale will be, and what content is necessary.

Faculty members are obligated to design learning activities that facilitate the students' efforts to meet the course objectives. That obligation may limit opportunities for freedom of choice, but it is quite likely that students can be given some choices without disrupting the learning environment. For example, if a formal paper or presentation about ethics is a class requirement, permit the student to choose from an array of topics in meeting that requirement. To avoid overlap, students might be required to select from a list of topics, but at least they have some choice in the matter.

Once the instructor acknowledges that there are various means for the students to gain the knowledge, attitudes, and competencies required by the course, then students can be open to flexible ways of facilitating that learning. In fact, students' ideas about what classroom activities are most efficacious may open a whole new world of learning.

If a course is required within a very structured curriculum or content allows little leeway, students can still be involved in making some decisions, even something simple such as the timing or length of class breaks.

---

11 What activities can I design to encourage students to prepare for each day's class?

Try take-home exercises or games, Internet-posted assignments, quizzes at the beginning of class (for which their outside reading prepares them), or a question-and-answer period to open the class. All of these may motivate students to prepare for class. Asking questions at the beginning to determine their level of readiness for the class will give them guidance about what your expectations are and reminds them that you are holding them responsible for their own learning.

Remember to prepare the syllabus carefully with time lines that allow students to predict with reasonable accuracy what each class session will include so that they can read ahead. Your positive responses to students who participate in class activities because they are prepared may stimulate other students to do the same.

Rehashing content that you have clearly expected students to learn will *not* be a stimulus to their continued outside preparation. Always end the class period with directions about how to prepare for the next one, or post instructions on-line about expectations or assignments for each class period.

---

12 What should I do if students are talking with each other enough to distract others in the classroom?

A related question is whether any conversations are appropriate during class. If you are presenting, whether in a large classroom or to a small group, conversations between students are likely to be disruptive. Unfortunately, if you are in a large auditorium, you might be unaware of the disruption even though some students are quite annoyed.

Among the actions you can take:

- Stop talking and wait. The silence often gains the attention of the offending students and makes them aware that you expect their attention.
- Suggest that if they must communicate with each other, they need to do it in writing rather than whispering or talking out loud. While passing notes may have been discouraged in grade school, it may be a reasonable solution in a college classroom.
- Gently remind the entire class to be courteous. This avoids embarrassing particular students but has the disadvantage of possibly annoying the majority of students who do not need a reminder to be respectful and who wish you would talk directly to the offenders.
- More assertively, call on the students who are talking, asking them if they have comments they would like to share with the class. You must decide whether you want to risk the personal embarrassment that may result when students are singled out in this way.
- If you use a wireless microphone or if the classroom is fairly small, move toward the persons who are talking as you continue the presentation; your presence near them is sure to remind them that you expect their attention.
- If the problem persists, speak to the offending students privately after class, explaining that they need to make

a choice: be prepared to listen quietly or not come to class, to avoid disturbing the other students. Usually, the problem will resolve itself once you make your expectations clear.

In addition, spend some time analyzing possible reasons for students' private conversations during class. Are they getting clarification from each other because you are not being clear? Are you confusing them by roaming too far from the presentation outline? Are you spending too much time talking rather than in interactive teaching strategies? Establish rapport with class members so they feel free to ask for clarification from you rather than from each other.

---

13 What should I do if students are being disruptive with a guest speaker?

This requires a more immediate and direct response than the previous question. Interrupting the speaker politely to ask if there is time for a brief break would give you the opportunity to approach the offending students quietly and remind them that they must either show polite attention or not attend the remainder of the class period. Stating expectations for proper classroom behavior at the beginning of the course and in the syllabus might help curtail such embarrassing incidents.

---

14 How will I know if I am holding the attention of the students?

You will know. When you hear lots of paper rustling, see students sleeping, see students leaving, or you simply note a general restlessness, something is wrong.

---

15 What can I do if I see the students' attention lagging?

Begin with a quick assessment. For example, be sure the microphone is working and that everyone can hear. Consider that you may be talking "above their heads" or "talking down" to them; ask for feedback. If you have turned down the lights to use PowerPoint, turn some of the lights back on to stimulate their reticular activating system. Walk around the classroom; do not just stand behind the podium. Change the pace, and interject a class activity. Ask questions to involve some active thinking, not just passive listening. Give examples of how your material can be applied, for example, to their clinical experiences so they can see the applicability of what you are discussing. Finally, just stop, and let students stand up and stretch, even if it is not yet time for a scheduled break.

What if lagging attention seems to be more the rule than the exception in your classes? Have someone videotape the class during one of your sessions, and check to see how much of the work *you* are doing and whether you are really involving the learners in the process or just letting them passively observe. Do not hesitate to ask the class to give quick, written feedback on what is assisting or inhibiting their learning in your classroom. Students will be glad to know that you care, and they may make suggestions that you can incorporate to the benefit of all.

16 Should students be allowed to bring wireless phones to class?

No, and neither should teachers. Cell phone etiquette has not been well defined for many settings, but a ringing wireless phone will be distracting to those within hearing range. Only in a dire impending situation should you make an exception and allow a student to bring a cell phone to class. Cell phones are particularly inappropriate during a testing situation, as they create a huge temptation for students to cheat.

17 How do I make sure students are comfortable about coming to see me outside of class?

The syllabus, with your phone number, office location, and office hours clearly listed, is the first step for student/faculty interactions. Having planned office hours tells students they are welcome during that time. Be sure to

remind students to make an appointment, if necessary, so
that you can devote time to their issues without interrup-
tion. Your office environment should provide for confidentiality and pleasant comfort. Your reception should
express warm, sincere interest in the student. Do not
expect to be a confidant to students, but rather make
appropriate referrals to other professionals when special
needs become apparent.

---

18 How can I help students prepare for examinations without teaching
"to the examination"?

- Give sample questions in class so students become
  familiar with the question format and difficulty level.
- Provide a list of study questions for each unit in the syllabus for self-study.
- Give quizzes early in the semester so that students
  can begin to identify any difficulties in preparing for
  examinations.
- Make sure students know how much time they will likely need to master new content, and have them log their
  study time for a few weeks to help them understand how
  productively (or not) they are studying. This reminds
  them to prepare consistently for examinations rather
  than cram.
- Suggest or provide tutors.
- Recommend study groups or study partners, letting
  stronger students in class help less-prepared students.
- Refer students to other resources on campus for assistance with study skills.

---

19 What can I do to prevent cheating during examinations?

- Be clear in the syllabus about what constitutes cheating
  in your classroom, leaving no room for doubt about
  what is appropriate.
- Use multiple versions of an examination to discourage
  cheating. Give the appearance of using multiple versions

(in two different colors), but recognize that such a strategy will work well only once.

- Provide an environment, if possible, that allows students to sit every other seat.
- Institute clear policies about taking tests (no backpacks, textbooks, notes, syllabi, cell phones or other digital devices, hats with visors, etc.)
- Use an adequate number of proctors to decrease the temptation to cheat.
- Remind students about professional integrity frequently; institute an honor code in your class.

20 Under what conditions should I cancel class?

Be sure you know and adhere to your institution's guidelines about class cancellations. Class should be cancelled only for the most compelling reasons, not just for your personal convenience and never because you are not adequately prepared. Inclement weather policies similarly serve as a guideline. Of course, a sudden illness or emergency may preclude making alternate arrangements for a substitute instructor, so class cancellations do happen. In this case, be prepared to notify students in a timely, reliable way so as not to inconvenience them. Group e-mail may work well for this purpose.

21 What should I do if students do not attend class regularly?

First, remember that students have other obligations. You have the responsibility to provide learning experiences that allow them to meet class objectives, but you cannot force them to attend class. Of course, if there is mandatory attendance and a student does not attend regularly, you will need to apply appropriate consequences. Your obligation is to have clearly stated expectations (written in the syllabus and stated verbally at the beginning of the semester), but having done that, it is not your responsibility to badger the student.

However, if many students are not attending class, you need to analyze the situation further. Are your learning activities problematic? A one-minute paper asking students to briefly evaluate the class may be very enlightening.

---

22 What can I do with a student who monopolizes the classroom discussion?

Structure classroom discussions to leave yourself reasonable control. For example, you might have a class rule that students must raise their hands to indicate they have something to say, allowing you to determine who speaks when and how often. If a monopolizing student continues to volunteer to speak too frequently, respectfully acknowledge his or her comments, but be ready to repeat that you want others to have a chance to participate. Another strategy is to have a soft ball (the talking ball) that, when tossed to a particular student, gives him or her the right to speak for a few minutes, but which must then be tossed to another student.

If the monopolizing student is asking too many questions, work with him outside of class to determine whether his knowledge base is truly deficient or whether there is some other motive, such as seeking attention.

Regarding questions during class, make sure students know that no question is too silly or superficial. However, if students' questions frequently indicate they are at a level of understanding below that of their peers, plan a remedial activity that does not impede the forward movement of the others. Always model respect for others. *Never* belittle a student.

---

23 Should I call on students to answer a question, or should I wait to see if someone can answer? How do I get a quiet student involved in class discussion?

It is usually best to give students an opportunity to volunteer an answer, but this may eliminate the less assertive students from the class discussion. One solution is to pose a question during the class discussion, but ask that students first write their answer down. This gives everyone a chance to check on their own understanding before someone else offers the answer. Then ask for volunteers to share what they wrote. At that point, the quieter student may have more confidence about responding verbally because he has had time to think about his answer before the bolder students have already answered.

Making class participation a part of the grade is another strategy for getting each student involved in class discussion, but this strategy is likely to be difficult in large classes and is a record-keeping challenge, at best. Too, students may make less than valuable contributions just to get credit for participating.

24   How do I respond to students who are disrespectful of others or of others' ideas?

Your professional example (modeled by your own response to students and interaction with students) is absolutely the best way to shape respectful behaviors. Guide classroom discussions to demonstrate appropriate ways to express contradictory views. Make sure that students know that you expect them to provide a rationale for their comments and ideas and that you also expect them to listen carefully to the ideas and rationales expressed by others. Create an atmosphere that not only allows for a variety of ideas but also establishes the expectation that thoughtful learners will disagree, respectfully, at times. If class discussions are a usual part of the course, include in your guidelines in the syllabus a reminder that students may not wage personal attacks on other students or on you. If a student's disrespect becomes a common pattern, a private discussion may be necessary to explore underlying reasons for the problem, to clearly state expectations for classroom decorum, or to suggest resources available in student services if necessary.

25 What should I do if a student asks a question and I do not know the answer?

If you teach for very long, it will happen. When you are a novice instructor, this is your worst nightmare, particularly if the student asks the difficult question in class. Nothing seems to diminish us more than being exposed as something other than the ultimate source of all knowledge related to our subject matter, just as we are trying to establish ourselves as polished instructors. Actually, more experienced instructors may be pleased about this event, because it can demonstrate that students are stretching their knowledge base.

Of the several responses that are appropriate, none of them include faking an answer. Then, in the following order:

- Commend the student for coming up with a good question.
- Admit straightforwardly that you do not know the answer. (The students will respect you for this honesty.)
- Suggest that the student seek the answer, and note all the resources available for seeking the answer.
- Promise to seek the answer yourself by taking advantage of those resources.
- At the next opportunity, ask the student to share what information was obtained, help to analyze the information and apply it, confirm and expand the information if knowledge gaps still exist, and encourage students to continue to ask questions.

Do not miss this opportunity to model good critical thinking skills as you ponder difficult questions posed by students.

26 What is the appropriate response to a student who answers a question but is completely wrong?

This is an opportunity to model respect for others. First, if there is anything correct in the answer, discuss that, and continue from there. Guide the student to a more fully correct answer. But if the answer is completely wrong, the challenge for you is somewhat greater. Never embarrass a student in front of peers. They may already know that the answer is incorrect and may be watching to see what you will do with the situation. In some way, commend the student for answering, and move on quickly to elicit other answers from other students. An opening might be to ask, "Does anyone have a different idea about this?" When the correct answer is offered, you can move on to provide a rationale for that answer, so that learning occurs in a positive atmosphere. Alternatively, sometimes it is effective to ask the student providing the wrong answer to give a rationale; the student may realize the error and be pleased to be self-correcting. While avoiding embarrassing the erring student, you also need to provide correct information to all of the students.

---

27 How can I help students understand difficult concepts?

- Restate the material in another way.
- Use diagrams.
- Use related Internet sites that present the material in novel ways.
- Relate the difficult concept to ideas the students already understand.
- Give an example of an application of the concept.
- Ask if someone understands what you are trying to communicate, and ask the person to rephrase it for the class. "Teaching is the highest form of understanding," according to Aristotle. Students realize quickly that if they can explain concepts to others, it also benefits them.

---

28 How will I know if students are understanding what is most important about the content?

In the final analysis, you will know what students understood when their performance on examinations or papers (and other outcome measures) is clearly not at the level that you expected. Your goal should be to determine problems prior to that point. Occasionally, at the close of class, ask the students to write down what they think were the five most important points about that class session and then to write down what questions they still have. Or ask them to quickly write down the "muddiest" point so that you can respond to that at the beginning of the next class meeting. If students feel welcome to e-mail questions to you, those questions will enlighten you about concepts that students are finding difficult to understand. You can then clarify those points for the whole class or send a group e-mail (protecting the identity of the questioner) to make sure the rest of the class members have the benefit of the same information.

29 What if the technology (microphone, PowerPoint, projector) does not work?

This is another of those situations where anticipation of problems can save you much anxiety. Get to class early, and get the technology ready. If something is not working, you will have time to call for assistance and still begin class on schedule. Being familiar with your material is crucial, because you may have to revert to chalk or whiteboard. You will be surprised at how creative you can be when you have to describe concepts with word pictures to supplement your notes or when you find yourself drawing freehand on a blackboard when your online images are unavailable.

30 Under what conditions should I grant permission for a student to take an examination outside the scheduled time?

Generally, makeup examinations are to be avoided, but obviously there are times when permission should be granted for a student to take a test early or late. There are several issues to be considered. One is the importance of examination security, which may be violated when students taking the test earlier may inadvertently give away important information by casual hallway discussion, unaware that others have not taken the examination. If possible, create at least two forms of each examination, so that students making special requests understand that they will be taking a different examination. For example, if you usually use multiple-choice questions, convert those to an essay form (simple sentence completion, fill in the blank, defining terms, or true essay) for students making up the test later.

Unless you have a testing center that can administer makeup examinations, recognize how much time and effort such examinations will require. Your syllabus should be very clear about your expectations regarding examinations; however, you should make exceptions to your general policy rarely, carefully, and fairly. Some of the valid reasons you might grant a request to take a test late (the usual request) or early (less frequently) include serious illness or surgery of the student or a family member, family emergencies (which can take an amazing number of forms), and other professional obligations. Be sensitive to legitimate requests, but be vigilant about spurious ones. Know the policies of your department, school, and university with regard to examinations (especially final examinations), and follow them scrupulously.

---

31 Under what conditions should I allow students to audiotape or videotape the class?

Within the guidelines and policies of your school, this is entirely up to you. For students who have difficulty absorbing material or taking adequate notes (particularly in a content-dense course), audiotaping a class gives them a chance to review the content. Some students with long commutes have noted that listening to class tapes is a good use of that time. Occasionally, students have asked to tape a lecture or presentation for a student who is unable to attend that particular class session. Obviously, any erroneous statements that you or others make in the classroom are recorded, so that adds an element of anxiety. Videotaping seems to offer little additional advantage to learning and might require the written consent of other class members as well as of the instructor.

---

32 What are some of the biggest mistakes instructors make in the classroom, and how can I avoid them?

Among the most significant mistakes instructors make are:

- Not caring about the students (or appearing not to care).
- Not showing respect for students.
- Changing the rules arbitrarily, especially when it disadvantages some or all of the students. (Actually, changing the class rules even with a good rationale will be met with ire in most situations.)
- Not being prepared, which seems to make a statement about how much you do not value the class.
- Testing unfairly.
- Showing favoritism.
- Treating adult learners like children.

The most important way to avoid the pitfalls listed is to spend adequate time in reflection about teaching and to think critically about why you do what you do. Student evaluations often remind us brutally of our classroom failures, but they can be an important starting point for quality improvement.

---

33 What are the best secrets of an effective classroom teacher?

Really care about the students. Make their learning your focus, not your teaching. Know your material. An effective teacher should have mastery of his or her discipline, although that alone is not sufficient. Be prepared. Pay attention to feedback from students. Start where they are. Keep current in your field. Acknowledge when you do not know something, and keep your promise to find the answer, and stimulate the students to seek the answer.

Make sure that your demeanor in every way suggests that your teaching is as important as your research or the service you provide to the profession and community. How you do you this? Getting to class on time is important, and it helps give the message that you have taken adequate time to prepare for class and that you respect the students and their time. Being early is even better because you can interact with students informally, and students are likely to come to class on time, too, for the chance to communicate with you without having to make a formal appointment. Be pleasant, even when you are having a bad day.

Good instructors are sensitive to what the class needs and are willing to stray from the usual format if necessary. Following even the best syllabus blindly will deter you from meeting the students' needs if something else will stimulate learning more effectively.

Good instructors are "real" to their students; that is, they reveal enough of themselves to be seen as more than just an expert in their field. They step from behind the podium and make sure that students understand that, ideally, the business of the classroom is not one person teaching and the others learning but everyone mutually involved in the teaching/learning experience.

Good instructors welcome student evaluations, both at semester's end and before. If midterm evaluations are sought, responses are actually used to shape the remainder of that semester's class, giving students the satisfaction of knowing that they are participating in a meaningful way in the format of the class. Good instructors value peer evaluations as well and talk with their colleagues about their teaching, both the high moments and those that are eventually forgotten. They regularly reflect on all aspects of their teaching experience and make appropriate changes.

Good instructors take teaching seriously and consistently work hard at it. Their commitment to teaching is characterized by the same passion they devote to their other professional roles of research, service, and administration.

In short, the best instructors are passionate about their subject matter, stay current in their topics, and care deeply about the students they teach, creating a teaching/learning environment that involves mutual respect and a profound love of learning that becomes a way of life.

Resources

Angelo, T. A. (1993). A "teacher's dozen": Fourteen general, research-based principles for improving higher learning in our classrooms. AAHE Bulletin, April, 3–7, 13.

Hipple, T. & McClam, T. (Mar. 11, 2002). Tips for better teaching (electronic version). The Chronicle of Higher Education. Accessed November 25, 2003, from http://chronicle.com/jobs/2002/03/2002031102c.htm

McKeachie, W. J. (2002). McKeachie's Teaching Tips, 11th ed. Boston: Houghton Mifflin.

Palmer, P. J. (1997). The heart of a teacher: Identity and integrity in teaching. Change, Nov/Dec, 15–21.

Shulman, L.S. (1999). Taking learning seriously. Change, July/August, 11–17.

12

Developing and Revising Curriculum

Debra P. Shelton, EdD, APRN-CS, CNA, OCN, CNE

---

1 What is curriculum?

Numerous definitions have been noted in nursing education. Over time, the term curriculum has evolved to mean "a course of study." The courses required for the program of study make up a curriculum. The curriculum needs to focus on the goals and outcomes of the program. How will the student progress through the course? Which courses are taken when and in what order? What skills do the students need to accomplish to progress through each course? These questions are just some of the elements of a curriculum.

---

2 What are the components of a curriculum?

The literature identifies numerous components. Basic components include the mission and philosophy of the nursing unit, the conceptual framework of the program of study, course sequencing and courses required for the program of study, program objectives, learning activities, outcomes or competencies of the graduate of the program, and a program of evaluation.

3 What is the relationship between the institutional mission and the program mission?

The institution's mission is what the university is and why the university exists. The nursing program's mission is developed using the institutional mission statement. The program's mission must reflect the institution's mission and the values and beliefs of the nursing program. Both mission statements should complement one another and provide the basis for the curriculum. Faculty members should be included in the development and any modification of the nursing program's mission statement.

4 What is a philosophy?

The philosophy is a statement of what the faculty and nursing program believe about nursing, the individual, health, society, and the environment. Some philosophies also include a statement on nursing education or teaching and learning. The philosophy should be developed and approved by the nursing faculty and needs to be reviewed and revised as necessary to remain current.

5 How does the mission relate to the philosophy?

The mission must be developed before the philosophy. These two statements complement one another and build on each other. The philosophy also takes into consideration the mission of the university, mission of the program, and the beliefs of faculty members.

6 Why do I need a philosophy?

Everyone has a philosophy of what nursing is to them and how to practice nursing. The nursing program also needs a philosophy to serve as a touchstone for the numerous faculty members with diverse beliefs, values, and philosophies. A common belief about nursing needs to be developed for the program so that all individuals, sharing that belief, demonstrate it as they go about accomplishing their mission.

---

7   What are program objectives?

Program objectives are statements of behavior that graduates should accomplish when they finish the program of study. The objectives address the curriculum (content) and not the instruction (methods) that will be used. Level, course, and unit objectives are progressively more specific than program objectives, which can be quite broad, identifying what the graduates will be able to know, think, and do.

---

8   I have read about program competencies. What are they?

After the program objectives have been developed, program competencies are identified. Program competencies identify the knowledge, skills, and attitudes that graduates of the nursing program must have to meet the program objectives. The competencies are written as a behavior and are student-focused.

---

9   Do I need goals and objectives? What is the difference? What does it mean to have level objectives?

All programs of studies and the courses in the program need goals and objectives. Many individuals state that there is no difference between goals and objectives. Others believe that goals are general statements about what the program or course is expected to accomplish and that objectives are more specific statements of what the learner should accomplish and by when. As students progress through the program, their knowledge and skills increase with each course. At entry into the program, what skill level is the student expected to exhibit? Upon completion of each course, what skill level is the student expected to demonstrate? These are important questions to indicate the increase in professional skills, the progression of objectives, and the increasing complexity of the curriculum during the course of study.

---

10 How do accreditation guidelines affect the curriculum?

Accreditation is a process for ensuring a quality program of study. Nursing programs undergo a self-study using accreditation standards developed by accrediting agencies. These standards are statements that identify what constitutes a quality program. Although accreditation is a voluntary process, most programs of study participate in the process as it confers formal recognition of the school's good work. The accreditation guidelines do not determine the curriculum per se, but they do denote that a program of study has met or exceeded the minimal standards of nursing education.

---

11 Do we have to follow the accreditation guidelines word for word?

Accreditation guidelines are not prescriptive; they are guidelines for developing a nursing curriculum for a particular type of program. Two nursing-specific accrediting bodies exist in this country:

- The Commission on Collegiate Nursing Education (CCNE), which accredits college and university nursing programs awarding baccalaureate, master's, and doctoral degrees
- The National League for Nursing Accreditation Commission (NLNAC), which accredits certificate, diploma, associate degree, baccalaureate degree, and master's degree programs of study in nursing.

Both accrediting bodies publish standards and guidelines for nursing programs and have Web sites with complete information.

---

12 Do I need to have a conceptual framework?

A conceptual framework is set of concepts/beliefs of a nursing program/curriculum. The relationships between the concepts become a blueprint of what the nursing faculty members believe about the curriculum. The blueprint shows how the curriculum will be structured, how content will be sequenced, how content will be taught, how the concepts relate to the program, and how evaluation will occur. The major concepts that are often present in a conceptual framework are person, environment, health, and nursing. The beliefs about the curriculum are often then described in a concept map or a graphic design.

---

13 How do curriculum theories fit into curriculum development?

Theories function to provide a description, prediction, and explanation of how the curriculum is developed. Tyler's theory is often used in nursing curriculum development and comprises four main components: purposes, experiences, methods, and evaluation. Knowles' Adult Education Theory and Watson's Theory of Human Caring are two other education frameworks that are used in curriculum development. Some learning theories that contribute to curriculum development are:

- Behavioral learning theories such as those of Skinner and Thorndike
- Cognitive learning theories such as information-processing theories, constructivism, and assimilation theory
- Cognitive development theories such as those of Piaget and Bruner
- Multiple intelligences theory of Howard Gardner

A number of nursing theories form the basis of a nursing curriculum, notably Roy's Adaptation Model and Betty Neuman's Systems Model. The nursing program can choose one theory or select a number of concepts from multiple theories to develop its own theory or model that underpins the curriculum.

---

14 What is an integrated curriculum?

Two types of designs are generally used for curriculum: blocking and integrated. Blocking course content involves structuring a curriculum around a practice setting or developmental stages or body systems. An integrated curriculum involves designing a curriculum around nursing concepts. The nursing concepts are integrated (or threaded) through each of the nursing courses during the entire program and are revisited at intervals and increasing levels of complexity as students progress.

15 I hear faculty members talking about curriculum threads. What are they?

Threads are concepts that are part of all courses within the curriculum. Examples of curriculum threads are the nursing process, nutrition, ethics, etc. Often, the concept will start at the basic level in the first course and progress to more advanced knowledge and skills in the last level of the curriculum.

16 Does developing curriculum include selecting learning experiences?

Yes. Carefully designed learning experiences prepare the graduate to handle the real world of nursing. The experiences should be varied and challenge students to apply their knowledge and the skills they have learned. Being a team member is part of the real world of nursing and, as such, collaborative experiences need to be integrated into the curriculum. Varied clinical settings should be included to provide the student with a wide scope of practice and to challenge the critical thinking and problem-solving skills required for graduates. The learning experiences must be designed so that students are able to meet the program of study's objectives and competencies.

17 Does the curriculum need to have teaching methods identified?

The content in a program may be relatively stable, but faculty members have flexibility in identifying how learners will interact with the content. Numerous teaching methods are used in nursing, and selection depends on the learners and the content taught. Some programs may select one primary teaching methodology, such as distance learning (Internet) or case study, supplemented with other methods as needed.

18 How are theory and laboratory hours devised?

Usually, state and accrediting agencies recommend a specific number of hours required for a degree; these are stated in credit hours. Deciding how many classroom (theory) and clinical (laboratory) hours are required for the curriculum will be a decision made during curriculum planning. Some programs have separate theory and clinical. Other programs combine both in one course. Generally, a three-credit theory course is just that: 3 hours a week for a specific number of weeks. A ratio of credit hours to clinical hours is used, usually a 1:3 ratio. This means 1 credit hour equates to 3 clinical hours, which means a 3–credit hour course includes 9 clinical hours per week. The program faculty will set the ratio during curriculum development. This ratio can be as high as 1:6.

19 How does the faculty decide how many hours of clinical for each course?

The nursing faculty must look at a couple of things when deciding the ratio and the number of clinical hours per course. One factor is the student workload for the semester. Another factor is the availability of clinical sites. Generally, students are going to spend anywhere from 6 to 24 hours a week in clinical. Some programs begin with 6 hours during the first semester and increase to 24 clinical hours in the final semester of study.

20 My state has a core curriculum. How do we incorporate the core curriculum in our nursing curriculum?

Most states have identified a core curriculum for an associate or baccalaureate degree. The core courses are those general education courses that all students receiving a degree must complete. These courses vary from state to state, but within the state the courses are universal for all degree programs.

21 How do I know the curriculum needs revision?

Curriculum revision usually occurs as a result of social forces and issues facing nursing and health care. Accreditation standards may influence a curriculum revision. Innovations in science and changes affecting health care within a community may instigate a curriculum revision. Teaching technology can also bring about a change in the curriculum.

22 Where do I start with curriculum revision?

A single faculty member or a group of faculty members can initiate a curriculum revision. The proposed change may be presented from the faculty, a committee, or the administration. Realize that any change within a curriculum is going to be a challenge for all involved. Hull et al. (2001) liken curriculum revision to moving a cemetery and propose six C's for success: commitment, compatibility, communication, contribution, consensus, and credit. Planning for a curriculum change is not an update of courses in the program of study; a curriculum revision involves time and effort from all faculty members. Administrative support and an organizational climate desiring curriculum change are essential.

23 How is curriculum linked to program evaluation?

Curriculum development is a dynamic process and requires continuous evaluation. The nursing program must participate in program evaluation in order to evaluate how well the program is accomplishing the specified outcomes and competencies. Internally, program evaluation provides the faculty and administrators with information on how the program measures up against state and national standards and identifies areas for improvement. Externally, program evaluation provides the public with information on the quality of the program or the success of its graduates on the NCLEX-RN examination. Nursing programs often do a program evaluation before an accreditation visit rather than completing ongoing evaluation on an annual basis. When done conscientiously, program evaluation provides the faculty with data on the program's effectiveness and how well the program is meeting its expected outcomes. The data gathered by the evaluation can provide the basis for curriculum revision and program improvements.

---

24 What is included in the program evaluation?

A program evaluation has a number of components, including all the aspects of curriculum development discussed, from the mission statement to the evaluation process. Resources (fiscal, physical, and material) within the nursing program are another important consideration. Part of the plan focuses on the students—their satisfaction with the nursing program, the graduation rate of the program, pass rate on the NCLEX-RN test, and job placement rates. Benchmarking, comparing one school with others, may be included in the evaluation plan. Another component is faculty information, including faculty qualifications, maintenance of expertise, and participation in scholarly activities. Employers of graduates and alumni will also be considered. Employers are typically asked to evaluate the graduates, how well they were prepared for the RN position, and how satisfied the employer is with the graduates. Alumni are often asked to provide data on how well they believe a nursing program prepared them for their position. Most programs will do this type of evaluation at 1 year post graduation and then at 3 to 5 years post graduation. Regular and systematic evaluation of the nursing program provides valuable information about the fundamental product of the program: the curriculum and how it translates to the proficiency of graduates to meet the needs of the public.

References

Bevis, E.O., & Watson, J. (1989). Toward a caring curriculum: A
   new pedagogy for nursing. New York: National League for
   Nursing.
Hull, E., et al. (2001). Moving cemeteries: A framework for facilitat-
   ing curriculum revision. Nurse Educator 26(16), 280–282.
Tyler, R.W. (1949). Basic principles of curriculum and instruction.
   Chicago: University of Chicago Press.

Resources

Diamond, R.M.(1989). Designing and assessing courses and curricula: A practical guide. San Francisco: Jossey-Bass.
Giddens, J.F., & Brady, D.P. (2007). Rescuing nursing education
   from content saturation: The case for a concept-based curriculum. Journal of Nursing Education 46(2), 65–69.
Mawn, B., & Reece, S.M. (2000). Reconfiguring a curriculum for the
   new millennium: The process of change. Journal of Nursing
   Education 39(3), 101–108.

13

Beyond the Classroom: Considering Distance Education Approaches

Helen R. Connors, PhD, RN, Dr PS (Hon), FAAN

1   What is distance education?

Distance education is organized education that occurs when the teacher and the learner are not in the same physical space at the same time. Distance education is not new. The concept of distance education emerged many years ago with correspondence courses. It later evolved into videotapes, satellite downlinks, television, and computer-assisted instruction (CAI). Although these learning methods had their place in the overall education process, their effectiveness was relatively low because the self-paced, noninteractive teaching often failed to retain the attention of students, resulting in very high attrition rates. Today, with the advancement of telecommunications technologies and Internet capabilities and emerging technologies designed for teaching and learning, distance education has rapidly moved to mainstream education (McGee & Diaz, 2007).

2   Why are academic institutions engaging in distance education?

Education is the single most important element in our nation's future. Old models of education no longer address the realities of most students' lives in our rapidly changing technological and multicultural society. Today's students approach academics with a set purpose: a desire for efficiency in learning, a perception of what they need to learn and, most important, a planned set of outcomes. They want and need accessible, flexible, learner-centered educational programs that fit their lifestyle and commitments. Academic institutions need to change to meet these consumer demands. Computers, the Internet, and other tools offer the promise of significant improvements in teaching and learning.

3 **What are the most common technologies used for distance education?**

The landscape of distance learning has changed significantly with advances in telecommunications and computing technologies allowing interactive, real-time education and training. The affordability and effectiveness of the new solutions have made them popular among a variety of user markets. The most prominent users of distance learning solutions include educational institutions (both K–12 and universities), the corporate market (including financial institutions, automotive companies, pharmaceutical/health care, and others), and the government. The most common technology for distance learning is the Internet and the worldwide Web. However, in the past 5 years the number of merging and emerging technologies supported by the Web has increased enormously, making it difficult for faculty members to keep up with the latest advances (McGee & Diaz, 2007).

4 **What pedagogical theories or concepts support distance education?**

Recent theories in education, such as constructivism (Brooks and Brooks, 1993; Cranton, 1994) and active learning (Myers and Jones, 1993), clearly support distance learning. These theories propose that learning takes place when learners reflect on their own experiences and actively create knowledge and meaning through active learning processes that include experimentation, exploration, and testing of ideas or concepts. Data support that learning takes place most effectively when it is connected with the personal experiences and knowledge base of the learner. Learning is reinforced and retained by generating knowledge from within, not by receiving information from outside. In distance learning courses, teachers can tailor their strategies to encourage students to use critical thinking and research skills to analyze, interpret, and predict information and to promote collaborative learning among students and between students and faculty. The use of technology to support group activities, simulations, gaming, and online discussion groups are only a few strategies for realizing these goals. The limitations of distance education make it impossible for faculty to be in charge of the learning; therefore, the principles associated with constructivism and active learning relate well to distance education and can create a powerful active learning environment.

---

5 | **How do I help students decide if distance learning is right for them?**

Distance learning is not right for all students. Faculty and other academic advisors need to help students determine if this is the right medium for them. Students who engage in distance learning need a certain mindset in order to be successful. Distance learners need to be highly motivated to succeed and disciplined enough to incorporate study time into their busy schedules. They must have a basic technology skill set and access to the appropriate hardware and software required to participate in the learning activities. Successful students are serious about their educational goals and willing to assume responsibility for their own learning. They are able to accept the faculty's role as a facilitator of learning and are comfortable with the lack of face-to-face (F2F) interaction with faculty and fellow students.

For an example of a self-assessment for distance learning, refer to:

http://elearning.kumc.edu/about.html#skill session
http://ittraining.iu.edu/workshops/deguide/de_student_primer.pdf

6 What are the common characteristics of successful distance learners?

Distance learners are people who, because of time, geographic, financial, or other constraints, choose not to attend a traditional classroom. They come from a wide variety of backgrounds and are all ages. Most commonly, they turn to distance learning for convenience, accessibility, and flexibility. Learners who do best in this environment are adult learners who are self-directed. Because of the increased use of advanced telecommunications technology, they must have the mind-set to embrace the new educational technologies and adapt to a new learning environment. These adaptations will be less of a challenge for the students who grew up in the digital age.

7 What are the common characteristics of successful faculty members who use distance learning strategies?

Just as distance education is not right for all students, it is not right for all faculty. Many teachers are being challenged to develop new skills and knowledge to use in technology-based distance learning environments. In this environment, faculty members must shift their teaching style and philosophy from that of a "sage on the stage" to that of a "guide on the side." The faculty and student become partners in the learning process, and the faculty serves as a facilitator of learning. This transition requires faculty members to develop an ever-evolving set of technical skills to support their teaching. In addition, they need development time and technical support to assist in course development. The technology should not be the focus of the teaching; it should be transparent to allow the pedagogy through. A design team consisting of faculty and an instructional design partner works well. Teachers need to be rewarded for their creativity and innovation in education. This can be done by adjusting appointment, promotion, and tenure criteria to support this type of scholarship and through teaching awards that recognize teaching excellence and innovation.

8 **What is the difference between a course taught in the classroom and one taught by distance education?**

The difference depends on what technology is being used to support the distance learning program. As stated previously, the most common platform used today to support distance learning is the Web. A course taught on the Web involves a great deal of planning before the course starts. The course needs to be ready to go when the students log on at the start of the semester. There is little opportunity for spur-of-the-moment teaching. Other than traditional syllabi, there are few similarities between the teaching strategies used in the classroom and the ones used online. Designing a course online requires the faculty to think differently and creatively in terms of meeting the objectives and covering the course content. The innovative technology available for online education provides for interactive learning and diverse strategies for meeting the varied learning styles of students. For the right students and the right faculty, online teaching strategies can be very powerful learning tools.

9 **How does distance education change my role as an educator?**

Distance education technologies change the way faculty teach. The overall goal of the faculty, whether in a F2F or online environment, is to ensure that some type of educational experience takes place. In the online environment, the instructor designs learning activities and provides guidance, which allows the student to interact with the material and use critical thinking to create new knowledge. The instructor then provides ongoing feedback and gently guides the learning experience. Most important, the instructor needs to provide learning experiences that require active learning, interaction or collaboration among students, and timely feedback. Some faculty resist the changes that technology-based course delivery brings. However, many of the resisters are converted once they have the experience of teaching with technology. On one hand, we must respect the fact that not all faculty can be successful at online teaching. On the other hand, faculty members need to consider that they may need to make this leap if online teaching is an integral part of their institution's mission.

---

10 What support services are required for distance learning students?

Distance learning students need the same support services available to all students, but they particularly need anytime/ anyplace access to these services. Student services include: marketing, admissions, registration, financial aid, advising, bookstore, library, career counseling, personal counseling, and services for students with disabilities. In addition, online students need technical support, orientation to the distance learning environment, and an opportunity to develop a sense of connectedness with faculty, other learners, and the institution. Many innovative methods using advanced telecommunications technology as well as software and design solutions are available to offer these services.

---

11 What support services are required for faculty who teach using distance education approaches?

Teachers need to have a certain basic technology skill set and embrace the use of technology in education. At a minimum, they need to be able to learn technical skills and pedagogical approaches to enhance education through technology. They need to be able to navigate the coursework and to troubleshoot common hardware and software issues. Faculty members who partner with an educational technologist/ instructional design specialist get the expertise, security, and support needed to develop and teach quality courses. In addition, faculty need the necessary administrative support to garner resources to sustain a quality program and need to be rewarded for innovation and strategic direction.

---

12 How do I ensure the same quality in a distance education course as in a traditional on-campus course?

As with all courses, the proof of the quality is in the learning outcomes. Proper use of technology and proven teaching strategies are essential for targeting those good outcomes. There is a great deal of research that demonstrates no significant difference in traditional courses versus distance learning courses, and in many cases the quality of the virtual courses in terms of best practices in education is better. The *No Significant Difference* Web site (http://teleeducation. nb.ca/nosignificantdifference/) provides excerpts from a variety of research studies: There is a companion site (http://teleeducation.nb.ca/significantdifference/) that does document significant differences. There should be no doubt that if the F2F and technology-based courses are developed with the same rigor, the learning outcomes can be met. The challenge we need to address is how to use the technologies to enrich the experience, to go beyond what can be done in the F2F or other delivery environment.

13 What are the "best practices" in distance learning?

Best practices are documented strategies or tactics employed by highly successful organizations. Because of the organization's drive for excellence, these practices have been implemented and perfected to make them most admired by others. These strategies or tactics are supported by evidence-based research to support their achievement. Best practices in education are documented strategies used to produce good teaching and learning outcomes, including customer satisfaction. The most widely used good practices in post–secondary education are those defined by Chickering and Gamson (1987) and later applied to technology-based education by Chickering and Ehrmann (1996). Currently, benchmarking surveys are available to study and compare best practices in online learning communities. These benchmarks can be used to create quality improvement initiatives within the organization or program to ensure best practices.

14 How do you evaluate distance education courses?

The Teaching, Learning, and Technology Group's Flashlight Program focuses on evaluating the outcomes of the use of technology in education. The framework for the evaluation is based on best practices in education (Chickering and Gamson, 1987). These are documented teaching and learning practices that have been demonstrated to be effective. Best practices include active learning, student-faculty interaction, student-student interaction, rapid feedback, time on task, high expectations, and respect for diverse ways of knowing. Focus your evaluation by thinking about the desired outcomes of your course, and determine what educational practices (best practices) promote these outcomes and what technologies provide support for the practices and outcomes. Again, do not let the technology be the driver. Do not use technologies because you can; use them because it is the best medium to foster best practices and good outcomes.

---

15 How do you evaluate distance education programs?

Methodologies supported by the Flashlight Program support program evaluation. Although the guiding framework for the evaluation may be the same, program evaluation usually involves a broader sweep because it may comprise a wider range of outcomes and include multiple views (those of faculty, learners, technical support services, potential learners, etc). The Flashlight Program uses a triad methodology to assist in establishing a framework for your assessment. See www.TLTgroup.org

---

16 What are the advantages to distance education?

Distance education makes learning accessible and convenient and, when taught asynchronously, allows for flexible scheduling. Distance education holds a lot of appeal for adult working professionals who are seeking career advancement as well as for the young single parent who lacks the resources to go back out at night after working all day and caring for children. It works well for both urban and rural learners who are able to squeeze virtual classes into their hectic professional and personal schedules because it brings education to them. A well-designed distance education program creates an active learning environment that engages students in the learning process. Many believe that students learn more in this environment. In addition, the self-paced nature of the environment allows students to learn at their own pace and demonstrates respect for diverse learning styles.

17 What are the barriers to distance education?

The biggest barrier to distance learning is getting faculty agreement. When faced with the challenge of creating distance learning programs, faculty members have concerns about a variety of issues, including intellectual property, a lack of incentives or rewards, a threat to tenure, and workload inflation. In addition, some teachers are intimidated by the use of technology for distance education. Involving faculty early in the distance learning planning processes and providing them with development and support services is essential to a successful program. Another significant barrier is the lack of infrastructure including support services and resources for maintenance and upgrading hardware and software.

18 How can students be socialized to the profession if they are not physically with faculty or other role models in the classroom?

Socialization to the practice role is an important component of professional education. Many educators are skeptical whether this socialization can occur without a physical presence. As virtual learning environments have not been in existence long enough to be able to determine the impact on socialization to the profession, this is a difficult outcome to support with evidence. Longitudinal studies that evaluate the technology in the context of socialization are recommended. When attempting to create a set of social experiences, it is important to be cognizant of the fact that the digital age requires us to think differently about how socialization might occur. This is where our experience and culture might get in the way of our imagination. The newer generation seems to have a different view of the effect of the digital world on socialization. We need to be open-minded on this issue and learn from the experiences and perceptions of students.

---

19 How can I ensure that students in the distant learning environment develop a sense of community or connectedness?

Today's online students tend to miss F2F interaction with faculty and peers. In addition, faculty tend to value these human interactions as well. Therefore, it is important when designing distance learning courses to consider how and through what technology you can achieve social presence for the students. The answer may be videoconferencing or mixed-mode delivery with some F2F meetings. This is often referred to as a hybrid or mixed-media course. Connectedness may also be accomplished by creating Internet spaces for discussion groups or sharing of personal information via a virtual student lounge or cyber cafe. As social network software advances in the marketplace, the possibilities for creating a sense of connectedness are not constrained by the technology but rather by our tunnel vision. A sense of presence may be defined very differently by this new generation of students, who are used to interacting with peers via the Internet. Some teaching techniques known to support virtual learning communities include personal Web sites, e-portfolio, e-mentoring, team-based learning, cooperative group learning, virtual world experiences, and professional learning projects. Second Life , a virtual world, opened to the public in 2003 and has grown enormously, even within the education market segment (http://secondlife.com/whatis/).

---

20 Does it take more or less time to teach courses on the Internet?

Faculty surveys reveal that about one-third of the faculty report that Web-based courses take more time, and one-third report less time than the traditional F2F teaching. The remaining third report that it takes the same amount of time. As with traditional courses, these differences may be due to the knowledge and expertise of the course developer. With Web-based courses, much of the time is "up front" time before the course begins. Other variables to be considered are the technology infrastructure, the support for faculty and students, the number of students in the course, the number of times the faculty has taught the course, the design of the course, and the teaching strategies employed. It is important to keep in mind that the rule of thumb for time on teaching tasks is 2 hours of preparation time for every hour of class. Therefore, a 3–credit hour course should take about 9 hours per week of faculty time.

21 How does copyright affect distance education?

Dramatic advances in communications technology have created many exciting distance education opportunities, which have played havoc with copyright issues and laws concerning the questions of fair use and ownership of newly created work. The easy access to information on the Internet, along with the ability to copy and circulate, makes it seem as though this material is not protected by copyright. However, this is not the case. In general, copyright law applies to works on the Web just as it does to traditional forms of copyrighted works. The Digital Millennium Copyright Act (1998) and the subsequent TEACH Act updated copyright law permitting the sharing of copyrighted works with registered students via digital technology. The law applies to the virtual classroom the same fair-use standards that are allowed in the traditional classroom. If you understand the Fair Use Doctrine and the TEACH Act, you have a good appreciation for copyright. The question of ownership of digital course materials is one that is answered by university policy. These policies can vary greatly across institutions and range from work-for-hire to academic freedom.

22 Is the distance education market saturated?

The distance education market is not saturated; on the contrary, most visionaries believe it is a growth market. With the increasing number of high school students graduating in the next few decades, the demand for post–secondary education will continue to grow. In fact, there is concern that the current higher education infrastructure will not be able to accommodate the future college-aged enrollments, thus fostering even more demand for distance education programs. This new generation of students will expect technology-based education at a distance or in the classroom. Also, growth will come from adult working professionals who desire a career change or advancement. Distance education programs tend to have great appeal for working individuals who cannot leave work to attend school.

23 Is distance education cost-effective?

The cost of distance education programs varies by the technology used to support the program. With the increase in advanced telecommunications technology for education, there is much interest and concern about the cost of providing these programs and the return on investment. Information technology services in higher education fall into two categories, those that build the infrastructure and those that provide the related support services. Services that are infrastructure-related involve aspects of acquiring, installing, maintaining, and replacing equipment on an annual basis. Support services are those areas whose budget components are largely staff-driven and provide support to users of the infrastructure. It is important when determining cost to move away from strictly assessing the cost of the technology and infrastructure to considering the educational value of the program or course. Unfortunately, various interactive technology systems for delivering distance education are seldom compared on a cost-benefit basis. The predominance of the Internet and interactive videoconferencing as a delivery system have resulted in large expenditures on technology with little critical analysis of the benefits of the systems in comparison with other potential systems, such as videotape distribution, audio-conferencing, and CAI.

24 What is the future of distance education?

Although no one can predict with certainty what will happen with distance education, there are many indications that it is a growth market. Currently, more than three million students are enrolled in online degree programs. In addition, Web-enhanced education is a central part of most traditional courses. The generation of students entering college today expects technology and innovation in education. They grew up with computers and other technology, so it is not considered innovative to them. It is a way of life. Advance telecommunications technology, which supports educating students in a virtual environment, will continue to expand, and bandwidth will increase in size and decrease in cost. These new telecommunication systems will create new learning paradigms and change the way knowledge is generated and information is transmitted and stored. They will allow educators to use an array of rich media, such as two-way videoconferencing, simulations, and virtual reality in wired or wireless environments. These trends, coupled with the projected increase in the number of enrollments in higher education, will have a dramatic impact on distance education. Familiarizing oneself with this trend and the technologies involved is time well spent by nurse educators both new and established in their career.

References

Brooks, J., & Brooks, M. (1993). In search of understanding: The case for constructivist classrooms. Alexandria, Va.: Association for Supervision and Curriculum Development.

Chickering, A.W., & Ehrmann, S. (1996). Implementing the seven principles: Technology as lever. Available at http://www.tltgroup.org/programs/seven.html

Chickering, A.W., & Gamson, Z.F. (1987). Seven principles for good practices in undergraduate education. AAHE Bulletin 39(7), 3–6.

Cranton, P. (1994). Understanding and promoting transformative learning: A guide for educators of adults. San Francisco: Jossey-Bass.

McGee, P., & Diaz, V. (2007) Wikis and podcasts and blogs! Oh, my! What is a faculty member supposed to do? Educause Review 42(5), 28–40.

Myers, C., & Jones, T. (1993). Promoting active learning: Strategies for the college classroom. San Francisco: Jossey-Bass.

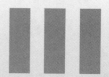

III

CLINICAL
TEACHING

14

Strategic Relationships With Clinical Agencies

Terry Misener, PhD, RN, FAAN

1 Whose responsibility is it to establish relationships with clinical agencies?

Establishing and maintaining relationships with clinical agencies is a shared responsibility of faculty, the dean's office, and the central administration. A relationship can be fragile, and each partner must feel valued. The key is to make sure the relationship is symbiotic and synergistic and reflects a mission match. This takes work and is an ongoing process. The dean must make sure that the academic enterprise does not take partnerships for granted.

2 What is the role of the dean and the chief nurse executive (CNE) of the agency in cultivating new relationships?

As the leaders of the two respective organizations, the dean and CNE are responsible for ensuring the infrastructures are in place for success. The two executives make commitments. They ensure that communications continue and monitor the quality and appropriateness of the relationship. Whereas the unit-level nurses (staff and managers) and the faculty are the day-to-day parties working with students to ensure quality education and safe patient care, the leadership of the two organizations ensure that visions and environments are poised for success. From a practical point of view, they must insist that legal contracts are in place to facilitate and protect all involved.

3 How is agency culture acquired?

All of us have worked in health-care facilities. We know that every agency, and often every unit within an agency, has its own culture. Shared beliefs, values, and expected behaviors may be explicit and written as formal policies, rules, and expectations, or the culture may be implicit and demonstrated through rituals, traditions, and informal understandings. It is important for the dean to allow faculty members new to a unit to be given time to orient themselves adequately to understand the culture of the unit; this is important as faculty members must model the behaviors they expect from their students. Students are likewise expected to learn and respect the culture of the unit. Orientation that includes the faculty member working on the unit even for a short period allows the staff to get to know the faculty person as a competent colleague, not merely as someone who drops in with unrealistic expectations. Although such an orientation costs money, it helps to ensure that relationships are established before students arrive. In these times of scarcity of clinical sites, it is unwise for the dean *not* to consider this approach.

4 What is the role of the dean in matching mission, philosophy, and outcomes with the clinical agency?

The dean is the person who deals with mission, philosophy, and outcomes at the highest level. These are used to judge the appropriateness of programs, clinical entities, and budget justifications. It is important that the dean use these variables as key factors in the assessment of all agencies that faculty recommend for placement of students. Faculty members may often overlook these variables in their zeal to find clinical placements and to respond to personal invitations of agency professional colleagues who want students.

5   How should faculty respond when agency personnel ask, "What's in it for me?"

One answer to the question is that most nurses find that they learn as much from the students as the students learn from them. If staff nurses delegate appropriately to students and provide supervision, the learner, except for the very newest student, provides quality care under the supervision of the staff nurse and the instructor and can actually help decrease certain aspects of the staff nurses' workload. For most of us (and the data support it), one of the primary rewards of the work environment for nurses is the relationships they have with their colleagues, and relationships with students are no exception. One of the most compelling reasons for hosting students is the recruiting potential. Graduates tend to go to work in the agencies where they had supportive and meaningful experiences as students.

6   What strategies support the development of collaboration between faculty and agency personnel?

Shared values are an important part of the foundation for establishing relationships between faculty and agency personnel. If mission, philosophy, and objectives are shared, then a firm base is present to foster the collaboration. As well, there are the "three" main ingredients for the success of the relationships: communication, communication, and communication. Relationships flourish and grow with healthy mutual communication. Factors that sabotage relationships are lack of communication, passive-aggressive behaviors, and negative power plays such as when one party makes another party look inferior. The dean and the CNE must constantly model exemplary behaviors and insist on communication that supports established chains of command while being consistent in "sending the right mail to the right address."

7   What is the impact of the nursing shortage on selection and use of clinical sites?

The nursing shortage makes it imperative that clinical facilities be used with purpose and plans. It is inappropriate to take students into acute care settings to learn communication patterns and skills that can be learned in less acute settings such as learning laboratories, simulation centers, and nonacute settings. As many schools of nursing increase enrollments to meet society and agency demands and to respond to the increased interest of students, new clinical sites must constantly be explored and cultivated. Faculty members must be willing to expand placements, take advantage of new opportunities, and take students not only to those facilities with which the faculty member has a history. Faculty will need to be responsive to a site's rhythms and needs, including placement of students on less traditional shifts such as nights and weekends. Nursing is a practice profession; nursing students need practice in the settings and environments in which they will eventually find themselves after graduation. The majority of new graduates will go to work nights and will be required to work their share of weekends. These shifts provide rich learning experiences and prepare students for the roles they will soon assume. We in education must be very careful not to take clinical agencies for granted.

8   Can employees of an agency be hired as part-time clinical faculty?

The answer depends on the policies of the agency and the academic institution. The dean must confirm that there is no policy in the clinical agency, collective bargaining agreement, or any cultural taboo against such a relationship. Deans and CNEs must ensure that agency employees, first and foremost, meet their obligations to the agency. It is not appropriate for employees to become so fatigued from working two jobs that they perform less than satisfactorily in either. The most likely candidates to work for both settings are those who work part-time in the agency. Dean and CNEs will have their own personal preferences. It can be a real advantage when staff in an agency can be hired as part-time faculty. Obviously they know the agency and the culture. They are trusted and respected by their peers. They do not have to learn a new culture while having students. Other deans and CNEs believe that staff can work as clinicians and as part-time faculty but that they cannot assume both roles in the same setting. In times of shortage, more CNEs will release nurses, even with pay, to serve as clinical instructors. Inevitably, it is only through collaboration with the educational institutions that CNEs will be able to develop new nurses.

---

9   What strategies encourage agencies to "donate" staff to serve as faculty?

Usually for a clinical agency to donate qualified staff to be faculty requires the visionary leadership that understands the ramifications of the nursing and faculty shortage. Agencies usually pay better than academic institutions, however. If the agencies do not share staff to be faculty, there is no way that the educational institutions can educate more nurses for the agencies. It is prestigious to be a faculty member, and most staff members appreciate the recognition of their excellence. Only a select minority of nurses is qualified to serve as faculty. Many agencies find that staff who serve as clinical instructors, even very infrequently, sharpen their clinical skills and critical thinking and often find the change of roles prevents burnout.

---

10   When students are in an agency, how are they covered under malpractice insurance?

Clinical agencies typically require academic institutions to carry malpractice insurance to cover faculty and students while they are in the clinical agency. This should be clearly and explicitly defined in the written contract between the agency and the school.

11 If an agency is unionized and goes on strike, what happens to the students' clinical experience?

Strikes are not surprises. The agency knows when a collective bargaining agreement is due to come up for negotiation. It is when negotiations fail that strikes occur. Therefore, when faculty and the dean know that a strike might happen during a clinical rotation, contingency plans should be in place. Sometimes, the school will choose not to put students in a particular setting when a strike is possible. This is a situation that is a very appropriate topic for the dean and the area CNEs to explore when they meet. It is not appropriate for faculty and students to cross a picket line. This sets up potential animosities that may never be healed after the strike.

12 In a competitive scenario, who determines which schools get which units and which days? Is it possible to have exclusive contracts so that only selected students can use a particular clinical facility?

Schools are the guest of the agencies. The agency may use any method it wishes to choose which schools get which units and when. It therefore behooves the schools to be good partners and stewards of the resources to ensure that the agencies continue to be willing to hear their requests for placements. If there are limited placements, several factors come into play. Many schools and health-care systems have formal agreements that have historical and even legal binding implications, such as that a certain school may have the right of first choice or refusal for available placements. Even where there are no formal agreements, most health-care systems have preferences based on longstanding informal relationships. In some settings, there are no relationships with selected schools. The hospital tells the schools which units, days, and shifts are available, and the schools are expected to work out who gets what. No matter the type of relationship, it benefits the dean to ensure that relationships are maintained, that faculty and students are good guests in a facility, and that faculty reciprocate the agencies in such ways as shared in-service offerings, invitations to academic offerings, and reduced tuition for staff, as a token of appreciation. Some schools also have an annual appreciation day when staff nurses who have served as preceptors are recognized formally and given certificates of appreciation or other signs of gratitude.

---

13 Whose responsibility is it that staff and faculty are oriented appropriately to the agency, unit, curriculum, course objectives, and other appropriate matters?

Many individuals are responsible for orientation, including faculty, unit managers, educational coordinators, and faculty coordinators. However, the ultimate responsibility belongs to the dean and the CNE, who are responsible for maintaining quality controls.

---

14 Are the faculty considered by staff in the clinical site as a guest, sage, resource, collaborator, colleague, or nuisance?

How the staff in the clinical agency view the faculty is a function of multiple factors and often centers around a series of questions. What relationships have been established between the staff and the faculty? Does the staff respect the faculty's knowledge and clinical skills? Does the staff view the faculty as team members or merely as people who have to be tolerated because higher administration has allowed them on the unit? When things are hectic, does the faculty member join in as a productive team member and, above all, as a role model for the students?

---

15 What are the mechanisms to ensure that there is a good match between faculty and the staff on a unit?

The dean sets expectations for the faculty and provides leadership to the faculty to develop cultural norms and expectations. Once the standards of behavior are established, they become the benchmark for faculty evaluation by students, peers, unit managers, and the dean. It is also appropriate for the unit manager to evaluate the faculty member so that continuous quality improvement occurs. If a faculty member is viewed as less than appropriate, tactful, appreciative, and collaborative, the dean needs to intervene to help the faculty member change behaviors or make changes before the clinical site is lost. The dean has a responsibility to support and develop faculty but also has an important obligation to protect the reputation and contracts so that subsequent students and faculty will be welcomed at a site.

16 How do faculty ensure that staff in an agency understand the teaching mission, philosophy, curriculum, and strategies?

Staff in the agencies understand these topics when the school communicates about them. Orientations may use multiple methods and media. Some components can be done in formal classes, some by other methods such as videotapes or audiocassettes. Staff nurses are busy. Ask them the best way to communicate basic information. Then follow up with question-and-answer sessions to ensure they are comfortable about the topics. Along the same lines, faculty need to know the mission, philosophy, and policies of the clinical agencies. This all gets back to faculty presence on the unit and contact with staff— communication, communication, and communication. This is best learned through the life experience of the faculty role model reflecting the mission, philosophy, and desired teaching strategies. A prime example is evidenced-based practice. If faculty expect students and staff to practice based on evidence, then faculty members are expected to use teaching strategies reflective of evidence and be able to document these to a variety of audiences not familiar with the educational literature.

17 Is it reasonable for faculty to expect agency personnel to serve on university committees?

Agency staff are usually better partners when they participate in the development of school curriculum and policies.

As members of the community, schools need to ensure that agencies have an active role in these domains. Sometimes they will not want to participate on faculty committees, but being asked to do so may be the important thing to them. Just being asked means a lot. However, school committees are strengthened when a clinical partner serves on committees.

18 How is funding sought that benefits both the university and agency?

Many of the foundations that fund initiatives to increase clinical capacity or to revitalize the curriculum want the academic institution to demonstrate partnerships. It is important that the partnerships be true partners. This can ensure that each entity is included in the budget process to support programs. Each institutional partner will have differing priorities for needs and wants from grant funds. The dean and the CNE should work out these agreements to the best advantage of both organizations.

19 When clinical research is being undertaken, whose review board is used for approval?

In most cases, each institution will require its own institutional review board (IRB), to review the proposal to ensure adequate subject protection. In some instances, one IRB will defer to decisions of another to decrease the workload of each. The IRB chairs of each organization should communicate to ensure that the appropriate paper trails are maintained in each agency.

20 How are the requirements for each agency, such as immunizations, malpractice insurance, CPR and HIPAA standards, and criminal background checks, decided and managed?

Each agency has its own unique requirements for its staff. The academic institution must abide by these requirements if it wants to use the clinical site. However, just because a

requirement is levied does not mean that it is not nego-
tiable. If a site requires that all students have an 8-hour orientation to its computer system and the students will only
be in a home health agency that is not computerized, rea-
sonableness should be negotiated. Requirements will be
part of the clinical contract with the agency. Sometimes
agencies become zealous in their requirements and when a
logical inquiry is made, everyone's work can be decreased.
For example, some agencies require a duplicate copy of documentation, which is already required by the agency contract.
Bring to their attention that these records are maintained at
the school and that duplicates should not be necessary. If any
accreditation agency needs to see proof, the school can provide it at that time rather than maintaining dual records. The
school must be very careful to maintain these records. All it
would take is one failure in maintaining diligent standards
for the school's reputation to be tarnished, thus affecting
clinical placements throughout the entire community.

---

21 Why is my dean so vehement about clinical contracts/agreements
being in place before we have students in the agency? Sometimes
we have to move quickly.

Whenever two legal entities (the clinical agency and the
university) do business, a contract is needed to outline the
responsibilities and legal authority of each. As mentioned
earlier, this is most important regarding malpractice insurance. Each agency wants to avoid litigation that is not
properly covered. The need for rapid access cannot replace
the legal necessities.

---

22 Why does it take so long for the approval of contracts in a clinical
agency?

These are legal documents with tremendous potential implications. Each partner may require its attorney to review the
contract. If any changes are made by a partner, the contract
has to go back to each attorney. Academic priorities and time
schedules are not those of the agency. Schools must plan

well in advance and should have more contracts than they will ever need. Also, it is important that frequency of contract renewals be appropriate. Most agencies are comfortable with a 3-year time frame for renewal or an open contract with a clause that allows for change and termination using stipulated procedures. Do not renew contracts every year if it is not required by the agency.

23   Who has to approve the contracts with the clinical agency?

The approval authority within each institution is different. However, in most cases a very high official in each must sign the contracts as the legal signatory for the agency. At a university usually a vice-president and at a clinical agency often the CEO signs. It is important for faculty members to know that the preceptor or individual provider of care is not the signatory in most cases for this contract, unless it is a solo practice where the provider is the owner, signatory, and preceptor.

24   How do key players get involved when the university or agency plans new programs that affect the other?

The answer depends on where the impetus is coming from. In some instances, staff and faculty members develop programs and ideas. In other instances, programs are envisioned and created by the dean or the CNE. It hardly matters whether it is a bottoms-up or a top-down creation. What matters is that the right people are involved at the right time, to ensure appropriate commitment and approval. Again, communication, communication, communication is the best approach.

25   Should faculty and staff hold joint appointments? If so, who pays the salary?

Joint appointments are often strong alliances because they indicate to the world and to the players that they are valued by each institution. In other situations, because of collective bargaining agreements and the like, this might not be a viable approach. How pay is negotiated is a matter that the dean and CNE have to work out within their unique organizations. The pay is often not the largest challenge. It is the benefits packages that are different between the organizations.

---

26 What are the concerns that agency staff and faculty have about each other?

Often the concerns are the same. Sometimes there is a difference in standards of care and expectations of students. Sometimes the staff and faculty do not understand the culture and workload of the other. Staff members sometimes believe that faculty members "dump" students. Faculty members sometimes believe that staff members do not understand the curriculum and actively participate in teaching the students. Again, communication is the answer.

Resources

http://www.phf.org/Link/Linkages-Award-San-Diego.pdf
Paterson, C., & Lane, L. (2000). An analysis of legal issues concerning university-based nursing education programs. Journal of Nursing Law 7(2): 7–18.

15

Developing New Clinical Experiences for Students

Susan Letvak, PhD, RN

1 What does it mean to "develop" a clinical site?

It means finding and promoting new clinical opportunities for students. Development consists of finding new clinical sites, determining if the new site can provide opportunities to meet course objectives, and determining if the site is willing and able to accept new clinical students.

2 Why is there a need to develop new clinical sites?

There is always the need to seek new opportunities for students to learn and practice clinical skills outside of the nursing school. Additionally, fewer opportunities exist in traditional hospital settings because much patient care has moved from acute care to outpatient settings, downsizing has closed units, and there is increased competition for clinical space from other schools and health-care disciplines.

3 Why is it becoming more difficult to find clinical sites?

There are more programs and students competing for the same clinical spaces. Schools are sending students further away for clinical experiences. Other health-care disciplines are now providing more bedside care, including physical and occupational therapists, clinical pharmacists, and physician assistants. Additionally, health-care environments are increasingly stressful, with higher patient acuity and staff shortages making the addition of students difficult for staff.

4 Who is responsible for choosing and developing new clinical sites for students?

All faculty members in schools of nursing are responsible for seeking out new clinical sites for students. The responsibility for choosing and developing new clinical sites primarily falls on the clinical faculty in a specific course. However, the dean is responsible for all community collaboration. Permission from the dean or dean's designees is required to place students in any new clinical agency.

5 How are new clinical sites found?

Nursing faculty members should always have their eyes and ears open for the opening of new agencies or new clinical opportunities within existing agencies. State boards of nursing and accrediting bodies can provide information on community agencies that provide health-care services. Additionally, join and become active in your professional and specialty organizations: networking and learning where your colleagues are employed is often the best way to find new clinical opportunities. Wherever nurses are employed, there may be an opportunity for a nursing student.

6 What type of clinical sites exist outside of inpatient settings?

If you have spent most of your nursing career in hospital settings, it is often difficult to envision what other sites may provide clinical opportunities for students. There are two types of sites other than inpatient settings that offer clinical opportunities: wellness sites and ambulatory sites. Wellness sites include day-care centers, schools, continuous care retirement communities, senior programs, and parish nursing programs. Clinical opportunities in these sites focus on health promotion and primary prevention. Ambulatory sites include surgi-centers, sick child centers, rehabilitation centers, respite centers, childbirth centers, occupational health clinics, public health and health-care clinics, and public and community health nursing agencies. Clinical opportunities in these sites focus on primary, secondary, and tertiary health promotion/prevention.

---

7 What are the most important factors to consider when choosing to develop a new clinical site?

The most important factor is the course objectives. Other factors you must consider include determining if:

- The philosophy of the agency is consistent with your school of nursing's philosophy
- The agency provides a high standard of care
- The agency is within a reasonable commuting distance for students
- The agency offers adequate parking and can ensure safety when students travel to and from the parking area
- There is food service or storage for students to bring their own meals
- There is conference or meeting space
- The agency staff is eager to have students

---

8 What would be considered an ideal clinical setting?

One that provides experiences that are relevant and timely to what is being taught in concurrent courses and that allows continued reinforcement and practice of what has been learned. Ideal agencies welcome students and actively assist in finding learning opportunities. They share resources, including meeting space, use of photocopiers, and supplies. Computers are readily available, and students receive training on the computer system along with passwords to access patient information. An ideal site may have a small library or current textbooks and medication and laboratory manuals. Additionally, ideal settings are similar to those for which your program prepares graduates.

---

9 Who should I call at an agency when considering it as a new clinical site?

Start with a call to the director of nursing. The director of nursing may refer you to other administrative staff. In addition, you may also wish to speak with a staff educator to determine orientation needs for students and yourself and to nurse managers of specific departments within an agency.

---

10 When meeting with the director of nursing or other agency administrator, what information do I need to collect to determine if the site is appropriate for my students?

Ask about the agency philosophy and goals, the type of clients the agency cares for, usual staffing patterns, average census (number of potential clients), hours of availability for your students, and any special restrictions (e.g., faculty must stay on site or teach a restricted number of students). Ask about a staff cafeteria, locker space, conference space, parking availability, access to the library (if one is on site), and if emergency medical care is available if a student is injured. Additionally, ask if other schools of nursing are utilizing the agency and if any conflicts in scheduling are anticipated.

---

11 What are possible barriers that a clinical site may impose?

Possible barriers include accepting too small a number of students, refusing to allow students to park on site, not allowing access to computers/client information, preventing students from providing all client care, and preventing students from practicing skills (especially medication administration). Clinical sites may also require background checks and/or mandatory drug testing to be paid by the students.

12 What information will I need to give to the agency when first meeting to discuss clinical opportunities?

Have the course syllabus with learning objectives for students, hours needed (days of the week as well as hours in the day), and whether a faculty member will need to be present with the students or if you are requesting staff to serve as preceptors.

13 Is a formal contract needed before I can bring students to a new clinical site?

Yes, a formal contract is required before students can begin clinical in a new agency. Most contracts are prepared and approved by attorneys. The contract is usually reviewed and signed by administrators of the agency as well as administrators of your school of nursing. Most schools of nursing have a standard contract form; some clinical agencies may insist on their own contract. As long as the agency contract provides content and protection similar to what is in the school of nursing contract and is approved by the school of nursing attorney, there is usually no problem with using the agency contract. While contracts are usually completed in a few weeks, they can often take months to develop as both parties negotiate questionable items. Thus, it is always best to start to negotiate contracts at least a semester before you desire to use a new agency. Once contracts are complete, the school of nursing and clinical agency will each keep a copy. Faculty should always review the agency contract prior to beginning clinical.

14 What is the clinical agency's responsibility in a contract?

The clinical agency generally retains control over patients. The agency will specify the number of students it can accept as well as the faculty/student ratios it may require. A clinical agency may also need to agree to be approved by the state board of nursing as an appropriate clinical site for student learning. Boards of nursing in most states review and assess the appropriateness of clinical experiences within nursing programs. Some states also require board of nursing approval of all new clinical agencies prior to their use as clinical sites. Even if your state board of nursing does not formally approve clinical agencies, it may still be a useful resource in determining the appropriateness of clinical agencies.

15 What is my school of nursing's responsibility in a contract?

The school of nursing retains control over the educational curriculum, health requirements and immunizations of students and faculty, and liability issues and insurance coverage for students and faculty. Additionally, the school of nursing faculty is responsible for the supervision and evaluation of students.

16 What information goes into a contract?

A contract includes dates and times of clinical experiences, maximum student/faculty ratio, health requirements of students and faculty, and, insurance information. Use of the clinical agency's facilities by students (such as library, parking, and cafeteria use/discounts) may also be included. Additionally, contracts are usually written to renew automatically each year unless one of the parties requests a change or termination of the contract.

17 After the contract has been obtained, what else will I have to do before bringing students into a new clinical agency?

- Attend new employee orientation, or arrange orientation for yourself at the agency.
- Become familiar with your specific unit or department. It is very helpful to accompany a nurse for a few days to become comfortable in the new environment.
- Know the usual clinical problems/issues, the average census, age ranges of the clients, average length of stay and acuity levels, and unit routines (including how report is given, breaks, shift changes, etc).
- Familiarize yourself with the general unit/agency layout, learning where supplies and emergency equipment are

kept, learning personnel (especially secretarial staff), and learning where information on policies and other reference materials are kept.

- Learn the required forms, including charting specifics. Will you have to co-sign all student entries? You may also need to obtain computer training to learn the computer system of the agency.
- Educate the agency staff on the learning needs of the students. Inform them of the level of the student (first-semester students are very different from last-semester students), an overview of student activities (will students be giving baths? just doing assessments? administering medications?), and how assignments will be made and posted. A course syllabus should also be provided.
- Determine how staff should communicate with you, especially when problems arise.
- Arrange for orientation of students to the agency. Will agency staff provide orientation, or will you need to provide orientation?
- Determine and resolve scheduling conflicts with other schools of nursing.

18 How will I know if the new clinical site met my students' learning needs and the course objectives?

When in a new clinical agency you will need to closely assess if learning objectives are being met. You should survey students early in the clinical rotation as well as at the end of the rotation when evaluations are routinely done. It is helpful if the clinical site staff are also asked to provide feedback on their experiences with the students. By being open with students and staff, problems will be avoided or solved early, and the new clinical site will be optimal for not only your current students but for other students for years to come.

19 What should I do to ensure that a new clinical site remains a site?

Once you have developed a new clinical site, you must work to ensure that the clinical site will continue to receive your students. In addition to ensuring that you followed all the agreements that were made in advance, be sure that students always followed the rules and regulations of the facility. You should arrive at the assigned time and depart at your assigned time. Students should complete all assigned tasks before they depart the site. Additionally, open communication with the staff and administrative team is very important. Feedback should be provided continuously during the clinical rotation as well as a summary report at the end.

---

20 What specific feedback should you provide to a new clinical site to continue the relationship for next term?

Feedback should be provided continuously to the facility staff and administration. Provide feedback on negative and, especially, positive events. Course objectives should be reviewed routinely to ensure student learning needs are being met. Agency staff must be encouraged to provide feedback to you as well. A formal face-to-face meeting should be conducted at the conclusion of the clinical rotation to openly discuss positive and negative events for students as well as the clinical agency.

---

21 If the new clinical site does not work out, what is the best way to conclude the relationship?

It is not unusual for a new clinical site to not work out; either learning objectives were not able to be met, or the facility and staff were not adequately prepared or willing to accept nursing students. You do not want to "burn any bridges" by being overly negative (and agency situations change), so you should remain as positive as possible. You can state that learning needs were not fully met and provide recommendations to the facility. You should also solicit recommendations from the facility on how staff could have better served student learning needs. You and your faculty colleagues will, ideally, be negotiating additional clinical sites, and you will have alternatives for student placement if the current agency does not work out.

Resources

Altmann, T.K. (2005). Preceptor selection, orientation, and evaluation in baccalaureate nursing education. International Journal of Nursing Education Scholarship 3(1), 1–16.

Chen, S., et al. (2002). Nursing home use for clinical rotations: Taking a second look. Nursing and Health Sciences 3, 131–137.

Eddy, C., Reinhart, S, & Warren, D.R. (2005). Preparing for community health nursing roles utilizing diverse community clinical experiences. Home Health Care Management & Practice 18(1), 10–14.

Gross, C., & Anderson, C. (2004). Critical care practicum: an essential component in baccalaureate nursing programs. Nurse Educator, 29(5), 199–202.

Kirkham, S.R., Harwood C.H., & Van Hofwegen, L. (2005). Capturing a vision for nursing: Undergraduate nursing students in alternative clinical settings. Nurse Educator 30(6), 263–270.

Kline, K.S., & Hodges, J. (2006). A rational approach to solving the problem of competition for undergraduate clinical sites. Nursing Education Perspectives 27(2), 80–83.

Otterness, N., Gehrke, P., & Sener, I.M. (2007). Partnerships between nursing education and faith communities: Benefits and challenges. Journal of Nursing Education 4(1), 39–44.

16

Managing Logistics of Clinical Experiences

Brenda Kelley Burke, MS, APRN, BC, and
Sue Ellen Van Nostrand, MS, FNP, BC

1 What should I do to prepare for the first clinical day?

Call the clinical site several weeks before the start date to set up a time to meet the nurse manager. Schedule a date to orient to the clinical unit. Spend several hours working with staff on the same shifts that students will be working. Bring a copy of the clinical objectives to review with the nurse manager. This is a time to discuss mutual expectations. Reserve a room for pre- and post-conferences. As the start date approaches, place a reminder call to the unit. Knowing when to expect you helps to start things off on a positive note.

2 How do I respond to a tardy student?

Students need to call/page faculty immediately if they are going to be late, and they must let the unit know as well. If a student will be significantly late (for an 8-hour clinical day, more than 1 hour is significant), you need to decide whether the day needs to be made up. Remember to record the time the student arrives.

3   What should I do with the students if I will be unavoidably late for clinical?

Students should not be in the clinical area without you. This information is an important part of the clinical orientation for students. You should call the clinical unit so that staff will be aware that students will not be caring for their assigned clients until you arrive. Students should remain off the unit until you arrive.

4   What should I do if the student does not follow the dress code?

Students have been sent home from clinical for inappropriate dress, as this is part of their adaptation to the professional role. The school's dress code must be followed, and enforcement needs to be consistent. It is essential that students wear an ID badge that identifies them as "student nurse." Clean, nonfaded, nonwrinkled uniforms and white shoes and socks are expected. Undergarments should not be noticeable. Most nursing programs/agencies also have policies on body piercings; some have policies on visible tattoos.

5   What happens if a student is injured on the clinical unit?

Student injuries should be handled as any employee injury. Follow the facility protocol and procedures. A physical injury to the student can be assessed by the student's physician or by a physician at the agency if the student agrees. However, the agency or school does not always cover the cost of being treated in the emergency department. This could be expensive for the student. Incident reports should be filed with the facility and the school. Injured or sick students should not drive themselves home.

6   If a staff member uses unsafe techniques in front of a student, what should I do?

Unfortunately, sometimes students learn through negative experiences. Take the student aside and ask, "What would you have done differently?" "What did you observe that might have been a break in proper technique?" If client care is compromised, a discussion with the nurse manager is appropriate. In some circumstances, students may learn techniques based on recent nursing research. However, evidenced-based practice is slower and at times difficult to integrate into clinical practice for a variety of reasons. Nonetheless, nurse educators should model and facilitate adoption of evidence-based practice in the clinical setting whenever possible.

7   How should I intervene if the staff acts disrespectfully to me or to a student?

Advise students that some staff members may not be as welcoming as others. Many things motivate behavior, and students should not react personally or defensively. However, students should report episodes of disrespect to you. If there is a pattern or if one particular staff member is a chronic offender, speak to the nurse directly saying," I notice that...." It is important not to start the conversation with, "The student tells me...." Comment on the behavior that you have seen. If this proves unsuccessful in solving the issue, then consulting with the nurse manager is appropriate. Do not let a problem get established. Speak with nurse manager after several student reports. Chances are the offenders are already known to nursing management.

8   Who can I talk to about clinical issues that are troubling me?

Professional supervision is a necessary resource when working with students. Ideally, you should have an assigned mentor from your faculty who can help you process issues, but any seasoned faculty member with whom you work can offer support and advice. Be sure to establish a regular time to meet to discuss your work. Know how to contact people when an emergency arises that needs their input.

9 How should I handle the chemically impaired student who comes to clinical?

Spotting a student with a substance abuse problem is not always easy. You may notice subtle things:

- Client care that is unfinished, of poor quality, or that shows a pattern of inconsistent care
- Absences from the unit
- Trips to the car for "forgotten" items
- Inappropriate affect (smiling, laughing, angry outbursts)
- The smell of alcohol
- Unsteady hands or gait

Behavior changes of any kind should make you suspect a problem. Check your school's policy to know how to handle the problem if it arises. Usually students are dismissed from clinical, and a ride home from a family member is secured. Never let a chemically impaired student drive. The situation should be written up and shared with the program director for follow-up.

10 How do I handle the emotionally impaired student who comes to clinical?

The care of clients leaves no room for a student who is emotionally upset. Students who you believe are emotionally distraught should be sent off the unit and dismissed from clinical. Makeup of clinical time can be arranged at a later date. The student should be encouraged to seek help from a professional who can help work through the issues. Do not counsel the student. The faculty role is not one of therapist.

11 What is involved in making clinical assignments?

Good communication with staff about clients' conditions and needs will aid in the selection process. Select clients who will allow students to meet clinical objectives. Factors that will help you determine this are the client's:

- **Medical diagnosis:** Does it coincide with what is being taught in theory?
- **Admission date:** Will the student be able to take care of the client for 2 days?
- **Medications/scheduled times:** Too many at the same time will make it difficult for you to supervise administration of all of them efficiently.
- **Treatments** (dressings, IV fluids, feeding tubes, etc.): Be sure students have been instructed on these skills before you assign them in clinical.
- **Scheduled diagnostic tests:** These can enrich student learning.
- **Consent:** Ask if the client will agree to have a student work with the primary nurse to administer care.

12 What do I do if there is a low census on the clinical unit when I make the assignments?

Be creative. Some strategies you can use are:

- Pair students to administer care.
- Co-assign students to a staff person to give care.
- Use other departments to provide an enrichment observational experience; for example, rotate students off the unit systematically to respiratory therapy, IV team, or endoscopy.
- Create a "just in case folder" with educational activities worksheets or case studies for students to do together or in small groups during downtime.

13 When should clinical assignments be made?

Assignments are usually posted on the clinical unit the afternoon before the clinical day. This allows students time to go to the nursing unit and gather information needed to care safely for clients. Keep in mind that most clinical units have a preferred time that students can come for their assignments. Collaborating with staff about anticipated discharges will help ensure that students will care for the client they have researched. Be aware that some schools expect faculty to bring clinical assignments and prescribed client information back to the school for the students to get there. Be certain to maintain client confidentiality as you distribute client information outside the clinical setting.

14 How do I maintain fairness in assigning clients?

Initially, assigning clients randomly is practical. As the rotation progresses, the assignments should be made based on the clinical objectives that the student needs to meet.

15 Should I give the weaker students the easier assignments?

Resist the temptation to do this. Doing so does not allow the student to develop higher-level skills necessary to meet the course objectives. Of course, this means that you will have to more closely supervise that student to ensure proper care is given.

16 Is there value to an off-unit rotation?

Yes, if the rotation enhances the learning experience. For instance: care of the surgical client is enhanced by an experience in the operating room (OR) or post-anesthesia care unit (PACU). During a psychiatric rotation, time spent teaching a client about electroconvulsive therapy (ECT), observing the procedure, and follow-up care brings concepts together.

17 How can I plan off-unit rotations?

Call or visit the unit you intend to use to inquire about an experience. Set up guidelines (what the students can and cannot do) and a rotation schedule. Give these to the students and unit personnel who will be working with the students. It helps to put the guidelines and schedule, along with any written objectives, in a folder to be kept on the unit for reference. Be sure to update the folder each semester and confirm that the unit is still willing to work with students. Include your business card and pager number in the information.

Some experiences that are useful during medical-surgical rotations are OR, PACU, emergency department, oncology clinic, IV team, or special procedures such as in cardiac catheter laboratory, endoscopy, or pain clinic.

During a mental health rotation, probable cause hearings, open speaker meetings of Alcoholics Anonymous/Narcotics Anonymous/Adult Children of Alcoholics, National Alliance on Mental Illness, and others that may meet objectives are appropriate to attend.

18   How should I manage clinical absences?

Keep a daily clinical attendance sheet, and record absences. Be aware of the nursing program's policy regarding absences. Some programs want you to call the school to report absences. Check the school's policy on how many absences a student is allowed. In some programs, if there are more than two absences, the student must petition the faculty in writing to be allowed to remain in the program. A written warning to the student after two absences is prudent on your part. Clinical makeup is often necessary to meet the required number of hours designated by state boards of nursing. Clinical absences are usually made up at the end of the semester. Ideally, the makeup should be scheduled on the same unit where the absences took place with the same faculty supervising.

19   How do I develop good rapport with staff?

Be friendly, be positive, and be there. Faculty availability is essential to good rapport. Let staff and students know when you are going off the unit. Carry a pager so students can contact you directly with questions and concerns.

20   How can nursing instructors earn the respect and support of nursing staff?

- Be organized in managing the student experience
- Make expectations of the staff clear
- Value members' time and expertise

- Give staff positive feedback
- Encourage students to assist staff when possible
- Be available to staff as a resource
- Share insights, articles, and other information

---

21 How I should conclude the clinical experience?

Usually students sign a card of appreciation to staff and complete an evaluation of the experience, the agency, and the instructor. An exit meeting between you and the nurse manager to discuss the clinical rotation is essential. This is a time for both you and the manager to offer feedback on how things went and to make plans for the next group. Sharing students' comments from their evaluations is useful. Discuss problem issues first, and always end on a positive note. Faculty should send a letter of thanks to the nursing unit and the nurse administrator when the rotation is over.

Resources

Allison-Jones, Lisa A., & Hirt, Joan B. (2004). Comparing the teaching effectiveness of part-time and full-time clinical nurse faculty. Nursing Education Perspectives 25(5), 238–243.

Forget, M.A. (2004). MAX teaching with reading and writing: Classroom activities for helping students learn new subject matter while acquiring literacy skills. Victoria, Canada: Trafford Publishing.

Hrobsky, P.E., & Kersbergen, A.L. (2002). Preceptor's perceptions of clinical performance failure. Journal of Nursing Education 41(12), 550–554.

Meyer, L.A. (2005). Teach! The art of teaching adults, 2nd ed. California: LAMA Books.

17

Teaching in Clinical Settings

Brenda Kelley Burke, MS, APRN, BC, and
Sue Ellen Van Nostrand, MS, FNP, BC

1 What should I do to prepare students for the first day of clinical?

Prior to the first day of clinical, the students should receive a letter outlining the specifics of the first clinical day; i.e., time of arrival, where to meet the instructor, dress code, your pager number (or how students can reach you if there is a problem), and the telephone number and name of the clinical unit. Students who will be assigned to a preceptor or mentor should write a brief note of introduction on school letterhead to that individual. This letter should contain the following points:

- A personal introduction
- Confirmation of the start date, time, and place to meet
- A gracious closing thanking the preceptor/mentor for the opportunity to work together.

These notes should be hand-delivered a few days before the actual start date. These serve as a reminder to staff that students are coming and delivery gives the students the opportunity to locate the site and parking. It is helpful on the first day to circulate a telephone call tree in case of inclement weather or other reasons you may need to contact students.

2   What constitutes a good orientation to a clinical unit?

A good orientation includes a clear statement of expectations and conveys a feeling of warmth, excitement, and a sense of belonging. In addition, you should review clinical objectives, your rules for supervising their practice, and required clinical paperwork. It is good practice to put all of this in writing in the event of concerns/issues later in the rotation.

If there is considerable orientation material, unit information, or policies that students will need throughout the rotation, it is helpful to put copies of all written information in a three-ring orientation binder. Students can refer to or copy this information and return the binders to faculty, who can update and reuse them with the next group.

A tour of the unit including introduction to the nurse manager and staff is essential. A scavenger hunt allows students to become familiar with the unit. (Do not start all scavenger groups on the same item as this causes too much congestion in each area. Start some of the students at the top of the list, some in the middle, and the rest at the bottom with the rule that items must be gathered in the order they appear on the list. This will spread the students out and eliminate congestion.)

3   By what title should the students address me ?

Professor or Doctor sets the tone that this is a professional relationship.

4   How should students address staff members?

Students may address staff by whatever title staff members prefer. You may want to discuss this during your orientation to the unit, or you can instruct students to ask the staff members with whom they work how they want to be addressed. This second action forces students to introduce themselves to staff, which is a valuable habit to acquire and sets a collegial tone for the day.

---

5 How should staff address students and me?

This is a personal decision. Many staff members use first names, and this feels comfortable. Staff members usually address students by their first name.

---

6 How can I manage multiple students on a busy clinical unit?

Begin by being organized. Prepare an assignment grid for yourself with student names and times you need to supervise them doing a particular skill. Try a sample grid like the one in Figure 17–1 in order to manage multiple students and events.

Students and their assignment obligations need to be managed. In most cases, the instructor-to-student ratio is 1:8. This makes it impossible for you to supervise all students doing all medication administration and procedures every day. Not all students need to give all medications all the time. For instance, divide the group in half, and have the first half give 8 a.m. medications and the second half the 10 a.m. medications. The next day, reverse the groups' times.

Before students call you to supervise them doing a procedure they should have:

- The chart open to the doctor's order
- Reviewed the facility's policy procedure protocol
- Read the last nurse's note
- Assembled all equipment at the bedside

This saves time and encourages the student to develop good organizational skills.

If you are already busy supervising a student and a second student needs to perform a procedure at the same time, you could have the second student assist the

Student	0700	0800	0900	1000	1100	1200	1300
Sue		IVPB		IV med			
Mary	Insulin		NG feed			Insulin	
Brenda		Dsg					

Figure 17–1. Multiple student assignment grid.

staff nurse with the procedure. Do not let a student perform a procedure under the supervision of a staff nurse unless the student has already been evaluated as competent on that procedure. Students may perform only procedures they have already learned and practiced in the laboratory.

---

7 | What can I do to safely oversee students when they are assigned to different units?

Supervising students on multiple clinical units can be done by following the preceding steps. You can also:

- Use different-colored paper to color-code the units.
- Alternate medication administration opportunities, e.g., have students on one unit give medications at 0800 and 1000 while students on another unit can give the medications at 1200 and 1400. Then reverse the times the next day.
- Designate a resource nurse for students to go to when you are not immediately available.
- Give students your pager number to use when they need you or when they are set up and ready to be supervised doing a skill.

---

8 | How do I help students correlate content with clinical practice?

Teaching moments can be accomplished in pre-conference or prior to a procedure or administering medication outside the client's room (if this is appropriate in your setting). For example:

- **Medication administration.** Ask the student to explain the medication's mechanism of action, nursing implications (including side and adverse effects), and how these relate to the medical problem.
- **Clinical skills/procedures.** Ask students why they think a procedure has been ordered and the expected outcome; e.g., a nasogastric tube is being inserted to decompress a bowel, which will relieve the client's nausea. Ask

students to summarize the steps involved in that procedure. Review the essential components of documenting the procedure.

- **Psychiatric rotation.** Have students focus on thoughts, feelings, and perceptions, and chronicle them with daily journal entries.

Daily individualized supervision sessions provide students with faculty guidance the opportunities necessary to develop personal and professional growth as well as correlate classroom theory with clinical practice.

---

9   What conference space is best for students?

A conference area off the unit works well. Students can conclude their clinical duties after a busy day and go to conference relaxed with minimal interruptions. A conference room with a white board, television, or DVD or VCR player is helpful. Because students will be discussing their day, the room must be secure so that client information may be kept confidential.

---

10   How do I conduct a pre-conference?

Pre-conference can be structured (with assigned topics/objectives) or unstructured (process-oriented). For instance, in a community rotation, in which students go to different sites, students may meet formally before the clinical day to discuss clinical goals for the day and present content material that meet clinical objectives. A sign-up schedule with topics and presentation dates can be circulated among the group so that all students share responsibility for the pre-conference.

For a novice group, the pre-conference may include reviewing care plans they have prepared for their assigned client. Choose one or two students randomly each day to present their care plan to the group. This should ensure that all students come well prepared.

For a senior group, a pre-conference may not be needed. Students may have multiple clients to get report on, and a pre-conference may logistically not be feasible. In this case, a post-conference is better suited to meet the learning needs of the group.

11 How do I conduct a post-conference?

Post-conferences can be structured (with assigned topics) or unstructured (process oriented). The last hour of the clinical day, after students have given report to their staff nurse and their responsibilities are done, is the usual time for the post-conference. Starting time for post-conference should be strictly enforced as the topics discussed can meet clinical objectives and if students are not present, they will not be able meet them. Also, enforcing the start time forces students to manage their clinical time on the unit.

Topics for a structured post-conference should reflect clinical objectives and, although may be presented by students, should be faculty directed. Post-conferences presented by students work well when presented by two or three students as a team. Short videos are sometimes helpful to reinforce concepts, as are field trips to different departments within the agency. Guest speakers who have different roles (i.e., diabetic nurse educator, IV nurse, ostomy nurse) are also a good choice. Concept maps or worksheets on presented topics reinforce content and give students an opportunity to help other students learn how to solve problems. Gaming is a good way to allow student interaction after a tiring day. Critical thinking or drill and practice format also work well.

Rounds on one or two of the students' clients are also a good way to encourage critical thinking and reflection. Faculty guide this review, pose questions, and offer insights as needed to the group.

12 How should I respond if a student chronically monopolizes conference time?

Setting limits on students who monopolize time is an important skill for faculty to develop. A simple "Thank you for your input . . . now I'd like to hear from someone else" is usually sufficient to move things along. For students who persist, speak to them outside of conference in a private setting. Address their behavior with positive statements like, "I know you are very enthusiastic about this topic but . . . . " or "I'm so glad you like to participate in the discussion but . . . . " Each student has a story to tell, and each deserves the opportunity to express it.

13 What happens when a student comes to clinical unprepared to care for the client?

Students who are unprepared are unsafe. Every client deserves quality care, and this is not possible when students are not prepared. Students should be dismissed and required to make up the lost clinical time. This zero-tolerance policy makes an impression and usually results in no one arriving unprepared.

14 How can I offer feedback/constructive criticism without embarrassing a student?

If a safety issue is involved and correction is needed immediately to prevent harm to the client, then the student should know that you will intercede without discussion until after the procedure is done. Sometimes gently guiding, cueing, or gesturing can be done at the moment. Taking a student aside to a private area is best when you need to give feedback that is not positive. Starting with the question, "How did you think things went?" will usually give the student a chance to explain his or her thinking and perspective. Then you can correct the student's reasoning or discuss a plan on how the student could improve in the area in question. Follow the rule, "Praise in public and correct in private."

15 When should I discuss clinical problems with a student?

Clinical problems should be discussed as soon as they are identified. A written summary of this student-faculty discussion along with any plan for remediation, is prudent.

16 What should I do if students accuse me of "picking on them"?

Students who suggest faculty members are picking on them are generally not assuming responsibility for a problem. Identifying students' feelings of personal reproach puts the focus on the student where it belongs and allows for dialogue between both of you. Validating feelings is important and is key to a satisfying working relationship.

17 What should I do if a student lies to me?

Veracity is an ethical principle that is basic to nursing practice. Students who lie, for whatever reason, lack an important fundamental value. Their clients' safety is compromised, and it becomes questionable whether these individuals should be working with clients. Check your school's policy for consequences and course of action. In some instances, this is cause for dismissal from the nursing program.

18 What is a professional boundary, and how do I recognize when it has been crossed?

A professional boundary is defined by legal, moral, and professional standards of nursing that dictate the conduct of the instructor as a professional in relating to the student while helping the student achieve identified learning objectives. It is important that you remember that you are not the student's friend or confidant. Boundaries make the relationship safe for the student and instructor. Warning signs that a boundary may have been crossed are:

- Giving extra time to certain students (picking a favorite).
- Visiting students in off-hours.
- Feeling resentment when other faculty members are professionally involved with the student.
- Putting the student in a position where he or she feels obligated to you.

19 Should students accompany their client for diagnostic tests or when they are transferred off the unit?

This depends on the setting, where the client is going, the client's wishes, and the physician's permission. In larger facilities that have multiple groups of students, it may not always be possible for students to accompany their client. However, if you believe it would be a valuable learning experience for the student, then you must obtain the permission of the parties involved.

20 How do I handle a student's medication error?

The medication error policies of the unit should be followed. This is an area of concern for instructors, and instituting a few rules regarding medication administration for your clinical group can minimize the potential for error. First, inform the primary nurse about the error. The student with your input usually completes the incident report. For beginning students, all medications must be double-checked by the instructor or, in some instances, the staff nurse. All parenteral medications must be given with the instructor present. This is usually a condition that is included in the contract between the school and the agency. Most student errors are errors of omission.

21 When should I make weekly clinical paperwork due?

Some rotations require daily paperwork, and this is usually turned in the following morning. In the authors' experience, work must be submitted by 1600 the day following clinical, thus giving students a full 24 hours to finish their assignments.

22 Should I grant extensions on written paperwork?

Circumstances occur in students' lives that make extensions on written paperwork reasonable. However, this should be the exception.

23 Should I keep detailed, written notes on my students?

Notes regarding students should be objective in nature. If you need to document an incident, an objective description of what happened and what the student said and did is sufficient. Keep in mind that students and their legal counsel have the right to see your notes. Therefore, be sure that there are no subjective or judgmental comments in them.

Resources

Clayton, L.H. (2006). Concept mapping: An effective, active teaching learning method. Nursing Education Perspectives 27(4), 197–203.

Lipe, S.K., & Beasley, S. (2004). Critical thinking in nursing: A cognitive skills workbook. Philadelphia: Lippincott, Williams and Wilkins.

Lowenstein, A.J., & Bradshaw, M.J. (2004). Fuszard's innovative teaching strategies in nursing, 3rd ed. Sudbury, Mass.: Jones and Bartlett.

Penz, K.L., & Bassendowski, S.L. (2006). Evidenced-based nursing in clinical practice: Implications for nurse educators. Journal of Continuing Education in Nursing 37(6), 250–254.

Raingruber, B., & Hoffer, A. (2001). Using your head to land on your feet: A beginning nurse's guide to critical thinking. Philadelphia: F.A. Davis.

18

Working With Clinical Preceptors

Barbara K. Haas, PhD, RN, and
Kathleen Deardorff, MSN, RN

1 What is a preceptor?

A preceptor is a registered nurse or other health-care professional who serves as a role model, resource person, and mentor for nursing students in the preceptor's clinical setting. As an expert clinician, the preceptor works with the faculty to facilitate, support, and supervise a student's clinical learning experiences while assuring safe nursing practice. Preceptors continue to work their usual schedule of weekends, nights, and holidays, providing assigned students with a "real-world" experience. This creates a unique relationship as depicted in Figure 18–1. Educational outcomes and activities are developed in collaboration between the faculty member and the preceptor, who both support and encourage the student.

2 Who can be a preceptor?

This varies among states; consult your state board of nurse examiners for the rules regarding selection and use of clinical preceptors in your state. Generally, a preceptor is a registered nurse or other licensed health-care professional who meets the minimum requirements of their title. They

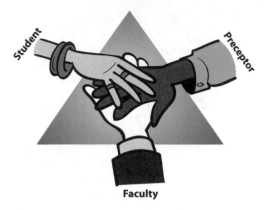

Figure 18–1. Preceptor relationship.

should have experience in the area and, ideally, be an exemplar in their profession. Preceptors must enjoy mentoring students and have a desire to share their knowledge and clinical expertise. You may want to have additional requirements of the preceptor, such as educational or experience requirements that are specific to your course or level of students.

---

3 Which students get preceptors?

Historically, preceptors were used only at the end of a nursing program as a capstone experience. Currently, preceptors are being used successfully at *all* levels of nursing programs, with novices in the first course to seniors in an advanced elective. It is up to the faculty of your nursing program to identify when and where preceptors will be used, staying cognizant of the rules of the state board of nurse examiners.

---

4 How do I select preceptors?

There are several means of building a pool of preceptors. You may find it easier if you have experience working with the nurses, either as a peer or in your faculty role, and have established credibility. We recommend that you first speak with the agency coordinators or unit managers and ask them to identify those who might be interested in and qualified to mentor one or two students for a specific period. Current preceptors are very good referral sources as they know the demands of the role and the strengths of their peers. You might also approach potential preceptors directly.

Sometimes students identify potential preceptors. If they do, it is important to verify the individuals' qualifications and their current relationship with the student. We do not recommend using relatives or good friends as preceptors, although they may be paired with a different student. Once a preceptor program has been established, it is not unusual for nurses who have observed their peers to approach you and ask if they, too, can be a preceptor!

---

5 How are preceptors oriented to their role?

There are two issues involved: *how* and *what*? For the first question, there are several means of orienting preceptors. Sometimes a one-to-one setup works best, in which a faculty member spends time with a preceptor orienting him or her to the program. Offering a program at the clinical agency may permit several preceptors at once to attend, although our experience has been that it is difficult for them to leave their work settings to attend sessions. We have offered full-day workshops with continuing education credit and asked our participating institutions to arrange for the preceptors to be given paid educational leave, an approach that attracted dozens of preceptors. Some institutions offer their own preceptor orientation, and if this is the case, review the orientation to see if it meets your needs. We have also instituted an on-line orientation program that permits flexibility for the preceptor and can be updated easily.

The second question, *what* to include in an orientation, is very important. The following information should be part of your preceptor orientation program:

- Objectives of the orientation
- College of Nursing philosophy

- Role and expectations of the preceptor, student, and faculty
- Characteristics of the adult learner
- Assessment of student learning needs
- Teaching strategies
- Supervision of students
- Evaluation as an ongoing process
- Problem-solving and conflict resolution
- Communication with faculty
- Specific course and clinical objectives, including skills checklist and course evaluation tool
- College-specific forms pertinent to the clinical setting

---

6   How are preceptors paid?

They are not paid by the academic institution but rather by their own employers while fulfilling their preceptor role.

---

7   Why do preceptors volunteer?

Preceptors volunteer because they recognize this service as part of their professional responsibility and they love working with students. They should be in the role because of the intrinsic rewards, not because they are given external enticements.

---

8   So what are the benefits to the preceptor?

There are numerous benefits. Those listed here are a compilation of comments made by our preceptors who were evaluating the benefits of their participation:

- Stimulated own professional growth
- Personal satisfaction; rewarding for preceptors
- Student actually provided help toward end of rotation
- Continuity—knowing what the student is capable of doing
- Gives nurses on evenings and nights an opportunity to participate
- Smaller institutions can participate (do not have to accommodate 10 students at a time)

- Preview of future employees; recruitment tool
- Increased professionalism among staff
- Increased collaboration with nursing faculty
- Renewed sense of pride in nursing

Since the development of our preceptor program in 1998, we have also chosen to provide our preceptors with specific benefits. These are offered, not as encouragement to participate, but rather as a means of thanking them for serving as a preceptor. The university gives the preceptor a nonbudgeted title of clinical education specialist. This provides these individuals with:

- Library privileges at the university
- Faculty discounts to the university's fine arts series
- Campus exercise facilities
- Faculty discounts at the university bookstore
- Free registration to continuing education programs offered by the College of Nursing
- Free tuition to one nursing course (toward a BSN or MSN) for each year of preceptor service

Since its inception, our preceptor program has spread to many nursing schools throughout the state. As a result of the widespread use of preceptors, the Texas legislature enacted an incentive program in 2006 that provides a stipend to preceptors and their children pursuing a baccalaureate degree in nursing. Therefore, our free tuition benefit is now limited to nurses pursuing an advanced degree. Other schools offer different benefits, such as faculty titles, name tags, or other signs of affiliation with the educational program. Some clinical institutions have rewarded their nurses for serving as preceptors through recognition in the agency's newsletter, gift certificates, or advancement on a career ladder.

---

9   What are the benefits to the student?

Benefits to the student (as identified by our students, faculty, and preceptors) include:

- Richer clinical experiences
- Increased confidence in their nursing skills

- Continuity
- Better time management
- Better awareness of and use of resources
- Understanding of real-world expectations of nursing
- Validation of chosen profession
- Flexibility in their clinical hours
- Increased responsibility for their own learning
- Development of a relationship with preceptor and unit
- Potential to do clinical rotation close to home
- Preview of potential employers

10 Are there benefits to the instructor?

The instructor also experiences benefits from this approach:

- Flexibility in hours
- Ability to spend increased time with students who need it
- Decreased stress wondering what other students are doing while you spend time with one
- Increased collegiality with personnel at institutions
- Opens up many additional clinical sites, such as clinics, specialty hospitals, schools, small acute care institutions, and alternate shifts at traditional institutions, that could not manage a full clinical group
- Easier to schedule meetings among faculty members

11 What kind of challenges are there to using preceptors?

As the faculty participant, you will need exceptional organizational skills to set up and track students and preceptors. There is much more time spent at the beginning of the semester arranging for preceptors, gathering preceptor agreement forms, orienting students (especially if their first experience with a preceptor), and pairing students with preceptors. Once that is done, you will need to track which student is in clinical on which day and at what time. We use various methods to help with this task, including grids, e-mail, and online calendars. An additional challenge is being available whenever students are in the clinical setting with their preceptor. A practical consideration is whether you will be reimbursed for travel if your students are spread out over a large geographical area, so you will want to talk to your dean about this. Managing a precepted clinical is not easier than a structured clinical, nor does it take less time. It is simply different. Faculty members who think they can relinquish their responsibility to the preceptors are quite incorrect.

---

12 What is my role when I use preceptors?

You will serve as the coordinator of the students' clinical experience. You will no longer be at the clinical site the entire time a student is there, but you will make rounds to evaluate students and teach in the clinical setting. You will meet with the preceptor and student on a regular basis. You will also hold clinical conferences or seminars, and you will still be responsible for evaluating the student's clinical performance.

---

13 If I am not at the clinical site the entire time, how do I know what the students are doing?

You may not know what the students are doing, but, if you think about it, did you ever really know what all the students were doing at a given time? In a structured clinical you may be responsible for 10 students, but you can be with only one at a time, leaving the others virtually unsupervised. In a precepted clinical experience, the student now has someone to work with on an individual basis, minimizing the mistakes the student may make when performing without supervision. You will still be able to evaluate the students by making rounds, observing and questioning them, consulting with the preceptor, evaluating written assignments, and listening to them in clinical conferences. Often preceptors are willing to communicate through e-mail, chat room, or phone to update you on student progress.

14 What do I do when I make rounds on students assigned to preceptors?

The preceptor now serves as the clinical expert and as a role model for prioritizing, communicating, assessing, and patient teaching. The preceptor assists the student with skills such as suctioning and injections. This allows you to focus on larger issues, such as evaluating the students' critical thinking skills, and become less task-oriented. When you visit the students, you will still go with them into patient rooms to observe them assessing patients, administering medications, communicating, and performing technical skills. You will still have the opportunity to be a role model. You will be able to delve into the student's understanding of the pathophysiology for a particular patient, for example, or explore options for referrals. You can help students understand laboratory values or discuss alternative ways to approach a problem. You can spend as much time as necessary with a particular student, reassured that your other students are adequately supervised. Your time is much more focused, with virtually no time wasted waiting for students to come out of morning report or returning from lunch. You will want to stop at different times of the day to observe students in different scenarios. You will also want to discuss with the preceptors each time you make rounds to hear their perceptions of the students' clinical performance and progress.

15 Can the students work with their preceptors on nights and on weekends?

Yes. One of the benefits of using preceptors is that students have the opportunity to work on different shifts. This provides them with a more realistic view of what nursing is like and, for some students, helps them deal with child care issues and other factors that may interfere with successful completion of a traditional structured clinical experience.

16 If the students are with preceptors on different shifts and all days, am I on call around the clock?

This is a very important question; the answer is: you could be. Because that is a potential risk, it is very important that you set limits. There are several ways to do this. First, you can simply limit the days that you will be on call and tell the students that they must schedule only on days when you are available. Even with that approach, you may find yourself on call very often. Second, use faculty partners or teams. Take turns being on call for one another's students. It is critical that students and preceptors know that, whenever a student is in the clinical setting, there is a faculty member available for consultation. As well, if you do not already have pagers, your college should invest in providing them for faculty.

17 Why would I want to use preceptors?

This depends on the school. If there is no requirement, there are several options for using preceptors, and one may be right for you. Depending on the objectives of the nursing course, the level of the students, and the availability of clinical sites and faculty, you may decide that a traditional structured approach is most appropriate. Other faculty members choose to introduce preceptors midway during clinical after spending structured time with their students. Others assign students to preceptors for the entire clinical experience.

The major reason you may want to consider preceptors has to do with the weaknesses that have been identified in the traditional structured clinical. Over time, it became apparent to us that structured clinicals were often unsatisfactory: Our students expressed a need for more clinical experience before graduation, and they complained about the limited number of patients they were able to manage because faculty members were not available. Managers at the institutions expressed a need for graduate nurses who were better able to prioritize, manage a larger load of patients, have realistic expectations of the workplace, and demonstrate better technical skills. Faculty can be overwhelmed by the task of trying to provide students with all the knowledge and skills they need to graduate, frustration due to the mandate to educate more nurses when clinical sites are limited and nursing faculty are scarce. Using preceptors addresses all of these concerns.

18 Do I still have clinical conferences? If so, how does that work?

Your clinical conferences will probably work better than ever. Because your students are no longer all in the clinical setting at the same time, schedule your clinical conferences at a time when everyone is available at a location that is convenient. When conferences are scheduled on a clinical day, the students may not work with their preceptors during that time so that all of the students are available for conference.

19 How do I know a student is competent before being assigned to a preceptor?

We still give medication administration tests to all students before they are allowed in the clinical setting to help ensure basic safety with medications. We still have our students in the skills laboratory learn technical skills such as initiating intravenous therapy before allowing them in the clinical setting. While this does not guarantee that students are proficient, it does give us insight into how they perform. The advantage of the precepted clinical is that students have more opportunity to perform clinical skills while increasing their confidence and competence because the preceptor is working one-on-one with them. They no longer have to wait for the instructor, who may be tied up with another student. For this reason, student weaknesses often become apparent more quickly than in a traditional setting.

20 Who evaluates and grades the student: the preceptors or faculty?

You are still responsible for the overall teaching and evaluation of the students. However, you will collaborate with the preceptor to complete the written and verbal student evaluations as the preceptor has spent hours working closely with the student and therefore has much valuable information. Because evaluation is an ongoing process, you should have a format detailing how you want this accomplished. You may want to use a daily log in which the student and preceptor comment on the student's daily performance. Some faculty make periodic rounds during which the student and preceptor discuss the student's progress. An evaluation may also be accomplished by telephone, e-mail, or chat rooms. It has been reassuring to us to find that the preceptor's perception of the student's performance has mirrored that of the faculty. This is a validation for both the preceptor and the faculty.

21 What if a preceptor and student do not get along?

We try to avoid this potential problem. Problems of relationships should be discussed during the orientation of the preceptors as conflict resolution is an important aspect of professional behavior. Preceptors should be free to approach faculty.

We ask students to complete a brief profile at the beginning of the semester to try and match student and preceptor personalities, schedules, and interests. For example, we will put a self-described shy student with a preceptor who works well with that type of personality. This presumes that you know the preceptors—one of the reasons we recommend that faculty who use this approach have a relationship established with the nursing staff. In the rare instances that preceptors and students do not work well together, the problem is usually the student's performance. We then deal with that issue, which usually resolves any conflict between the preceptor and student. Very rarely have we chosen to reassign a student to a different preceptor on a different unit.

22 What do I do if a preceptor is ill or otherwise away from work unexpectedly?

This is a potentially frustrating experience for the student, but you can often work around it. The first step is that the student pages the faculty member on call. If the student has been in the clinical setting and there is another nurse working that day who has had the preceptor orientation, that nurse can be requested to serve as the student's preceptor for the day. Because the student has often become an integral part of the unit, this is usually not a problem. We make sure that there are extra preceptor agreements on each unit and that each student has a copy for the purpose of covering situations like this. If, however, it is the student's very first day or if there is not another qualified preceptor available, the student cannot be allowed to remain in the clinical setting. The day will either need to be rescheduled or the faculty will have to have an alternate clinical experience available.

---

23 Suppose I sense the preceptor is "covering" for the student?

Preceptors often take "ownership" of their students and may want to cover for them, ensuring that their students perform well. It is best if this can be prevented. Part of the preceptor orientation includes addressing the roles of the different participants and making sure that the preceptors understand their own role as a member of the educational team as well as everyone's responsibility in helping produce safe and competent nursing graduates. If, in spite of this preemptive move, the preceptor covers for the student, it becomes important for you, as faculty, to spend additional time with the student to closely evaluate the student's competence (not the preceptor's). If a deficit is noted, meet with the student and preceptor together to develop a plan to address the weakness. You may need to reassure the preceptor that early identification of and intervention due to student weaknesses are critical to the student's eventual success.

---

24 What if the preceptor is being too strict or has unrealistic expectations of the student?

This situation is also best handled preventively. If you thoroughly communicate clinical objectives and expectations of students, the preceptors will have a better sense of the student's capabilities. If, in spite of this information, the preceptor has unrealistic expectations, meet with the preceptor to explore the issue. Sometimes it is just a matter of helping preceptors remember how it was when they were students.

---

25 Do the students like this type of clinical?

Nearly all students prefer having a preceptor. They enjoy the personal relationship they develop with the preceptor, the flexibility, the enriched clinical experiences, and the sense that they are real nurses. The students who struggle with this type of clinical are those who have trouble with time management or who are not motivated. They are likely the students who would also struggle in a more traditional clinical experience.

---

26 Are there any disadvantages for the student?

Students may be limited to one particular patient population, providing them with less exposure to other potentially interesting specialty areas. Scheduling their hours can sometimes be difficult and may be frustrating when a day is scheduled but the preceptor is sick or has a schedule change due to unit needs. The students also put in long days that may not be ideal for learning, but then that is part of the real-world experience.

---

27 Do the agencies really like this approach to clinical?

Agencies have been overwhelmingly in favor of using preceptors. They appreciate not having to try to schedule all the various nursing students into a Monday-through-Friday day shift, which burdens one particular shift. They like having the opportunity to evaluate potential employees and actively recruit those who impress them.

---

28 Who evaluates the preceptors?

Students are given the opportunity to evaluate their preceptors every semester, just as they evaluate the faculty and the courses. In addition, the faculty evaluates preceptors' performances. On the rare occasion that preceptors do not perform as anticipated, they are not assigned additional students.

---

29 I think I would like to try using preceptors. Is there anywhere I can get additional information?

Our first recommendation is to visit the Web site for your state board of nursing to see what particular guidelines apply to you. A literature search will also lead you to articles that describe the use of preceptors in nursing education, either anecdotally or in terms of research outcomes. Talk to faculty members who have used preceptors, clinical staff who have served as preceptors, and students who have worked with preceptors: they are all ideally suited to give you practical advice.

Resources

Altmann, TK (2005). Preceptor selection, orientation, and evaluation in baccalaureate nursing education. International Journal of Nursing Education Scholarship 3, 1–16.

Haas, B.K., et al. (2002). Creating a collaborative partnership between academia and service. The Journal of Nursing Education 41,518–523.

Krugman, M. (May 8, 2006). Precepting: The chance to shape nursing's future. Nurseweek, 32–35. Retrieved February 12, 2007, from http://www.nurse.com/ce/course.html?CCID=3685

Myrick, F., & Barrett, C. (1994). Selecting clinical preceptors for basic baccalaureate nursing students: A critical issue in clinical teaching. Journal of Advanced Nursing 19, 194–198.

Öhrling K., & Hallbert, I.R. (2000). Nurses' lived experience of being a preceptor. Journal of Professional Nursing 16(4), 228–239.

Yonge O., et al. (2002). Supporting preceptors. Journal for Nurses in Staff Development 18(2): 73–79.

Yonge O., & Myrick, F. (2004). Preceptorship and the preparatory process for undergraduate nursing students and their preceptors. Journal for Nurses in Staff Development 20(6): 294–297.

19

Utilizing Clinical Simulation

Debra Spunt, DNP, RN, FAAN, and
Barbara G. Covington, PhD, RN

---

1 What is clinical simulation?

Clinical simulation is the replication, as near to reality as possible, of a clinical setting and/or situation. This can encompass the emergency room, critical care, labor and delivery, pediatrics, psychiatry, home care, or clinical office. Regardless of clinical context, it is a strong bridge between theory and practice. This unique, safe environment is flexible, and it can be altered to model a specific situation, use particular equipment, or replicate a unique patient. The clinical simulation environment is constructed to allow the student the opportunity to learn and integrate "basic parts" into the whole clinical situation (Infante, 1985). As such, it can be the golden thread through the curriculum. Clinical simulation develops learners who are self-directed; provides an interactive environment where students can learn at their own speed, review skills or equipment as needed throughout their program rather than being tied to just one course, and perform in a safe environment to apply their knowledge/rationale in practice. The faculty is able to use the clinical simulation to provide experiences missing from clinical or classroom time and build in the same experience for all students. Clinical simulation is one step beyond the classroom and one step before the full clinical experience.

---

2 How does clinical simulation prepare students for the clinical arena?

Clinical simulation provides opportunities for the students to apply their didactic knowledge and problem-solving, critical-thinking, and time management skills to clinical situations. By having these experiences, students are able to bring to the real clinical setting more self-confidence in their own abilities. Research also shows that the active learning process used in clinical simulation has an advantage in that students retain the knowledge longer (Johnson, Zerwic, & Theis, 1999). Low- and high-fidelity simulators enable the student to experience simple or complex, stable or unpredictable clinical situations before encountering real ones in the clinical setting. Low-fidelity simulation might be as simple as a scenario that a student hears or reads and uses as a basis to plan actions. High-fidelity simulation offers the most realistic clinical experience possible, short of caring for a real patient, and may involve advanced equipment that interacts with the learner.

Simulation can offer students very valuable problem-solving opportunities that may not be obvious to an expert clinician. For example, in learning a procedure, the student may want to use an over-bed table to set up for the procedure. But in the clinical setting, these tables are often filled with items and not available for use. Setting up the scenario in the laboratory for the student following a problem-based scenario allows the student to consider various options. A more complex cardiac arrest situation can be replicated with a high-fidelity simulator to not only allow the students to care for the victim with realism but also to fulfill various response team roles and react appropriately if the "patient's" family or visitors are present.

3 What are the advantages of using clinical simulation over the clinical setting?

There are a number of advantages. Simulation:

- Allows students to learn at their own pace.
- Provides a setting to which learners can return for remediation or re-education throughout their program.
- Offers flexibility in timing so students can fit it into their busy schedules.
- Provides the opportunity for students to experience repetitive practice. This practice may allow students to master tasks more quickly, improving performance before they go to a clinical setting where they need to locate and do their assignment in a shorter period.
- Enables the learner to participate in a whole experience or focus on subparts or tasks.
- Lends itself well to problem-based learning that can begin in a simple format and increase in complexity.
- Can include team efforts, even interdisciplinary teams.
- Enables study of patient care scenarios and diagnoses that do not frequently or consistently present themselves in clinical learning.
- Can serve as a focal point for the development and integration of competency-based skill evaluation within the health-care curriculum, including evaluations too risky to take place in a live clinical setting.
- Students have time to review and analyze their own performance and, through reflection, develop various critical thinking abilities and skill proficiencies.
- Offers a safe clinical simulation environment in which students can be allowed to be unsuccessful in a skill and faculty does not have to feel responsible for patient safety, stepping in to correct the student or finish the skill or task.
- Allows for a larger faculty-to-student ratio than allowed in many clinical settings.
- Provides opportunities for the faculty and students to actually use equipment and supplies that are not available for teaching in the clinical setting, such as code carts.

4   What are the disadvantages of using clinical simulation over the clinical setting?

Disadvantages do exist and need to be addressed when building the laboratories or integrating clinical simulation into a curriculum. For many institutions, space is a shrinking commodity, and there are specific space needs for the simulation laboratory, disposable supplies, and equipment storage. The equipment needed may require technical support, maintenance agreements, and contracts that increase the annual operating budget. The cost of supplies can be prohibitive for some schools. Once purchased, the items may eventually no longer be state-of-the-art. Additionally, an individual is needed to set up the equipment and assist faculty in developing the class lesson plans, scenarios, and evaluation and practice approaches. Clinical simulation laboratories may require additional staffing, possibly during evening or Saturday hours. Finally, students and faculty using simulation can gain a false sense of security in that both may believe students are more prepared than they actually are.

5   What are the adult learning principles involved in clinical simulation?

There are many theories and principles of adult learning that are involved in clinical simulation, most notably those of Malcolm Knowles and Carl Rogers. Malcolm Knowles (1970) is perhaps one of the most recognized authors addressing the adult learner, describing both how they learn and their unique needs, and offering principles to be applied in adult learning situations. Knowles describes adult learning as a process of self-direction and emphasizes the adult preferences for an interactive environment and using hands-on skills (O'Brien, 2007). Clearly, simulation offers both a hands-on approach and an interactive nature to the scenarios.

Carl Rogers' (1969) experiential learning or learning by doing is also seen in clinical simulation. The teacher is a facilitator, not a director. The simulation laboratory offers a positive environment for adults to gain knowledge, learn skills, and enhance their critical thinking abilities. Rogers' view of adult learning also supports access to learning resources set up in an organized manner. The simulations can easily build in the needed balance of intellectual and emotional learning. For example, a simulated code or patient death that includes debriefing time allows learner needs to be addressed on the spot. Difficulties and emotions can be addressed before the learner walks into the first actual cardiac arrest or death in the clinical setting.

The adult learning process is facilitated by learner participation and results in faster learning if the student does not feel personally threatened. The self-initiated learning for adults also lasts longer. The addition of self-evaluation as the prime method for adults to assess progress and success also shows a shift in focus from child to the adult, who needs both the external and internal motivations.

---

6   What types of clinical simulation are available to enhance the clinical experience?

Equipment and models cover all areas of nursing practice, all levels from entry-level to expert practitioner, even such roles as nurse researcher. They exist for inpatient to home care settings. Simulators range from specific task trainers with changeable parts for simulation of various conditions of the eye, ear, skin, and so forth, to virtual reality trainers connected to computer programs that can be scripted to have the necessary vital signs, heart sounds, bowel sounds, cardiac rhythms, or even to give birth. Regardless of the patient care experience being simulated, it is essential to orient learners to the adult learner role of demonstrating responsibility, accountability, and active inquiry in clinical simulation—just as in-patient care situations.

---

7   How do I help learners translate clinical simulation into clinical practice?

The goal is to have the clinical simulation match the objectives and to be scripted so that it provides the quality and consistency for each student that the faculty would seek in clinical rotation or final clinical practice. The process of backward chaining allows faculty to look at the expected level and type of clinical practice demanded of the student in clinical practice. Then those expectations are divided into objectives, and scenarios are developed with full scripts and evaluation approaches. This process allows the simulations to replicate the care population, environment, correct level and extent of complexity, or unstable environment where the clinical practice must be performed.

---

8 Where should clinical simulation be placed in the nursing curriculum?

Clinical simulation should be placed throughout the curriculum, beginning with the first undergraduate semester and progressing through graduate programs with clinical specialization and in doctoral studies for research projects. Frequently, clinical simulation is seen simply as nursing process applied to physical assessments, nursing scenarios, and environmental assessment. Because health-care education is a practice-based profession that integrates theory and research into clinical practice, clinical simulation can also serve as a focal point for the development and integration of competency-based skill evaluation at any point in the curriculum.

---

9 Why would I want to integrate simulation into the curriculum?

Simulation allows faculty to adjust variations among clinical sites and variations in clinical experiences within sites. When clinical experiences are not available to meet the objectives of a course, those experiences, regardless of complexity, can be created using simulation. If evaluations show that a group demonstrates weakness in an area, the faculty can reassess the clinical site for the students or build in remediation or simulations to fill the gap. Using simulation provides the faculty new opportunities to objectively assess students' psychomotor skills and critical thinking abilities.

There are many patient care experiences available in simulation that could not be performed in the classroom or the clinical setting for reasons of patient availability and safety. Simulation also offers a reflective aspect not always available in real-time clinical. Students gain more insight about their level of performance and progress over the semester if they are encouraged to analyze their simulation experiences. All learning styles can be addressed because simulations can be set up using computers, videos, auscultation sounds, or equipment to reinforce concepts or the operational steps for a procedure.

10 What is my role as faculty in clinical simulation?

This differs with the faculty position and program. If you are a clinical coordinator, your role will include working in collaboration with course faculty as a facilitator to develop and structure the clinical simulation to mesh with the didactic content being taught. As a clinical simulation laboratory faculty member (this could be a number of different personnel), you will ensure supplies are available and, possibly, that the class is set up properly and taken down at the end, based on laboratory policies and the clinical simulation for each specific class. If you are the actual clinical simulation faculty/facilitator for the session, you will ask and answer questions to motivate the students to succeed and go to the next level. As a faculty member, you have the responsibility for setting up and maintaining a positive climate for adult learners to feel safe as they work on gaining knowledge, skills, critical thinking abilities, and self-evaluation and making mistakes or failing without serious consequences to the patient. The faculty role includes being able to clarify the purposes of the clinical simulations.

11 What is the role of the student in clinical simulation?

Students have the most important role in clinical simulation. They are responsible for identifying their preferred learning styles and what strategies work best for them.

They are expected to be active learners and to come prepared to the clinical simulation. They need to decide what they want to work on. For example, students:

- Develop the team for a clinical simulation exercise or scenario, serving as team leader and team member in addition to working independently
- Work with peers to facilitate and promote themselves in the learning process
- Are responsible for quality self-assessment or evaluation following a simulation

Applying adult learning principles and guidelines, you can see easily that students are responsible for four areas, consisting of the personal, social, emotional, and administrative aspects of the simulation experience. They need to experience making mistakes or failing but be motivated to improve and willing to put in the time and effort to meet challenges successfully.

---

12 How is clinical simulation used for clinical remediation?

Because clinical simulation provides a positive, safe, structured adult learning environment, the fit is natural for clinical remediation for individuals or groups. Clinical simulations can be structured for specific psychomotor or critical thinking skills, depending on what must be mastered. Clinical faculty might identify that a student (or group of students) needs clinical remediation before returning to the clinical setting or needs to strengthen skills, procedures, time management, or critical thinking skills while continuing in clinical. The clinical faculty should request help in writing to the simulation faculty, being specific about student needs. The simulation laboratory faculty then can work with the students on a baseline assessment and develop an individualized plan for student growth.

Students are responsible for their learning and practice while the clinical simulation faculty serves as facilitator. Students perform ongoing self-assessment to monitor how they are progressing. They have debriefings with the simulation faculty to monitor progress, plan for future learning and evaluation, and modify needed clinical simulation activities as they close in on required goals.

In the case of group remediation, a student group may be weak in communication skills with other disciplines, slow in procedure preparation, or weak in collection of assessment data. In clinical simulation, scripted scenarios could be created for the student group, and students could repeatedly practice the scenario as well as complete periodic self-assessments and debriefings with the simulation faculty. This provides the clinical faculty with time to focus on the objectives for a clinical rotation with other students, not being concerned with weaker students.

---

13 How can critical thinking be incorporated into clinical simulation?

Critical thinking, according to Ennis (1987), involves both the skills and process utilized in making rational decisions regarding what to do or what to believe. The health-care literature identifies several distinct aspects to critical thinking: defining and clarifying the problem, judging information related to the problem, solving problems, and drawing conclusions (Costa, 1985). Critical thinking can be incorporated into clinical simulation in any number of ways, ranging from simple learning activities to problem-based learning scenarios that ask students to apply their new skills and knowledge and selected processes to make rational decisions in different environments. One example is when the students learn a basic skill in the laboratory and then have to transfer that skill and knowledge to a totally new environment, like a particular care setting or to a specific patient population. By their nature, simulations, case studies, problem-based learning scenarios, and critical analysis of exercises and content all utilize critical thinking skills and can assist students to evaluate and transfer knowledge and skills to new situations.

Ideally, faculty and the clinical simulation staff work together to develop clinical scenarios, tasks, and instructional procedures to meet instructional objectives. They should address how critical thinking skills can be incorporated into students' clinical simulation time.

14 How can leadership skills be included in clinical simulation?

The needed delegation, team-building, and leadership skills commonly employed by health-care providers can be deliberately written into communication exercises or clinical simulation experiences such as a cardiac arrest situation. With faculty guidance, learners can successfully incorporate leadership and delegation approaches as group exercises are undertaken. The skills can be further practiced and refined in subsequent simulation classes and in student practice sessions. Some of these skills include team communication, providing guidance and direction to others, time management, completing tasks within given periods, prioritizing the steps and actions to be completed, and team problem-solving approaches. Also included are multidirectional communication skills, including written, verbal, and nonverbal; collaboration; task identification; and individual task assignment. The learners also need to work well with other members of the team, evaluate their own performance and that of others, and assess the outcomes of the simulation.

From the first day, students can be teamed in pairs or small groups that can be rotated or maintained. They work together to prepare for a skill or procedure they either are assigned or for which they volunteer or for a role they assume in problem-based scenarios designed to focus on specific delegation or leadership skills. These leadership simulations allow learners to experience success and failures, increased speed and facility with the skills over time, and comfort with taking charge in increasingly complex scenarios. The goal is for the delegation and leadership skills to transfer to real-life clinical experiences.

Interdisciplinary team-building skills can also be taught and refined through clinical simulation. Interdisciplinary specialty team rounds, a discharge planning meeting, or an emergency response exercise can increase student awareness of the strengths and contributions of all team members and help students work and communicate effectively as a team.

---

15 What teaching-learning strategies are utilized in the clinical simulation laboratories?

These strategies utilized in the clinical simulation laboratories are limited only by faculty and student imaginations, hardware and software availability, and, to an extent, budget. The explosion of new technology, multimedia, software, the Internet, high-fidelity simulators, standardized patients, and animations allow schools, teachers, and learners to select single or combination strategies to use in clinical simulation.

Computers are no longer only for the computer laboratory or to watch skill videos in the learning resource center. By bringing this hardware and software into clinical simulation, a student can be at a bedside caring for a "patient" while reviewing a computer-assisted instruction program, an equipment tutorial, or a skill video. One benefit of this strategy is that the student repeats the exercise as many times as necessary to learn.

Having the simulation laboratory connected to the Internet and the school intranet and using video and DVD equipment allows faculty to mix the learning strategies. For example, in learning physical assessment, a student listens with a stethoscope to a heart sound simulator while watching a video that shows the flow of blood through the heart and the valve actions responsible for the different heart sounds being heard.

Electronic health record systems now being made available to health-care academic settings incorporate many teaching-learning strategies that can be used in class, in the clinical simulation laboratory computer systems, and also over the school network out to remote sites or students' homes. These systems provide the educator and student with opportunities to participate in tailoring the system to their curriculum needs, and each semester can offer new teaching-learning strategies.

16 What measures are used to evaluate students doing simulated skills?

Evaluation in simulation is like traditional evaluation. That is, it arises from the school's evaluation philosophy, adult learning principles underpinning the student learning experience, the design of the simulation, and the evaluation plan itself. The outcome measures to be evaluated in the clinical simulation laboratory include those that are assigned to the student but that cannot be done in an actual clinical setting for a variety of reasons.

It is important to distinguish between formative and summative approaches when considering what and how to evaluate. At the formative evaluation stage, the focus is on the learner's progress toward a goal, and you evaluate a partial task or a whole series of events, an individual or group effort, and provide feedback for corrective action. The feedback allows students to improve their performance or you to change your teaching, if necessary, while the semester is in progress. This is not meant to be graded. In addition to your formative assessment of your students, students can use skills checklists, self-reflection notebooks, peer/faculty feedback, anecdotal notes from the faculty's observations, and videotaped self-assessments. At this stage, the measurements may be broken down into broad categories, with faculty or students filling out the form displaying the student progress level 1, 2, or 3:

- 1 = The skill was not performed within the time frame
  - Inconsistent proficiency
  - Requires prompting
- 2 = Performance within the time frame
  - Consistently proficient
  - Without prompting
- 3 = Performance within the time frame
  - Competent, independent
  - A resource for peers

The focus of summative evaluation is the learner's final achievement of identified objectives and, typically, the teacher's assignment of a score or grade. These evaluation procedures are more carefully planned, tools to measure the achievement are thoughtfully selected by the simulation team, and evaluators are trained on the tools to help ensure consistency (and therefore fairness) in evaluations across students.

There are now many outcome measure evaluation tools available in the clinical simulation laboratory. They even permit evaluation of behaviors in the cognitive domain. Students can be observed or videotaped and then evaluated by the faculty against predetermined standards in the areas of knowledge, comprehension, and application. Also, students can evaluate their own performance after doing the scenario. The same video protocol may allow students to talk through their analysis of the scenario, describe the plan they are going to carry out, and provide rationale for their actions. In the clinical setting, evaluation may be less objective because information on student performance may come from multiple preceptors or faculty and be influenced by personality dynamics. The use of standardized patients and computerized outputs available from simulators, for example, enable faculty to evaluate students more objectively and consistently than ever before.

17   How are student performances evaluated in the clinical simulation laboratories?

From the first semester, the students are taught that they are key players in the evaluation of their performance. They also learn the value of having others providing input into the evaluation. Initially they experience uncomplicated skill(s) verification by carrying out problem-based clinical scenarios with peers videotaping them. The videotape is evaluated by faculty and student self-reviews, and the student is allowed to redo the unsuccessful component (or the entire event). The student's performance is also evaluated with faculty-developed skills check sheets to ensure specific objectives are met.

The evaluation of students' performance progresses through the semester from formative to summative. Their performance has to stay consistently in the safe area and not backslide in the areas of timing or performance in either the clinical simulations or the clinical setting. The students, their peers, and the faculty are all active in the evaluation process at each stage.

18 What measures can evaluate teamwork in the clinical simulation laboratory?

The procedures, events, and actions to evaluate teamwork are structured for two or more students to carry out. In fact, most simulation exercises or scenarios are written for at least two participants, and most simulated procedures can have two or more students involved. The teamwork activities they perform provide data for student evaluation. The evaluation measures and appropriate tools are selected by the faculty in collaboration with the clinical simulation staff during the design phase of the course and classes. As teamwork is evaluated from three perspectives (individual performance, team performance, and the amount of success in achieving the objective), more than one tool is employed. The scenario being carried out for the evaluation may be videotaped with a clock in the frame for timing, or the student teams do a problem-based scenario at a station and are evaluated according to predetermined criteria by faculty or a student evaluator taught by the faculty. A number of stations can be set up in one clinical simulation room, and student teams rotate around the room for evaluations on a number of scenarios, all stressing an aspect of teamwork. These might include completing a task correctly, problem solving, prioritizing skills, assessment and communication skills, and flexibility in the face of scenario changes.

19 How can clinical simulation foster interdisciplinary education?

Most clinical situations involve more than one discipline. A carefully planned simulation can encourage students to integrate basic knowledge and skills from their own specialty education into the whole clinical situation (Infante, 1985). If the clinical scenario script is for a mock code, nursing students can be assigned to different discipline team roles, or students from other health-care professions can fill their own roles. For example, a team could include the nurse caring for the patient, crash cart nurse, scribe nurse (nurse/manager/supervisor), team leader, representatives from respiratory/anesthesia, IV team, runner, patient representative, clergy, and security. The active learning includes collaboration from student to student, between student and faculty, and interdisciplinary student collaboration. In this case, it is especially important to allow time for debriefing and reflective thinking at the end (time equal to the simulation activity). This gives team members a chance to gain insight from each other and their faculty while providing direction for improving their performances. Because clinical simulations can be scripted with endless possibilities for situations and settings, interdisciplinary teams can go on rounds together, deliver a baby, care for a postoperative patient, respond to emergency room situations, or communicate with patients and families.

20 How do you adapt simulation to individual learning styles?

So many learning styles can be addressed within the simulations. Four common learning styles—visual, auditory, tactile, and kinesthetic—can be accommodated by carefully constructed simulations. Faculty often are surprised by how many of the simulation environmental elements, processes, and student roles and interactions (between students, students to simulation, students to the material, students to the teacher, students to themselves) support one or more of the four learning styles.

Because simulation is the replication of the clinical setting, the sights, sounds, equipment, materials (verbal, written, videos, CAI, images), and real-time tracking (clock) accommodate the visual learner. The auditory learner benefits from the sounds in the setting and by having verbalized instructions, team member communications, faculty clarification, audiotapes, videotapes, sound simulators, and computers with multimedia applications. The tactile learner benefits from having mannequins or models with real heart or lung sounds or with different conditions the student can assess or treat. These students also benefit from touching the computer or video screen to trace an image or the path of blood flow through the body. The kinesthetic learner benefits by having the real supplies and equipment to handle and use in the simulation. Learning style is important to all students but may be especially so for the student having academic difficulty. When a student is referred from a clinical rotation to the simulation laboratory for remediation, the remediation objectives and simulation activities are designed to include activities that complement the student's learning style as much as possible.

21 How do you ensure equal participation among all members of groups working in the clinical simulation laboratory?

Equal participation is desirable but difficult to ensure without some planning. Participation can be improved by informing all participants what is expected of them and how they will be evaluated and by having them agree on student responsibilities for group work. The faculty can structure group experiences that include more members in a variety of roles during group work and by scripting the experiences with sufficient opportunities for all members to participate. The physical activity of some learners should be considered equivalent to the mental effort of the observers. The NLN/Laerdal Simulation study showed that faculty members need to work at constructing the role for the observers in a way that draws them into group collaboration efforts (Jefferies, 2007). It is important to build in periods throughout the simulation when observers can provide feedback to the team and make suggestions.

22 What should my faculty colleagues and I consider if we want to create a clinical simulation laboratory?

Creating a clinical simulation laboratory parallels in process steps to creating a health-care environment:

- **Vision.** Carefully consider the laboratory's use now *and* in the future. Will the resource be shared or dedicated to nursing? Will the space be used for general or specialty practice? What anticipated educational programs will require simulation in the future?

- **Support.** Be sure you have administrative support and the necessary approvals to proceed. Clinical simulation settings and required resources are time-consuming and often expensive, and you will need support all along the way.

- **Space.** Determine how much space you will need, using available benchmarks of successful laboratories, and individualize the measurement to your vision, including use and support. The floor area required per inpatient bed is 85 square feet. In the laboratory, this allows four to six students to work in each bed unit. A six-bed simulation laboratory with teaching space, storage, and preparation area averages a minimum of 988 square feet.

- **Infrastructure.** The functional infrastructure of the simulation laboratory should include:
  o Computer networking and connection to the Internet
  o Electrical supplies sufficient for the equipment load
  o Utilities: water, air, heat
  o Headwall units (lighting, call system, air and suction equipment with compressors)

- **Supplies.** The space and use plans drive the supplies and equipment needed for laboratory operations and any special classes or scenarios. If your space is limited, you might want to outfit the room as a multipurpose space and build in storage for equipment that is not always used or for future growth. One example would be if you are teaching physical assessment or code techniques. You may decide in advance that the space will be for one specialty, such as operating room or critical care. You can order equipment and supplies from a variety of vendors or check with your local hospitals. The supplies for a course can be purchased by the student with the course fee or supplied centrally from the clinical simulation laboratory into student bins for use throughout the semester.

23 What clinical simulation resources are available for faculty?

- **Books.** Among the several references in this chapter, one particularly helpful resource is the book on simulation in nursing education written by the nurses who participated in the NLN/Laerdal eight-site research study on simulation in the United States (Jefferies, 2007). The authors offer realistic evidence-based information and share their knowledge of how to approach every step of the implementation process.
- **Associations.** These connect you with the international community of educators interested in clinical simulation in nursing education and across disciplines. The organization focusing on nursing is the International Nursing Association for Clinical Simulation and Learning (INACSL). The Web site, www.inacsl.org, has both open pages and a members-only portal that opens to a wealth of information on a wide variety of topics, resources, and hosted discussions. The online journal is filled with current simulation topics and new simulation research and lessons learned. The listserv is open for anyone interested in this area and can be subscribed from the Web site. With hundreds on the list, it connects in real time with nurse and health-care simulation professionals from all settings (clinical, educational, and service) and institutions together to share concerns, questions, ideas, and offer guidance and support. A second association, dedicated to interdisciplinary simulation in health care (including nurses), is the Society for Simulation in Healthcare (www.simulationinhealthcare.com), and it also has an excellent journal and listserv.
- **Conferences.** There is an increasing number of conferences specifically focusing on clinical simulation in education, held annually or periodically. There is an updated list on the INACSL Web site for conferences throughout the United States. Conferences often offer CD-ROMs, audiotapes, or DVDs during or after the conference to expand the reach of the educational offering.
- **Companies.** This may be one of the most promising resources. Medical simulation and health profession

education companies are developing particularly helpful resources. Faculty can learn about how products or equipment can enhance the simulation experience and gain more general information about simulation, constructing simulation laboratories, creating scenarios and simulations using templates, and approaches that are being used successfully to integrate simulation into nursing and health-care curricula. Simulation is an increasingly important way to approach nursing education as the nursing role becomes more complex and as clinical resources shrink.

Resources

Costa, A. (Ed). (1985). Developing minds: A resource book for teaching thinking. Arlington Va.: Association for Curriculum and Supervision.

Ennis, R. (1987). A taxonomy of critical thinking dispositions and abilities. In Baron, J., & Sternberg, R. (Eds.). Teaching thinking skills: Theory and practice. New York: W.H. Freeman.

Infante, M. (1985). The clinical laboratory in nursing education, 2nd ed. New York: Wiley Press.

Jefferies, P.R. (Ed.). (2007). Simulation in nursing education: From conceptualization to evaluation. New York: National League for Nursing.

Johnson, J.H., Zerwic, J.J., & Theis, S.L. (1999). Clinical simulation laboratory: An adjunct to clinical teaching. Nurse Educator 24(5), 37–41.

Knowles, M.S. (1970). The modern practice of adult education: Andragogy versus pedagogy. New York: Association Press.

O'Brien, G. (2007). What are the principles of adult learning? SHCN Postgraduate Bulletin. 20 March 2007 Online at http://www.southernhealth.org.au/cpme/articles/adult_learning.htm

Rogers, C.R. (1969). Freedom to learn. Columbus, Ohio: Merrill.

IV

EVALUATING STUDENTS AND LEARNING

20

Evaluating Teaching and Learning

Jackie McVey, PhD, RN

1   What are the characteristics of evaluation systems in nursing education?

The evaluation process answers important questions in three categories:

- What are the real priorities of a particular learning topic or clinical placement?
- How can I communicate to students what these concepts help to accomplish?
- Is it possible to use evaluation to foster a sense of mutuality and teamwork in order to get agreement on a learning project?

We need a balance of all three of these components in order to achieve success in positive and effective student learning.

2   How can I help the evaluation process live up to its potential?

The way to capture the special gift of evaluation is to discover the ways it can enhance the lessons for which it provides a supportive framework. Here are two questions to ask at the beginning of any project:

- What do I hope to accomplish?
- How can I decide whether the project is successful?

Planning begins with objectives and includes how to measure outcomes. When evaluation is included in objectives, then continual assessment supports the whole learning process. Evaluation that facilitates learning is more positive than its traditional end use to reward success or punish failure.

---

3 Who are the primary stakeholders in successful outcomes for nursing education?

Every component of nursing education benefits other healthcare professionals, health agencies, communities, educational institutions, legislators, and taxpayers. Nursing's strongest commitment is to improve the human situation, so society at large is the ultimate stakeholder regarding the quality of nursing program outcomes.

---

4 How can I develop a philosophy of evaluation that integrates an emphasis on program outcomes with genuine respect for all persons?

Nurse caring has become a dynamic theme that supports individuals as well as their positive educational and health outcomes. Use every opportunity you can to reflect on ways to develop teaching and evaluation strategies that promote both excellence and human caring. Be sure to include holistic self-care measures so that your stamina and optimism are maintained in the process of learning how to become a really good teacher.

---

5 How can I learn about types of evaluation required in my nursing program and who is responsible for them?

Study your school's curriculum plan, faculty and student handbooks, master evaluation plan, committee reports, and summaries of findings from state board and accrediting agency reviews. Every program has its own master evaluation plan that includes ways to assess the curriculum, compliance with policies for admissions and progression, student academic and clinical performance, quality of faculty work, budget and financial resources, and the satisfaction of health-care agencies with the program's graduates. Procedures for all these types of evaluation are reviewed at least once a year by committees and the faculty as a whole. Periodically, the program has a required review by its state board of nurse examiners and a voluntary evaluation by one of the national nursing education accrediting agencies. All faculty members are expected to participate to some extent in all aspects of evaluation.

---

6   Are there other mechanisms of evaluation in nursing education?

Nursing programs are held to very high evaluation standards because of their legal and ethical commitment to safe standards of health care by their graduates. In addition to state and national reviews, each college or university constantly monitors its nursing program for quality of instruction, student satisfaction, graduation rates, and employment of graduates. Statistics on how many graduates pass national standardized tests, including the NCLEX-RN licensure examination, have a big impact on program approval and accreditation as well as funding, recruitment, and reputation.

---

7   What do I need to know, and what do I need to do about how I am evaluated as a nursing teacher?

Your job description gives a basic list of your responsibilities for teaching, clinical supervision, and other faculty roles. You can find more specific information in the faculty evaluation form used to document your role performance at least once a year. The experienced faculty member designated to supervise your job orientation can explain the evaluation process and how to keep records such as student reviews of your teaching and reports of your participation on committees. You will submit annual goals and write a self-evaluation of your accomplishments. Include your vision for professional development and your contributions to nursing education. Remember to stay realistic.

8 How can I positively influence my overall evaluation?

Your main participation in evaluation during your first years of teaching will be to clearly document your work in assigned courses. Find opportunities to let others know what you are doing to promote student success. Other faculty may want to try some of your methods or to collaborate with you in finding other innovative ways to support student learning. Negotiate being assigned to committees that really engage your interests and abilities. Show interest in issues affecting the entire program, and reflect shared values when stating your opinions in faculty meetings. Find ways to promote and publicize your program in the community. Consistently keep evidence of your activities and ideas to serve as documentation material for your own annual faculty evaluation.

9 How can I stay enthusiastic about the evaluation process so that it does not become just another boring chore?

Every teacher has to live with the basics of what accountants call "counting the beans" in using evaluation to check the bottom line on planned outcomes. Stay aware of the intent of these standard evaluation procedures, and try new ways to improve results. If you can discover new opportunities in everyday tasks, your evaluation will reflect your active and vital engagement in your work. Remember that no one else can make the unique contributions you are making as a nursing teacher.

10 When does the evaluation process begin for nursing students, faculties, and programs?

The answer is, "Yesterday, today, tomorrow, and always." Evaluation started when the nursing profession began and when your program was initiated. Because evaluation is constantly changing, it is also new every moment. Tune in to the history of evaluation in your school, and discern trends in current evaluations. Reflect on the types of evaluation you are expected to use, including understanding the difference between merely doing things right and attempting to do the right things. Decide evaluation approaches, and write evaluation tools as early as possible in any planning process. Remember that evaluation statements are promises of anticipated results.

11 Do I need better evaluation skills in ongoing and interim evaluation of students or in calculating final grades for academic or clinical performance?

These two evaluation components are part of the whole student evaluation picture. A final grade is a clear statement of student success or failure. However, periodic feedback, correction, and acknowledgment of progress teach learners the meaning of evaluation. You can encourage students to seek consultation on how they are doing on tests and assignments in order to learn about their work styles, strengths, and areas for improvement. One of your jobs is to teach students to be skilled in self-evaluation and to become accountable for their own success.

12 How can I encourage students to be more autonomous in the evaluation process?

Your first challenge is to help students understand what each type of evaluation tool is attempting to measure. For example, written examinations are intended to evaluate the quality of nursing judgment, not merely how well facts are recalled. Clinical evaluations have the same aim, along with the responsibility of furnishing good rationales for nursing actions. You can build student ownership of evaluations by writing good self-evaluation tools. Test reviews need to include explorations of individual study and test-taking styles. Clinical self-evaluation forms can require a student to rank relative strengths in specific competencies rather than just list a self-rating score for each area.

13 Are there ways I can consider individual learning styles in evaluating students without having a different evaluation plan for each person?

A well-written evaluation form for a final course grade or for an academic or clinical assignment can measure overall meeting of standards as well as individual abilities, especially if individualized comments are added. One way you can incorporate each student's special gifts and potentials is to provide self-tests on personality traits, learning styles, and challenge areas such as time organization. Faculty can help students discern ways to integrate their personal styles with required standards. Group and individual reflective exercises in classes and clinical conferences can show students' wide diversities of styles. This awareness can help them manage their own work habits and negotiate effective collaboration with other individuals.

14 How can I be a good coach and mentor for student nurses when I am also their teacher, clinical supervisor, and evaluator?

Teachers have always had a reputation for finding opportunities for "teachable moments" in almost any situation. You can develop a whole collection of ways to be a good academic and clinical coach for your students. Learn to use performance flowcharts, informal evaluation consultations, reflective assignments, and interim grades to alert and advise students on the quality of their work. True mentoring relationships may not occur with every student, but you can teach all of them how to seek and use support networking during their professional careers. Even difficult situations that require boundary setting, corrective measures, or notification of failure can be based on trust and good communication.

15 How can I help students see class and clinical evaluations as having the same values and goals?

Both classroom grades and clinical evaluations are part of the unified task of assessing the quality of demonstrated nursing judgment. When you become expert in making all classes application-based and all clinical experiences supported by rationales, students will experience this vital overlap of classes and nursing practice. Do not permit a student to "coast" by overemphasizing either academic or clinical abilities. Challenge all students to balance and bridge these areas with principles of good reasoning, focused judgment, and holistic caring practice. Informed caring is the primary aim of all nursing.

16 What can I do as a teacher to promote communication and unity among the many stakeholders who care about having good nursing education outcomes?

One great form of faculty service is for every nurse educator to develop a sense of community with individuals and groups outside their own nursing programs. Such efforts can be incorporated naturally into your other teaching responsibilities through scheduled and informal contacts with health agency staff, individuals in the community, and expert consultants and policy makers. You can invite them as guest speakers for classes and clinical conferences or find opportunities to explore shared concerns on nursing and health care. Join other nursing organizations in order to build and support a unified voice to advocate for nursing, nursing education, and health-care causes.

17 How do I know if my evaluation approaches are effective?

Here are some ways to check your own level of expertise in evaluation:

- **Comparisons:** Every nursing teacher can use the strategy of continuous comparisons to gain better perspectives on evaluation planning and implementation. Read nursing education literature on evaluation, and talk with faculty in other programs. Compare your evaluation of students with their performance in other nursing courses or clinical areas, including grades on standardized tests.

- **Committees:** Learn how to work effectively on faculty committees structuring evaluation tools and conducting periodic program evaluations. Evaluation methods, policies, and protocols need periodic review and revisions, including testing procedures, clinical grading, grading scales, and requirements for student admission, progression, and graduation.
- **Consultation:** Ask for feedback from your supervisors and mentors on your own evaluation abilities. Set goals on improving evaluation skills and monitor progress.

---

18 How can I find out what nursing students and graduates think about their experiences with nursing education evaluation?

More research needs to be done on the development of evaluation tools that emphasize student learning and development of learner autonomy in self-evaluation. Many evaluation approaches only ask for student or graduate opinions about textbooks, media resources, and faculty teaching styles rather than how well learning was supported. Such methods can produce evaluation data that are skewed toward extremes of very good or very bad judgments on program, course, and faculty performance. Look for opportunities in your school to influence the development of evaluation processes that focus on what helps students learn nursing judgment. Successful students who have been taught the meaning of effective evaluation are more likely to give informed and accurate feedback on how well they were evaluated.

---

19 How important is it for me to join other nurse educators in letting the public know how serious we are in self-regulating our profession?

When we become good evaluators of students, ourselves, faculty colleagues, nursing programs, and our contributions to nursing and health care, we gain the right to credibility as professionals. However, we gain credibility only when we let others know that we are actively seeking to develop and maintain high standards and outcomes. Many people do not know what nurses learn beyond doing simple technical procedures. Take advantage of every opportunity to clarify roles in nursing and nursing education and to answer questions about how we evaluate ourselves. Join with others in public forums and participate in professional organizations concerned with nursing education issues. See yourself as an example and promoter for the idea, "Those who care, teach; those who teach, care."

20 What hope is there to have student nurses graduate with solid skills in evaluation of learning and with enthusiasm for evaluation processes?

Evaluation skills offer hope for improved performance in present and future nursing settings. Well-written performance assessment tools are promises that informed and honest evaluation processes can enrich and facilitate learning. You can teach your students the meaning of metacognition, meaning "knowing that you know." If you empower your students with good self-evaluation skills, they can respond more positively and more comprehensively to being evaluated by others. You will have equipped them with ways to improve shortcomings and explain the "why" of their performance outcomes. As a teacher, you will have given them a gift of valuable self-guidance that will last a lifetime.

Resources

American Association of Colleges of Nursing. (1998). The essentials of baccalaureate education for professional nursing practice. Washington, DC: Author. www.aacn.nche.edu/ Education/essentials.htm

Benner, P. (2001). From novice to expert. Commemorative Edition. Menlo Park, Calif.: Addison-Wesley.

Billings, D., & Halstead, J. (2005). Teaching in nursing: A guide for faculty, 2nd ed. Philadelphia: W. B. Saunders.

McVey, J. (2006). Critical thinking in novice nurse clinical learning. In M. Jackson, D.D. Ignatavicius, & B. Case (Eds.) Conversations in clinical judgment and critical thinking. American Association of Critical Care Nurses. Sudbury, Mass.: Jones & Bartlett. Originally published 2004. Pensacola, Fla.: Pohl Publishing.

National League for Nursing Accrediting Commission: http://www.nlnac.org/home.htm

Oermann, M.H., & Gaberson, K.B. (2006). Evaluation and testing in nursing education, 2nd ed. New York: Springer.

Overbay, J.D., & Aaltonen, P.M. (2001). A comparison of NLNAC and CCNE accreditation. Nurse Educator (26)1, 17–22.

Paul, R.W., & Heaslip, P. (1995).Critical thinking and intuitive nursing practice. Journal of Advanced Nursing 22, 40–47.

Rayfield, S., & Manning, L. (2006). Pathways of teaching nursing: Keeping it real. Bossier City, La.: ICAN Publishing.

21

The Importance of Objectives

Jackie McVey, PhD, RN

1 What primary purposes are served by written objectives for theoretical courses and clinical experiences in nursing education?

Objectives serve as a road map for the goals and activities in nursing education. Classroom and clinical learning both have the same destination. Their mutual aim is to develop graduate competencies that demonstrate high professional standards in nursing care, research, and knowledge building. When faculty, students, and administrators use shared maps, learning teams arrive at their destinations with a minimum of disagreement and delay.

2 In what ways do course and clinical objectives form an educational, legal, and ethical contract between nursing programs and students?

Objectives based on program graduate outcome goals let students and other stakeholders in student success know the content and competencies that students are required to master. The objectives also serve as promises to students that faculty will use effective teaching strategies to help students actively learn what they need to know.

3 How can faculty use objectives as gatekeeping standards for progression in a nursing program without eliminating potentially successful students?

When all types of nursing education objectives are effectively written, they serve as binding agreements that students can progress in the program when they show proof of mastering designated outcomes. Good objectives also protect the faculty and program if students fail one or more courses by documenting areas of learning deficits. When evaluation methods use objectives as the basis for ongoing evaluation that includes student coaching and tutoring, faculty can often save failing students who merely need extra guidance.

4 To what extent should I expect student nurses to understand, explain, and effectively use course and clinical objectives?

Students need to comprehend very well how their learning performance will be judged. If you have the opportunity to write objectives, then you can learn to make them clear, concise, and very practical. On the other hand, you will often inherit objectives that you cannot change, either due to time or faculty protocols. In this case, you should interpret the intent of each objective in your own words so students are actively engaged in learning. Avoid accepting text chapter objectives as printed because they rarely express your own program's curriculum plan and unique strengths.

5 How can I use course and clinical objectives to promote student accountability and growth in meeting academic and clinical performance standards?

Most nursing education objectives are written as learner outcomes, not as teacher activities. Interpret objectives for students in terms of how outcomes will be evaluated. For example, class objectives are usually evaluated by written tests, assigned papers, or student presentations. Clinical objectives are evaluated by assessing nursing care behaviors and clinical assignments. Link objectives to evaluation by giving example test questions, furnishing sample student assignments, and discussing grading measures very early in a course or clinical experience. Then the contract is clear, and students can be held more accountable for reaching expected performance outcomes.

6   How can clear and effective learning objectives promote successful outcomes on written course examinations?

When your written examinations are based on nursing judgments for actions and evaluations, there is a clear link with application-based questions on your tests and graduate licensure tests. Such practical objectives will guide your teaching so that you give students previews of the type of judgment that is required on an examination. This flow from objectives to teaching and learning experiences to testing builds a "no surprises" learning climate. Students can respond to missed test items with a willingness to consult with faculty on study strategies rather than placing blame on flaws in teaching.

7   What elements of clinical objectives are essential for planning nursing care experiences for diverse groups of students in a wide variety of settings?

You need to build your clinical objectives around core competencies that include required outcomes with flexible ways to fulfill them. For example, an objective can state that students will effectively plan care for a patient with chronic oxygenation problems, but without listing exact types of medical diagnoses. The setting may be an outpatient clinic or a critical care unit. The student may decide to seek experiences with older adults or families of uninsured children. The plan itself may be a concept map, a computerized flowchart, or a critique of a health agency's standardized care map. Teachers do need to agree on grading criteria for such varied assignments.

8 How can objectives form bridges for students between theory courses and clinical experiences?

The shared road map as a characteristic for classroom and clinical objectives can give some clues about how to build student competencies that apply to both areas. Students should have multiple very similar learning opportunities provided in theory and clinical experiences. Active learning classroom work such as case studies and clinical assignments that require rationales can help students realize that all nursing practice involves both abstract learning and practical application. If learning objectives are well planned, students will often have "déjà vu" experiences due to the links that faculty help them form among class, reading, evidence-based practice literature searches, and their clinical practice.

9 How do effectively written objectives support systems of regular interim student feedback on learning progress as well as final evaluations?

When every objective includes some evaluation subcategories, then students can more clearly understand how to navigate the road to positive final evaluations. For example, a clinical objective that requires students to show teaching competencies for individuals with diabetes should specify glucose self-monitoring, diet, and reporting complications. Merely requiring overall patient-teaching competency in the objective can end up in a game of "Guess what I am thinking" when it comes to evaluation. With performance qualifiers, interim evaluations can focus on component skills, not just entire objectives.

10 Which objectives in my school do I have the freedom to revise, and which are more permanent?

Generally, you have the most freedom to write your own objectives for your lectures and for unique clinical experiences that allow flexible implementation. Course objectives are part of official agreements with the academic institution and are revised only every few years. Outcome objectives for graduates form a part of curriculum design and are revised only with major program changes. You do have substantial creative freedom in finding ways to build learning experiences based on all these types and levels of objectives.

11 What are my choices on using the three learning domains to be sure my objectives cover all the types of required nursing competencies?

Explore the wealth of professional resources available on writing objectives so that you understand and use each of the three traditionally recognized domains of learning: cognitive (thinking), psychomotor (doing), and affective (valuing). As an application discipline rather than a purely academic one, nursing is expected to develop not only levels of intellectual ability referred to in the cognitive domain. Nursing students are taught psychomotor skills in procedures and technical actions. The affective domain covers the human communication and caring elements of nursing, characterized by personal values and beliefs. Often the steps of the nursing process are used to describe the levels of complexity for all three types of learning. The nursing process expresses all learning domain levels, from simple knowledge and comprehension through analysis, application, and evaluation.

12 What principles of clear writing are especially important in developing effective objectives in nursing education?

Move away from the principles of creative writing to the more direct styles used in education, technology, and science. Newspaper front-page stories jump right to their topics in their first few words. Start with an action term that fits the method that will be used to evaluate nursing competencies in the objective, such as a written test or clinical performance. Clearly written objectives usually also include the highest relevant nursing process step, the component of health care addressed, and competency subtopics.

13 How can my class objectives help students sort through the enormous quantity of facts and concepts in order to develop nursing judgment for effective practice?

Consider doing some preliminary planning even before you begin to write objectives. After a basic review of the material you plan to cover, list the mastery concepts that address why the topic is important for nurses, the types of human problems represented by the topic, and the unique contributions nursing care can make. Build your objectives and teaching plan around those mastery concepts. Condense all review material on problems and pathophysiology. This saves time to integrate the content as supportive evidence for nursing decisions and actions.

14 To what extent can course and clinical objectives emphasize mastery concepts and competencies without the pitfall of giving too much information?

The potential pitfall is more likely to be giving too little information in objectives rather than too much. We are so conscientious about challenging students to learn concepts and skills that we often withhold vital information. This does not mean we ought to write wordy objectives. Our objectives are promises to students that include a focus on relevant learning, clear preparation for evaluation, and an overall sense of fairness. Good objectives create an environment in which faculty and students are on the same team and devoted to student success.

15 How can outcome measurements including grading criteria be included in objectives?

Your first action word in an objective specifies what you expect a student to do to receive a passing grade. For example, in a clinical objective, use a phrase such as "Implement effective nurse teaching to promote good self-care measures." For a theory class graded by a multiple-choice examination, different action terms must be used, such as "Critique effectiveness of example nurse teaching...." The other way to include grading criteria in an objective is to list the key evaluation areas for a topic, such as the diabetic teaching example that requires inclusion of glucose monitoring, diet, and reporting of complications.

---

16 Are there some less obvious uses for objectives or strategies I should know about?

Course objectives (class and clinical) serve not only as a blueprint for student evaluation but also as a framework for deciding what should be taught and learned. They also provide the basis for teaching/learning strategies, which include meeting professional standards as the potential for creativity. Good objectives promote holistic care, a scholarly nursing education community, and perhaps even reduced stress for students and faculty.

---

17 What are some of the biggest pitfalls to avoid when writing objectives in nursing education?

The biggest problems with objectives include lack of skill in how to write them, overemphasis on abstract vocabulary, and a belief that the process is a disagreeable chore that has no practical uses. Teachers tend to write too many objectives, make them too long, and explain them too quickly to students. Look at your own objectives to see if your writing style wanders, giving a long preface before you get to action terms. The biggest mistake teachers make is a failure to trust their own clinical wisdom on the topic or competency being covered and to rely too strongly on texts and other content resources.

---

18 What are some examples of how learning objectives become more complex as students progress through a nursing curriculum?

When you think of objectives for beginning nursing students, remember when you were learning to drive a car. You had to learn new terminology, memorize related concepts or procedural steps, and be able to know what to avoid in your thinking or actions. Beginners in nursing have similar tasks; they are expected to begin learning how to appropriately apply judgment related to safe and effective care. Students in mid-level courses are ready for strongly application-based objectives with immediate and long-term implications for nursing judgment. Advanced students preparing for graduation need objectives that require them to synthesize multiple concepts into a whole and identify ways to develop their own strengths for transition into future nursing roles.

19 How can objectives written for a whole class allow for individual creativity and judgment?

The best way for you to accommodate individual expressiveness is to decide when it is appropriate and when it might endanger critical outcomes. Set boundaries for students when practice matters require strict protocols, such as situations involving public health safety. Then in many other learning areas, you can actively encourage students to explore their styles in figuring out their own conclusions and unique way of doing things. You will need to know your own values, fears, and strengths in order to respond to student approaches very different from your own. Achieving this balance between the group and individuals forms the heart of a genuine community of experienced and novice nurses who want to discover the real potentials of the profession.

20 How can I participate with other nursing teachers in evaluating all types of objectives across a nursing curriculum?

Evaluating the clarity and effectiveness of objectives requires a sort of double vision. One part of you continues to use objectives in their current state, no matter how well or how poorly they are worded. At the same time, you develop skills in learning how to decide when objectives really work to facilitate learning. Courage is necessary to seek help with your own objectives, and considerable diplomatic skills are required for you to critique objectives written by your fellow novice teachers or by very experienced educators and resource experts. Keep on believing that what you know as a nurse clinician and as a teacher qualifies you to join with others in the task of developing great objectives for optimal student understanding and program success.

Resources

Bloom, B.S. (Ed.) (1956). Taxonomy of educational objectives: The classification of educational goals. Handbook I: Cognitive domain. White Plains, N.Y.: Longman.

Dave, R.H. (1970). Psychomotor levels. In R.J. Armstrong (Ed.) Developing and writing behavioral objectives. Tucson, Ariz.: Educational Innovators.

Fink, L.D. (2003). A taxonomy of significant learning. In Creating Significant Learning Experiences. San Francisco: Jossey-Bass.

Krathwohl, D., Bloom, B., & Masia, B. (1964). Taxonomy of educational objectives. Handbook II: Affective domain. New York: Longman.

Mager, R.F. (1997). Measuring instructional results, 3rd ed. Atlanta: CEP Press.

Mager, R.F. (1997). Preparing instructional objectives, 3rd ed. Atlanta: CEP Press.

Oermann, M.H., & Gaberson, K.B. (2006). Evaluation and testing in nursing education, 2nd ed. New York: Springer.

Rayfield, S., & Manning, L. (2006). Pathways of teaching nursing: Keeping it real. Bossier City, La.: ICAN Publishing.

22

Developing Trustworthy Classroom Tests

Mary E. McDonald, MA, RN

1 | I have to administer several tests this semester. Where do I begin?

Because teacher-made tests are the measurement instruments that are the basis of effective classroom assessment, careful planning is essential. As Robert Mager (1962) said, "If you don't know where you're going, you're liable to end up someplace else—and not even know it..." (p. vii). Using a systematic approach for developing comprehensive classroom examinations ensures that your assessment plan is comprehensive.

2 | What are the components of a systematic classroom assessment plan?

- **Identify course objectives.** Describe what you expect from the students by writing course objectives in terms of student behavior that will demonstrate mastery at the end of the course.
- **Identify course content.** Detail exactly what content is to be included in the course and in what time frame.
- **Identify teaching/learning activities.** Determine what opportunities you will offer the students to enable them to meet the objectives and master the course content.

- **Identify assessment strategies.** Carefully examine each objective and each unit of content, and decide what type of measurement instrument is most appropriate to measure student ability.
- **Develop measurement instruments.** A systematic approach will help to ensure that your examination results are trustworthy; that is, they are reliable and have evidence of validity for the decisions you make based on your assessment procedures.

3 What are the characteristics of a reliable test?

Reliability refers to the consistency of test results. Reliable tests provide consistent results that are reproducible, which means that if you were to give the same test a second time to the same individual, you would obtain the same result.

4 How is reliability measured?

A test itself is not reliable. Reliability can be estimated by several statistical formulas. Test development software programs can provide you with a reliability coefficient. Reliability coefficients range from zero to one: one indicates perfect reliability, and zero indicates no reliability.

5 What reliability coefficient should I expect for my classroom tests?

All measurements contain error; therefore, you will never see perfect reliability. The amount of error you can accept depends on the level of confidence you require for the decision you are making based on that test result. This is why you would not want to base a pass/fail decision on the results of one classroom test. The more information you have, the more confidence you will have in your decisions. Whereas a standardized test should have a reliability coefficient greater than 0.85, experts suggest that an acceptable classroom test reliability coefficient range between 0.5 and 0.85 for a 50-item multiple-choice test. Reliability is not the only issue. A test that has reliable results is not necessarily a good test.

6   **Why is a reliable test not necessarily a good test?**

Test results can be reliable for one purpose but not for another. For example, a test that is administered for the purpose of selecting candidates for entry into a police academy would not necessarily be useful for admission to a nursing program. Validity is the most important component of a classroom test. Every interpretation of a test score must be supported by evidence of validity.

7   **What is validity evidence?**

Validity evidence refers to the extent of the evidence that justifies the decisions you make based on the results of your classroom tests. Before you can judge whether a student has mastered a content area based on the results of a test, you have to show evidence that the test assesses that content. For example, a test that measures whether a student can safely administer a blood transfusion has to contain questions about blood transfusions.

8   **Why is validity evidence so important?**

The most critical element of an assessment program is fairness. Validity evidence ensures fairness. The greater the validity evidence for a test, the greater your confidence will be in the inferences you make based on the results of the test. As a faculty member, you have to make decisions that affect the lives of students. A test that demonstrates a high degree of validity evidence will increase the confidence you have in making those decisions.

9   **How can I establish validity evidence for my tests?**

Validity evidence for classroom assessment is a matter of judgment; it cannot be quantified. Because you cannot test everything that is included in a course, the key to establishing validity evidence for a test is sampling. You have to demonstrate that the items on the test address the objectives and comprise a representative sample of the content of your course.

---

10 How do I select a representative sample of content for a test?

A blueprint is a test plan that guides the selection of questions for a test. Selecting items from a blueprint provides you with the validity evidence that you need for making decisions based on the test results. The blueprint also serves to link the course objectives to the course content.

---

11 How do I set up a blueprint?

Your blueprint should be a two-way grid, with the course objectives represented on the horizontal axis and the content on the vertical axis. This type of blueprint provides evidence that you are evaluating your course objectives as well as the content of the course.

---

12 How do I decide how many questions are assigned to each box?

Most faculty sample the content to test based on the number of classroom hours devoted to each content area. Carefully examine your course objectives, and decide which ones are conducive to being evaluated by a classroom test. There is no magic formula; your judgment is what is important when deciding how to weight the objectives on the blueprint. Note that the items in each box represent a range. This is not an exact science. Once you have your blueprint, you are ready to start developing your measurement instruments.

	OBJECTIVE 1	OBJECTIVE 2	OBJECTIVE 3
Unit I	5–7	5–7	5–7
Unit II	4–6	4–6	7–9
Unit III	4–6	4–6	4–6
Total (50)	15	15	20

---

13 Should I share the blueprint with my students?

Yes. Students find a well-planned blueprint to be a helpful study guide. Include with the blueprint a sample of examination questions in each box as shown. You do not have to share the exact final distribution of the questions.

---

14 What types of measurement instruments can be used for classroom assessment?

There are many measurement instrument formats for classroom assessment. The challenge is to select the most appropriate format for the area of student achievement which you are assessing. The two most frequently used formats for classroom achievement testing are:

1. Selected-response or objective items, which provide answer options for the student to select. Examples include:
   - True-false type items require the student to decide whether a statement is correct or incorrect.
   - Matching columns require the student to connect a choice in one column to an option in a second column.
   - Multiple choice; items require the student to select the correct answer from a list of options. This format is widely used in nursing classroom tests.
2. Constructed-response items, which are open ended. They require the student to provide an answer. Examples include:
   - Completion or short-answer items require the student to provide a word, phrase, or brief statement to answer the question.
   - Essay questions, which require the student to develop an original composition to answer the question.

---

15 What are the advantages and disadvantages of selected-response items?

Although some criticize selected response items for providing the student with an answer and the ability to guess, these items allow testing of a broad range of content. The scoring of these items is objective, and the questions can be scanned electronically. Several software programs provide statistical analyses, which yield valuable information for increasing the trustworthiness of your selected-response tests.

16 What are the advantages and disadvantages of constructed-response items?

Guessing is limited with constructed-response items. They assess the student's ability to think because the student must provide an original answer. Whereas these items are relatively easy to write, they can be tedious to score, they can test only a narrow range of content, and they can be open to subjective scoring.

17 Why is the multiple-choice format widely used for nursing classroom achievement tests?

Multiple-choice tests facilitate testing the broadest sample of course objectives and content. They are the most compatible type of item for statistical analysis, which means they can be analyzed, improved, and banked for future use. Whereas they can be time-consuming to write, they are easy to score, and they can be developed to assess higher-order thinking. The nursing licensure test and most certification tests are in the multiple-choice format.

18 What are the essential attributes of a trustworthy multiple-choice test?

Good tests consist of good test items. The items on the test must address the blueprint. Every item must address both content and an objective. Every item should be relevant to clinical practice and should be written according to a style guide that is agreed upon by the faculty.

19 What suggestions can you provide about writing multiple-choice items?

Becoming a good item writer takes time and practice. For example:

- Avoid trivia; test only what is important.
- Make the questions clinically relevant. Have a nurse and/or a client in every stem. Ask yourself, "How would a nurse apply this concept in a clinical setting?"
- Avoid writing items that simply require the students to recall information from a textbook or a lecture.
- Use your objectives to frame the questions. For example, if setting priorities is an outcome for one of your objectives, write a question that requires a nurse to set priorities.
- Write the stem and the correct answer first. Then model the distractors (the incorrect options) on the correct answer.
- Keep the options homogeneous. If the correct answer looks different from the distractors, the uninformed students will have a better chance of guessing correctly.
- It is not enough for the distractors to be wrong; they have to be plausible. They have to be attractive to the uninformed. You do not want to trick the students, but you do want to identify those students who are not achieving.
- Make sure that there is only one correct answer. Double-check all the distractors to make sure they are wrong. Write a rationale explaining why the answer is correct and why each of the distractors is incorrect.
- Be meticulous about spelling and grammar. Nothing is more carefully scrutinized than the test questions you write. Write clearly and unambiguously. You want the students to spend time figuring out how to answer the question, not trying to figure out what the question is asking.
- Ask a colleague to review an unkeyed copy of the test to check the answer key, identify problem questions, and verify that the test meets the test blueprint.

20 Can you show me a example of a multiple-choice question that is at a higher cognitive level?

Here is an example of how to transform a recall-level question into one at the application level:

RECALL

A nurse should monitor a client who has had a thyroidectomy for signs of:

A. laryngeal edema.*
B. increasing intracranial pressure.
C. carotid artery distention.
D. hypercalcemia.

APPLICATION

Which of these measures should a nurse include in the care plan for a client during the immediate postoperative period following a thyroidectomy?

A. Asking the client to speak.*
B. Checking the client's pupillary response.
C. Palpating the client's carotid arteries.
D. Instructing the client to flex and extend the neck.

The application-level question not only requires the nurse to know the information questioned in the recall-level question, it also requires the student to use the information in the clinical setting.

21 How can I determine if an item is of high quality?

The quality of a multiple-choice item is directly related to its difficulty level and its ability to discriminate between the high and low achievers on a test. Item analysis software reports the difficulty level as the percentage of test takers who answer the item correctly (p-value) and the discrimination ability as the point biserial index (PBI) for each item.

22 What p-value should my questions have?

Because the difficulty of the individual items determines the overall difficulty of the test, the p-value of the items should reflect the mean of the test. If the mean of the test is 75%, the items should be within a close range of 75% to 80%. Generally, the p-values of items on a classroom test should range between 0.5 and 0.85, with a few items as difficult as 0.3 to identify the high achievers in the group. Items that have p-values greater than 0.85 contribute nothing to the reliability of the test, and an item that is too difficult (p-value below 0.3) usually indicates a problem with the question.

23 How do I interpret the PBI for the items?

The PBI ranges from –1 to +1, with –1 meaning no discrimination and +1 being perfect discrimination. Most test development software programs report the PBI for every option in a question. A high-quality item will have a negative PBI for every distractor and a positive PBI for the correct option. This simply means that the low achievers on the test selected the incorrect responses, and the high achievers selected the correct response.

24 Can you show an example of data for a question?

Here is an example of a question that has acceptable data:

Correct Answer: A
p-value: 0.71
PBI: 0.37

This question worked well statistically: 71% of the students answered it correctly. The PBI is 0.48, which means that the high achievers selected the correct answer more

OPTION	p-VALUE	PBI
A	0.71	0.48
B	0.07	−0.20
C	0.03	−0.10
D	0.19	−0.48

frequently than the low achievers. The negative biserials for all of the incorrect options mean that the low achievers were not able to guess the correct answer.

25 Should I review a test with the class after it is given?

It is very important to review a test with the students. Wait until after you examine the item analysis. Suppose a distractor has a positive biserial, which means that some high achievers selected it. You would be able to ask the students to share their reasoning so that you could determine if the item is flawed. Post grades after the review, and use the student input to adjust the grades. You may decide to accept two answers as correct based on student input, for example.

26 What are the advantages of using test development software?

Test development software has numerous advantages. For example:

- It streamlines the process of test development. Once an item is entered into the bank, it never has to be retyped or keyed again.
- It stores items with their item analysis data for future use. You can use the data to identify flawed items and fix them before you reuse them.
- It allows you to code items by several categories so that you can search the bank to find questions to meet your blueprint.

Once you master a test development software program, you will be amazed how you ever managed without it!

27 Where can I find out more about test development software?

Take a look at these Web sites:
www.assess.com (Fast Test)
www.lxr.com (LXR Test)
www.scantron.com (ParTEST)
www.softwarefornurses.com (A+ Test Manager)

28   When should I use other types of question formats?

True-false, matching, and short-answer questions are useful for testing students' comprehension of material. Use these types of questions for quizzes or to identify if students are reading the textbook, for example. Essay questions are valuable for assessing a student's critical thinking ability. However, essay questions can be time-consuming to develop and score.

29   Do you have any suggestions for using essay questions?

It is important to use a variety of strategies in your assessment plan, including essay questions. When developing the question, first write an outline of the main points that you want to include in the question. Then write the question clearly, with careful attention to spelling, punctuation, and grammar. Several short sentences are easier to understand than a long complex one. Once you have the question written, write a sample answer, and make a list of the points that you require the student to make. Then decide how you will weight each point, which will provide you with a scoring rubric. Finally, ask a colleague to review the question and your scoring rubric. When you score the students' essays, use the rubric, but be flexible. The students may have some ideas that you had not considered. Correct each essay, and record the grade on a class list. When you finish grading all the papers, read each one again without looking at the grade list to see if your second grade coincides with the first. If not, read the paper again, or ask a colleague for an opinion.

30   Why is it important to use a variety of classroom assessment strategies?

The key issue in classroom assessment is trustworthiness. You make critical decisions about students based on the results of your assessment instruments. The more information you have, the more confident you will be. Offering students a variety of assessment opportunities is important because, just as students have different learning styles, they also respond individually to different assessment strategies. In addition, all of your objectives will not lend themselves to assessment by multiple-choice or essay tests. Use your objectives as a guide. Ask yourself, "How can I best determine if the students are achieving this objective?" Include journals, class presentations, Internet searches, concept maps, care plans, and so on. Be creative. Your students will thank you.

Resources

Gronlund, N.E. (2000). How to write and use instructional objectives, 6th ed. Upper Saddle River, N.J.: Prentice Hall.

Haladyna, T.M. (2004). Developing and validating multiple-choice test items, 3rd ed. Mahwah, N.J.: Lawrence Erlbaum Associates.

Haladyna, T.M. (1997). Writing test items to evaluate higher order thinking. Needham Heights, Mass.: Allyn & Bacon.

McDonald, M.E. (2002). Systematic assessment of learning outcomes: Developing multiple-choice exams. Sudbury, Mass.: Jones and Bartlett/NLN Press.

McDonald, M.E. (2007). The nurse educator's guide to assessing learning outcomes, 2nd ed. Sudbury, Mass.: Jones and Bartlett.

Trice, A.D. (2000). A handbook of classroom assessment. New York: Longman.

23

Beyond Tests: Other Ways to Evaluate Learning

Debra P. Shelton, EdD, APRN-CS, CNA, OCN, CNE

1 In addition to tests, how can I evaluate student learning?

Evaluation of learning has gone beyond the use of multiple-choice examinations. The trend toward identifying the learning styles of students has placed the focus on utilizing a variety of methods to evaluate (or assess) that learning has taken place. The literature cites numerous methods of evaluating learning. Following is a list of some of the methods currently in use:

- Portfolios
- Group projects
- Role play
- Case studies
- Concept maps
- Concept papers
- Journals
- Research critiques
- Socratic questioning
- Videotaping

2   What are portfolios?

A portfolio is a collection of student work. According to Linn and Gronlund (2000), portfolios can serve a variety of purposes. They can be used to show student progress through a nursing course or a program of study, with students presenting portfolios at the end of a semester. Portfolios also provide documentation of an individual's work for placement in a program. Portfolios also document competency and career activities for a job search.

3   How do I use portfolios in evaluation?

You need to identify the specific purpose of the portfolio. Will it be a formative evaluation or a summative evaluation of student work?

A formative use of portfolios involves the student collecting and submitting papers/course work as the course progresses for the instructor to assess the student's progress. This examination of student products is not for the purpose of grading but rather to assess student progress and to actually modify content and teaching-learning strategies to maximize student learning.

A summative use involves evaluating a collection of student work, selected either by the student or the faculty, for placement at the completion of the program. The portfolio is used as a gradable outcome and may measure multiple aspects such as writing skills, mastery of specific content, and/or information literacy.

4   How do I design group projects for evaluation purposes?

A group project requires positive interdependence, individual accountability, interpersonal skills, face-to-face promotive interaction, and group processing or effective functioning (Johnson & Johnson, 2005). Before developing a group project, you will have to teach group behavior and principles so that the students know how to act and work in a group. The group project should be designed to ensure that the students have enough time to complete the project. Identify the purpose of the project (what the students will be learning), how many individuals will be in each group, what criteria will be used to group the students, and how much time the group project should take to complete (one class session, a number of class sessions or weeks, or the entire semester). A group project should have a number of objectives. Evaluation criteria should be specific: each group, for example, will submit a paper, presentation, or poster as a means for assessing student learning. One example of a group project is a community teaching project. Students work in groups of three or four, select a community group, and assess, plan, develop, and evaluate a teaching plan for that group.

---

5   If one or two members of the group did all the work, how do I grade the group?

This situation occurs frequently—one or two members of the group do the work and submit it on behalf of the entire group. One way to prevent this from happening is to have the group evaluate the performance of each individual. You will need to develop a peer evaluation tool. Average the peer evaluations for each student, and use the average as a percentage of the group grade. Faculty members have based 30% to 40% of a group's grade on the peer evaluation. You may want to have the group members identify duties for each member and have a contract for completing the project. Some instructors have a rule that a group can vote to terminate members who are not completing their portion of the project or not participating and that those members have to complete an individual project. Encourage groups to work out any conflicts without including the instructor.

---

6   Can role play be used for evaluation purposes?

Role play is a teaching strategy as well as being a useful evaluation tool for evaluating students' therapeutic communication and interpersonal relationships. Students are asked to assume the role of a specific person and then act out how they would respond in a situation. For example, in a leadership class, one student might assume the role of an employee being counseled for tardiness on the job, and a second student would play the manager or supervisor. The other students in the group critique the performance of the manager. During the discussion, the students share their insights on the role play, analyze feelings that were expressed by both players, critique strategies for handling the situation, offer insights from their observation, and add strategies that might have been useful. Role play can be time-consuming, so setting time limits is essential. You may initially feel awkward when using role play, but being prepared and familiar with the evaluation strategy can ease tension and increase the comfort zone for all involved.

---

7 How can case studies be used to evaluate learning?

Case studies are an excellent strategy for evaluating learning, especially critical thinking. Real nursing situations make good case studies. In fact, it is important to use *only* real situations because making them up often results in unanticipated omissions, inconsistencies, or errors that can sabotage the experience. A case study presents a realistic situation that a nurse might reasonably encounter. Case studies can be a short statement of a situation or a longer summary, with detailed information including laboratory data and assessment findings. You might want to try the unfolding case study, in which questions are posed and, as the questions are answered, more information is presented to the student. The case study bridges the gap between knowledge and application and should contain directions and questions to guide students in finding the information needed for the solution without guiding the students to the correct solution. A good case study will generate questions for both the student and instructor. Case studies often will not have one correct solution. Rather, they evaluate students' ability to think critically and find their own answers by considering many options and providing the rationale for a chosen solution. Be sure to review the case studies with the students, giving them feedback on their answers and thinking processes.

8   Are care plans still being used for evaluation?

Yes. The format may have changed over time, but the principles of developing care plans are still used in nursing programs. Care plans demonstrate a student's ability to utilize the nursing process in the clinical setting. It is essential to use a standardized care plan format and evaluation criteria throughout the nursing program. This allows nursing faculty to evaluate student progress and improvement on care planning. Nursing programs use several formats: long, short, and mini. Faculty might have the students do one long care plan for the clinical rotation and then do mini care plans more frequently. Some faculty have students submit a one-page care plan of the patient's primary problem. Some programs integrate nursing diagnosis, nursing intervention classification (NIC), and nursing outcome classification (NOC) into the care planning/nursing process. Regardless of the format you or your school adopt, clear, predetermined evaluation criteria are essential.

9   What are other ways to evaluate students' application of the nursing process?

Koehler (2001) identifies nursing process mapping as a tool to replace nursing care plans. The purpose of the maps is to have students develop critical thinking skills, and studies have shown that the use of mapping improves student performance. The clinical pathway is another tool that can be used to evaluate nursing process and clinical learning. Clinical or critical paths are used in some practice settings to guide health-care teams as they care for patients with particular diagnoses meet predetermined patient outcomes.

10   What are concept maps, and how are they used to evaluate learning?

Concept mapping has been used as a teaching strategy but can also be an evaluation tool. Concept mapping is a visual representation of the relationship between concepts.

Maps can be used in any clinical setting and require only paper and pencil to complete, although software is available for developing maps. One undergraduate nursing program uses concept maps in place of nursing care plans and incorporates nursing diagnosis, NIC, and NOC into the maps. A graduate pathophysiology nursing course uses the principles of concept maps in which students submit for grading three schematics based on articles in nursing literature, each schematic representing the relationships presented in the articles.

11 Are papers still a good way to evaluate learning?

Papers can be used to evaluate students in both theory and clinical courses. Writing assignments can be used to evaluate students' ability to think critically and to integrate and apply nursing theories and concepts. The writing-to-learn paradigm "reconceptualizes the relationship between critical thinking and writing process as mutually dependent" (Poirrer, 1997, p. 11). Papers can be used in any nursing course or setting. Writing-to-learn activities are short, informal writing tasks that help students think through key concepts presented in a course. The activity has the student integrate information already known with new information learned into a written product. Often, these writing tasks are either done in a certain amount of time in class (5 to 20 minutes) or out-of-class assignments to be turned in. An example of a writing-to-learn activity is a political letter. In a transition course for the RN to BSN students, students identify a current nursing problem or issue that affects nursing in the legislative arena, either regionally or nationally, and write a letter to a legislative individual. The purpose of this letter is to promote political activism and to demonstrate application and synthesis of a health-care issue. The students are evaluated on the content and format of the letter.

12 What is a rubric, and should I use one when grading?

A rubric is a scoring guide used for subjective assessments. The rubric lists the criteria for an assignment. For example, a rubric for a presentation might tell students that their presentation will be evaluated on organization, subject knowledge, graphics/teaching tools, mechanics, eye contact, and voice. For each criterion, a rating scale of 1 to 5 is used, with 1 being a beginning level of achievement to 5 being exemplary behavior. Rubrics can be used for subjective assessment: papers, presentations, projects, portfolios, or some of the other evaluation tools. Rubrics have also been developed for clinical evaluation.

---

13 How do I use qualitative and quantitative criteria in grading written assignments?

A qualitative approach to evaluation views the whole assignment; for example, how well the student was able to integrate knowledge in the written paper. An example of qualitative grading is A, A-, B+, B, and so on, without numbers being assigned to each of the letters. Another example is Excellent, Very Good, Good, Fair, and Poor. Faculty who use qualitative grading typically have some idea of what they are looking for in an A paper, but this subjective type of evaluation can be a major headache when students ask why they received a certain grade. Faculty must justify what the criteria are for each grade, and they risk inconsistency in grading across students. Quantitative grading assigns numbers to an assignment. The paper as a whole constitutes a certain percentage of the course grade, and each section of the paper is assigned points. For example, in a writing assignment for a community health course, students write a global issues paper worth 100 points, broken down as follows:

- Introduction = 10 points
- Body of the paper = 60 points (with specific criteria based on the objectives and purpose of the assignment. For example, discuss the following, worth 15 points each):
  - the population's health from an international perspective
  - health-care system trends

- o the role of the health-care provider/nurse-related to these trends
- o the challenges faced by health-care providers/nurse-related to these trends
- o Conclusion = 10 points
- o Minimum of 5 references from a variety of sources = 10 points
- o Format and writing style (APA format) = 10 points

---

14 What are some alternatives to long papers?

Rather than have students write a long paper, break up the assignment into a couple of shorter papers. Each paper can stand alone as an assignment. In a research course, for example, the first paper might be to write the introduction, stating the nature of the problem and the research questions. The second paper might be a literature review. Another example is from an information literacy course requiring two short papers. One paper focuses on developing a research question and a search plan for resources, and the second paper focuses on the outcome of the search, a mini-review of the literature. Each is usually not more than five pages in length. You can also have students write in class, no more than a page, what was discussed in class, what were the most difficult concepts, and any questions they may have and want addressed during the next class. This exercise would be an informal (not graded) way of evaluating learning and can give you excellent feedback on whether you are achieving your goals for the class as it progresses.

---

15 Can journaling be used to evaluate learning?

Journaling is an informal examination and reflective process for the student. It is usually a written assignment about a specific learning activity or clinical experience. The student reflects on events that occurred and gives meaning to the experiences. This approach provides opportunities for self-awareness and self-evaluation as well as developing critical thinking skills. Journal entries may describe experiences; feelings and thoughts; questions for inquiry; patterns and relationships; alternative actions or plans of care; and beliefs and values. You may require students to turn journals in weekly or at intervals during the course, and you should read and respond to the student's journaling. Evaluate students' work using criteria such as content, level, depth, completeness, validity, and insightfulness. Journaling can be used in any clinical setting, but it is particularly recommended for beginning-level nursing students.

---

16 If my students are intimidated by verbal questioning, how can I make students more comfortable with questioning to evaluate their learning?

Questioning is used primarily in the clinical setting, and students are nervous anyway when faculty members start questioning them; their self-confidence drops. Ideally, questioning is used to assess a student's ability to think critically, provide a rationale or justification for answers, and apply knowledge learned in theory to the clinical setting. One form of questioning is Socratic questioning, which is used by faculty members to analyze a student's ability to think. Socratic questions can focus on clarification, justification, reasoning, implication, or consequences. Faculty need to be patient when using Socratic questioning and allow students enough time to process questions. Use open-ended questions to promote critical thinking rather than closed-ended or yes/no questions, which do not promote student thinking or discussion. Questioning should be nonthreatening to students. Use the questioning period to enhance students' critical thinking ability with your guidance. Offer cues to students to guide them in the right direction for figuring out the answer. During questioning, tactfully identify weaknesses or errors in students' critical thinking skills so students gain skill in this important process as well as the content area.

---

17 I need to evaluate psychomotor skills. What are some options?

Psychomotor skills are not evaluated by a written test. Evaluation is usually done in a laboratory setting where students perform routine demonstration of the procedure or skill for the nursing instructor. A clinical simulation laboratory with mannequins is an ideal and increasingly common way to teach and evaluate students. Newer technology simulates realistic clinical situations, allows more realistic nursing interventions, and enables the learner to change care based on "patient" responses. Simulations can be used to evaluate not only performance of procedures or tasks but also assessment skills, therapeutic communication, and critical thinking skills. When using simulations as an evaluation tool, clearly identify both the purpose of the simulation and performance criteria.

18 Are teaching plans still used for evaluating student learning?

Many programs still use them. As teaching is a basic aspect of a nurse's functions in everyday practice, a teaching plan is an excellent way to evaluate the student's ability to assess patient learning needs, consider cultural and development attributes of the patient/learner, and develop a plan for teaching the patient. The teaching plan can be a formal written paper, or the faculty member can observe the student's ability to answer questions, communicate with the patient, and handle unexpected situations that arise in an actual teaching session.

19 Can you give me an example or two of a creative way you evaluated students that worked and that they really liked?

In an information literacy course, I have the students do a Web site critique. A class session focuses on the various components on a Web page and how to evaluate the usefulness of the site for either patients or health-care providers. Students use a Web site critique tool. Another example is a staff development project used in the RN-to-BSN program. The focus of the project is to assess learning needs of nursing staff and then develop, plan, implement, and evaluate a teaching session. Students use educational principles discussed in the leadership course and develop a continuing education packet for the session. Students like and appreciate evaluation methods that allow them to demonstrate more than "just the right answer." With some creative thought, teachers can and should develop a variety of ways to evaluate student mastery of the various aspects of nursing practice: skills, knowledge, attitudes, and clinical judgment.

References

Johnson, R.T., & Johnson, D.W. (2005). Cooperative learning center. Accessed February 20, 2007, at http://www.co-operation.org/

Koehler, C J. (2001). Nursing process mapping replaces nursing care plans. In A.J. Lowenstein & M.J. Bradshaw (Eds.) Fuszard's innovative teaching strategies in nursing, 3rd ed. Gaithersburg, Md.: Aspen Publications.

Linn, R.L., & Gronlund, N.E. (2000). Measurement and assessment in teaching, 8th ed. Upper Saddle River, N.J.: Prentice Hall.

Poirrier, G.P. (1997). Writing-to-learn: Curricular strategies for nursing and other disciplines. New York: NLN Press.

Resources

Billings, D.M., & Halstead, J.A. (2005). Teaching in nursing: A guide for faculty, 2nd ed. Philadelphia: Saunders.

4teachers.org. (2006). Create rubrics for project-based learning activities. Accessed February 20, 2007, at http://rubistar.4teachers.org/index.php

Mezeske, R.J., & Mezeske, B.A. (2007). Beyond tests and quizzes: Creative assessment in the college classroom. Jossey-Bass: San Francisco.

Moskal, B.M. (2000). Scoring rubrics: What, when, and how? Practical Assessment, Research & Evaluation 7(3). Accessed February 20, 2007, from http://PAREonline.net/getvn.asp?v=7&n=3

Oermann, M.H., & Gaberson, K.B. (2006). Evaluation and testing in nursing education, 2nd ed. New York: Springer Publishing.

Schuster, P.M. (2002). Concept mapping: A critical thinking approach to care planning. Philadelphia: F.A. Davis.

24

Clinical Evaluation

Marilyn H. Oermann, PhD, RN, FAAN

---

1 What is clinical evaluation?

In clinical evaluation, you make a judgment about the quality of a student's clinical performance. You evaluate how well a student plans and provides direct patient care, carries out other activities in clinical practice, performs skills and procedures, and interacts with patients and others. Students' clinical performance can also be evaluated in simulated experiences and in the learning laboratory.

Most frequently, clinical evaluation involves observing performance and arriving at judgments about the student's competence. You observe students and collect other data about their performance; then you draw conclusions or make judgments about the quality of that performance. In contrast to tests that are objective measures of learning, clinical evaluation is subjective because it involves *judgments* about how well the student is performing (Oermann & Gaberson, 2006).

2 What is the difference between clinical evaluation and grading clinical performance?

Clinical evaluation is the process of collecting data about how well the student is performing in clinical practice. At certain points in time, for example, midterm and at the end of the term, you summarize the evaluation data and use the data as the basis for determining the grade, such as pass-fail or A through F, for the clinical course. The grade is the quantitative symbol that represents the quality of the student's performance over time. You should never grade clinical practice without sufficient evaluation data to support that grade. However, you can evaluate performance without grading it (Oermann & Gaberson, 2006).

3 How do I offer feedback to students and evaluate their performance?

Feedback is a type of evaluation that is called formative evaluation. With formative evaluation you evaluate performance and give feedback to students about how well they are doing in clinical practice and how they can improve. Formative evaluation is diagnostic and for this reason should not be graded (Nitko, 2004). The goal is to give feedback to students for their learning and development of clinical competencies. The second type of evaluation, summative, is done at midterm, at the end of the term, and other specified points in time for the purpose of grading clinical practice. With summative evaluation, you compile the evaluation data you have collected and then indicate a grade that represents the student's performance.

4 How can I give good feedback to students so they learn from it?

Most of the evaluation you give should be in the form of feedback (formative evaluation) because this helps students improve their performance. For feedback to make a difference in learning, you should give *specific* information that tells students exactly what areas of their performance they should work on and how to develop those competencies further. Give students immediate feedback at the time you are observing them. The longer you wait, the less effective the feedback is because students cannot remember the specific clinical situation. Feedback should be positive, what the students are doing well in clinical practice, and include areas for improvement.

---

5 **Evaluation of clinical performance seems highly subjective. What can I do to make it more objective?**

Clinical evaluation involves judging student performance. Because of this, you need to examine your own values and attitudes so they do not interfere with the judgments you make about students. For example, if being organized is important to you, when a beginning student is having difficulty with organization on the unit, this should not interfere with your judgments about the student's competencies in other areas of clinical practice. Also, keep your evaluation focused on the clinical competencies or the outcomes of the clinical course, not on what you personally think the goals should be. The observations and judgments you make should relate to the competencies students are developing in clinical practice. Do not expect students to practice at the same level as a new graduate or staff nurse—students are learning to be nurses.

---

6 **Students appear to be very stressed in clinical practice. Has any research been done on this; if so, what does it show?**

There have been a number of studies done on student stress in clinical courses. The research shows that students in both associate and baccalaureate nursing programs are stressed when they are in the clinical setting (Gaberson & Oermann, 2007). A major stress for students is concern that they will make an error and harm the patient (Oermann & Lukomski, 2001). Other stresses are feeling inadequate to care for patients because of a lack of knowledge and skills, interacting with the teacher and others in the clinical setting, being unsure of what to do as the patient's condition changes, and having the teacher observe one's performance.

7   What can I do as a teacher to relieve some of this stress?

First, you should be aware of how stressful clinical experiences may be for students. Second, it is critical to spend time developing positive and trusting relationships with each student in your clinical group. Make it clear to students that your role is to help them learn, not to create more stress for them. A positive relationship will help to diminish the stress students experience from teachers observing them in the clinical setting. Third, feedback should be instructional, not demeaning and overly critical. Students should understand that your feedback is to help them develop their competencies further. Fourth, you should be alert to stresses students may be experiencing from staff and others in the setting. These are good to discuss individually with students or in postclinical conference, as students often need help solving problem situations with staff.

8   How do I use the clinical competencies or outcomes of the clinical course in my evaluation of students?

Some faculty members write one set of outcomes for a nursing course without designating the ones to be met in the classroom, online component of the course, or clinical practice. Other times there are specific outcomes for students to meet in the classroom or online component and different ones for clinical practice. In some schools of nursing there are separate theory and clinical courses, each with their own course outcomes (or objectives). Regardless of the method, the outcomes specify the knowledge, skills, and values that students should be able to demonstrate at the end of the course and on which they should be evaluated in clinical practice. Another approach is to specify clinical competencies that students should be able to demonstrate by the end of the course. Regardless of the format, clinical evaluation is always based on the outcomes or competencies to be achieved in the course.

9   How do students know what I am going to evaluate in clinical practice?

The outcomes of the clinical course or competencies tell students what they should be learning in the course and the knowledge and skills they should develop by the end of it. These are the outcomes or competencies that you observe, document in anecdotal notes, give feedback on, and grade at midterm and, finally, at the end of the course.

10   What methods can I use for evaluating clinical performance in a nursing course?

Clinical evaluation methods are the strategies you use to collect and record information on student performance in the clinical setting. Some evaluation methods, such as anecdotal notes, are best for giving feedback to students, whereas others, such as rating forms, can be used for grading performance (or summative evaluation). The predominant clinical evaluation method is *observing* students in the clinical setting as they provide care; interact with patients, staff, and others; and carry out activities related to patient care (Oermann & Gaberson, 2006). Your observations can be recorded in anecdotal notes, which can then be discussed with students throughout the clinical experience. Other evaluation strategies are checklists for skills and procedures, rating forms, pre- and postclinical conferences, concept maps, written assignments, journals, portfolios, simulations, standardized patients, clinical examinations, and self-evaluation.

11   When selecting clinical evaluation methods, what factors should I consider?

First, you should select evaluation methods that provide data on the specific clinical competencies students are to develop in your course. These competencies guide your clinical evaluation. Second, rather than rely solely on observing students and rating performance on the clinical evaluation tool, it is preferable to use multiple evaluation methods in a course. Observations can be flawed, and every observation is only a window of time in the student's clinical experience (Oermann & Gaberson, 2006). If you observe the student the following hour, your impressions might differ. Another reason to vary the method is that some students are more proficient in certain areas of practice than others, e.g., they may not do as well with writing assignments as they do with methods that involve interaction with others. Third, you need to explain to students which evaluation methods are for feedback only and which will be graded; not every method needs to be graded. You should always consider how much time you have to evaluate, and remember to give immediate feedback to the students.

12   What are some problems I should be aware of when I observe students in the practice setting?

As discussed earlier, your observations of students can be influenced by your biases, so be aware of them, and be careful that they do not skew what you see. Some experts have suggested that teachers often rely too much on first impressions of a student, which might change if the teachers observed the same behaviors another time. When a student is caring for a patient, particularly in a busy clinical setting, there are many different observations you could make. If the student is changing a dressing, you might focus on the technique to the exclusion of observing the student's communication with the patient. Another teacher might focus more on the interaction with the patient than on the actual technique. You might have sufficient data about a student's performance but then misinterpret the information. For example, a student who is unable to answer a question may not lack knowledge about the answer but be unsure of your question.

13   How can I make my observations more reliable?

One principle in clinical evaluation is to focus your observations on the outcomes or competencies to be met in clinical practice. These should be clear in your mind so you know what to look for when you are with a student. Do not rely on first impressions; instead, collect information on a number of occasions before arriving at conclusions about the student's performance and rating it. It also is important to discuss your observations with students and share notes about their performance with them. By sharing your impressions with students, you can get their perceptions of their performance, which may lead you to change your view of the student's competencies.

---

14 What are anecdotal notes, and how do I write them?

Anecdotal notes are your records of your observations of students in the clinical setting. There are different ways of writing anecdotal notes. Some faculty members record only the specific observations they made about a student; others also include their interpretations or judgments. Because anecdotal notes are intended to provide feedback on clinical performance, they should be shared frequently with students. Box 24–1 provides an example of an anecdotal note.

---

15 If I have 9 or 10 students to evaluate in a clinical course, how can I possibly write anecdotal notes about each student every clinical practice day?

The goal is to write a similar number of anecdotal notes for each student. You should decide first on the competencies you want to document in anecdotal notes, and then plan an

---

BOX 24–1
Sample Anecdotal Note
12/10: Observed explaining procedure for scan to Mrs. S. Began by assessing patient's understanding of the scan and why she was having it done. Asked appropriate questions. Explained procedure clearly, stopping frequently to ask patient if she understood. When done, asked her a few questions to see if she understood. Had eye contact with Mrs. S during teaching. Documented in record that teaching was done prior to scan.

approximate number of times you want to observe student performance of those competencies. That planning helps you to be more specific about the type of observations to make and the number of times to record those observations. Some faculty members write a short note about each student every day; other teachers might do this weekly. The principle is to use your notes as a record of significant observations related to the outcomes (objectives) or competencies so you can see a pattern of clinical performance.

16 What are checklists, and how do I use them in my clinical evaluation?

A checklist is a list of steps to be followed in performing a procedure or skill, with a place to check off if they were carried out correctly (Oermann & Gaberson, 2006). Checklists are good to use when observing students perform a procedure in the clinical setting or simulation/ learning laboratory because the checklist indicates the steps to follow and their order. The teacher, however, should not be rigid in observing procedures and checking off each step; the principle is that students can perform the critical steps in the procedure.

17 The course I am teaching has a rating form (i.e., clinical evaluation form or tool) to use at midterm and the end of the term. What should I know about rating forms for clinical evaluation of nursing students?

Most nursing courses use ratings forms for compiling the judgments made about the performance of students over time, for example, through midterm and at the end of the term. Rating forms have two parts: (1) a list of the outcomes or objectives to be met at the end of the course or of the competencies to be developed in clinical practice, and (2) a scale for rating students' performance of each objective. Ratings scales are best for grading because they are designed for compiling judgments over time and then rating performance.

18 What types of rating scales are used in nursing programs?

Most schools of nursing use rating scales that are pass-fail or satisfactory-unsatisfactory. With these scales you observe clinical performance and decide whether it is satisfactory. Other schools have multidimensional scales in which faculty rate performance as A, B, C, D, E or A, B, C, D, F; use numbers such as 1 through 5; use qualitative labels (excellent, very good, good, fair, poor); note frequency (always, usually, frequently, sometimes, never); or use other scales that combine standards (independent, supervised, assisted, marginal, dependent) (Oermann & Gaberson, 2006). With multidimensional scales, you have more categories to use to rate performance, but differences between categories, such as A and B or excellent and very good, are not always clear. Faculty should discuss what each label means in the rating form so that there is more consistency across faculty in their ratings.

19 When rating performance of nursing students, what are common errors that can occur?

Some of the errors that can occur with a rating scale that has multiple dimensions are: *leniency error,* which is a tendency to rate performance toward the high end of the scale; *severity error,* which is a tendency to rate students low; and *error of central tendency,* which is a tendency to rate students toward the middle of the scale (Nitko, 2004). A *halo effect* can influence your judgment with any scale. This is a tendency to rate a student's performance based on a general impression of the student rather than on the actual data you have collected. *Personal bias* can also affect ratings.

20 How can I prevent these errors and make my ratings for clinical evaluation more reliable?

When rating students' clinical performance, make sure you have collected enough data from your observations before drawing conclusions and rating performance. You should observe students over time; one observation of a skill is not enough to use for rating performance at midterm or final evaluation. If you find that you cannot observe students sufficiently to rate certain competencies on the form, then use other evaluation methods to collect those data. Table 24–1 describes some of the principles for using rating scales for clinical evaluation.

Table 24–1
Guidelines for Using Rating Scales for Clinical Evaluation

1. Be alert to the possible influence of your own values, attitudes, beliefs, and biases in observing performance and drawing conclusions about it.
2. Use the clinical outcomes, competencies, or behaviors to focus your observations. Give students feedback on other observations made about their performance.
3. Collect sufficient data on students' performance before drawing conclusions about it.
4. Observe the student more than once before rating performance. Rating scales when used for clinical evaluation should represent a *pattern* of the students' performance over time.
5. If possible, observe students' performance in different clinical situations, either in the patient care or simulated setting. If that is not possible, develop other strategies for evaluation so performance is evaluated with different methods and at different times.
6. Do not rely on first impressions; they may not be accurate.
7. Always discuss observations with students; obtain their perceptions of performance; and be willing to modify your own judgments and ratings when new data are presented.
8. Review the available clinical learning activities and opportunities in the simulation and learning laboratories. Do they provide sufficient data for completing the rating scale? If not, new learning activities may need to be developed or behaviors may need to be modified to be more realistic considering the clinical teaching circumstances.
9. Avoid using rating scales as the only source of data about a student's performance— use multiple evaluation methods for clinical practice.
10. Rate each outcome, competency, or behavior individually, based on your observations of performance and conclusions drawn. If you have insufficient information about achievement of a particular competency, do not rate it—leave it blank.
11. Do not rate all students high, low, or in the middle; similarly, do not let your general impression of the student or personal biases influence the ratings.
12. If the rating form is ineffective for judging student performance, then revise it. Consider these questions: Does the form yield data that can be used to make valid decisions about students' competence? Does it yield reliable, stable data? Is it easy to use? Is it realistic for the types of learning activities students complete and available in clinical settings?

From Oermann, M.H., & Gaberson, K. (2006). Evaluation and testing in nursing education, 2nd ed. New York: Springer, p. 222. Reprinted by permission of Springer Publishing Co., New York.

Some forms are too long, and you may find that you do not have sufficient data to judge each competency particularly when there are multiple items about the same area of practice. For example, there may be three competencies related to communication. If you have data to rate only one of these, do not rate all three; leave the others blank.

---

21 I want to carefully select the written assignments that students complete in my course. Which assignments are best for promoting and evaluating critical thinking and problem solving in clinical practice?

For critical thinking and problem solving, consider developing short assignments that ask students to identify multiple perspectives, to discuss different approaches that could be used in a clinical situation, and to weigh the options and provide a rationale for the "best" decision given that situation. As an example, students could write a few paragraphs that compare two different approaches they could use with a patient and discuss how they would decide on the best strategy to use.

Oermann (2006) suggests that short written assignments, e.g., a few paragraphs up to one or two pages, be used in clinical courses to encourage thinking about patient care "rather than summarizing what others have written about the topic" (p. 228). For example, students could identify a nursing intervention they used with one of their patients and write a one-page paper on the strength of the supporting evidence. They could identify a patient problem and write a paragraph about the data they would collect to verify that problem. Other written activities that are good for critical thinking are short cases in which students analyze and identify possible problems and approaches; position papers; and papers requiring analysis of issues and development of a supporting rationale.

---

22 Can portfolios be used for clinical evaluation?

With a portfolio students collect projects they have completed during a clinical course that demonstrate their achievement of the outcomes and competencies. You should establish guidelines for developing the portfolio and criteria for evaluating the examples that students place in them. Portfolios work well when you need to evaluate the outcomes of clinical courses where you are off-site; for example, when students are learning at a distance or are in a variety of community agencies. Portfolios can demonstrate the students' best-work (for grading purposes) or be used for growth and learning (Nitko, 2004).

23 How can I use journals in my courses, and should they be graded?

If you want students to have an opportunity to describe how they feel about their clinical experiences, journals are an effective strategy. Journals work well for outcomes that are affective or value-based because students can express their feelings that are shared only with the teacher. Be clear to students about the journal's purposes, provide guidelines for what they should write in their journals, and give prompt feedback on their entries. Journals are intended for formative evaluation, not for grading clinical practice. Across clinical courses, journals demonstrate a pattern of accomplishment for students and their development of knowledge and skills over time (Ruthman, et al., 2004).

24 What is a clinical examination?

A clinical examination is a structured evaluation of clinical performance in a simulated or laboratory setting for grading purposes. The clinical examination is usually given at the end of a course to assess knowledge and competencies in a more structured setting than a hospital. Students might be asked to analyze a scenario and to demonstrate skills, which are then evaluated by the examiner. Sometimes the performance by students is videotaped for evaluation and scoring.

25 What about asking students to evaluate their own progress in clinical practice? Is this reliable?

The long-term goal of your clinical teaching is to help students develop the ability and willingness to evaluate their own clinical performance and to seek to improve their knowledge and skills. When you meet with students to review your anecdotal notes and you ask them for their own perceptions about clinical practice, this helps them develop self-evaluation skills. Often, faculty will ask students at midterm and the end of the term to write a brief evaluation of their performance. This strategy encourages students to identify their strengths and weaknesses and gives you an opportunity to suggest ways to improve their performance. Self-evaluation strategies are not graded but used only for feedback.

26 When evaluating and grading clinical performance, should I accept input from the nurse manager and nurses who are working with my students?

Yes. However, the input may not be valid and may suffer from all the problems identified earlier with observations and performance ratings. Also, the individuals giving input may not understand the goals of the clinical experience, and their expectations of performance may not be consistent with the level of the student. It is important to share any input with students, use it as a basis for discussion, and problem-solve with students if needed, but be cautious about using the input in grading clinical practice. If you are working with preceptors and have prepared them for their role, their input can be used for clinical evaluation, but the final responsibility for grading is yours.

27 What are differences between pass-fail and a letter system for grading clinical performance?

One way of grading clinical courses is to indicate if students passed or failed clinical practice. In this system, if students met the outcomes or objectives of the clinical course, they pass the course; no letter grade is given. Alternatively, letter grades such as A through E or A through F, which may be combined with "+" and "-", can be given for the clinical component of a course (Oermann & Gaberson, 2006).

28 Tell me what I should do if a student is failing my clinical course.

Failing the clinical course should not be "news" to the student. If a student is not progressing in clinical practice, you should be meeting with the student, providing feedback, and suggesting learning activities to help improve performance. The teacher should develop an instructional plan with students that includes a time frame for completion of remedial learning activities. Meetings with students should be documented to provide a record of how you tried to help the student improve performance. It also is important for students to sign their rating forms and clinical evaluation documents, indicating that they have read them even if they do not agree with your comments. Teachers should keep these materials for at least a year.

Every nursing program has set policies for how to handle students who are not performing satisfactorily in the clinical setting and those with unsafe clinical performance. Those policies must be in writing, reviewed with students at the beginning of the course, available to them, and followed by the teacher.

29 How do I balance my role as evaluator with my role as teacher in the clinical setting?

Your role is teaching—guiding students to meet the outcomes of the course and to develop essential clinical competencies. Evaluation is part of that role, giving feedback to help students improve their knowledge and skills. Your role is not to catch the students when they are doing something wrong. Your role is to guide the students so that they learn in clinical practice.

References

Gaberson, K., & Oermann, M.H. (2007). Clinical teaching strategies in nursing, 2nd ed. New York: Springer.

Nitko, A.J. (2004). Educational assessment of students, 4th ed. Upper Saddle River, N.J.: Prentice-Hall.

Oermann, M.H. (2006). Short written assignments for clinical nursing courses. Nurse Educator 31, 228–231.

Oermann, M.H., & Gaberson, K. (2006). Evaluation and testing in nursing education, 2nd ed. New York: Springer.

Oermann, M.H., & Lukomski, A.P. (2001). Experiences of students in pediatric nursing clinical courses. Journal of the Society of Pediatric Nurses 9(2), 65–72.

Ruthman, J., et al. (2004). Using clinical journaling to capture critical thinking across the curriculum. Nursing Education Perspectives 25(3), 120–123.

Resources

Case, B., & Oermann, M.H. (2004). Clinical teaching and evaluation. In L. Caputi & L. Engelmann (Eds.) Teaching nursing: The art and science. Glen Ellyn, Ill.: College of DuPage Press, pp. 126–177.

O'Connor, A.B. (2006). Clinical instruction and evaluation: A teaching resource, 2nd ed. Sudbury, Mass.: Jones & Bartlett.

Oermann, M.H. (2004). Basic skills for teaching and the advanced practice nurse. In L. Joel (Ed.) Advanced practice nursing: Essentials for role development, pp. 398–429. Philadelphia: F.A. Davis.

Oermann, M.H., Truesdell, S., & Ziolkowski, L. (2000). Strategy to assess, develop, and evaluate critical thinking. Journal of Continuing Education in Nursing 31(4), 155–160.

Profetto-McGrath, J., et al. (2004). The questioning skills of tutors and students in a context-based baccalaureate nursing program. Nurse Education Today 24, 363–372.

Walsh, C.M., & Seldomridge, L.A. (2005). Clinical grades: Upward bound. Journal of Nursing Education 44, 162–168.

25

Resolving Grade Disputes With Students

Paula W. Boley, EdD, RN

---

1 How likely is it that I will get sued by a student?

You are very *unlikely* to ever get sued by a student. However, this is a fear that many new faculty members have. Following some simple guidelines, as discussed below, will help you avoid getting sued.

---

2 How can I determine and justify if a student is failing clinical as clinical grades are partially subjective?

You are an expert nurse, or you would not have been hired to teach. You know good and poor nursing when you see it. If a student is not providing the nursing care you expect or is not meeting the course requirements, document the specific behavior. Students make errors, but a pattern of errors, omissions, or poor nursing care should indicate that the student is unsatisfactory. Be cognizant, however, of the student's level of expertise (i.e., you expect more expert behavior from a senior than from a sophomore); refer to the course requirements.

3   What is due process?

Under the 14th Amendment, no person may be denied the right to life, liberty, or property without due process of law by a government institution, which includes universities. This means that if there is a dispute about grades, the student has a right to tell his or her story. Each university must have a published grade appeals due process that describes to students the formal mechanism for telling their side of the story. Once a university, either public or private, publishes its due process procedures, the policies should be followed, or the university may be at risk for losing a lawsuit should one be filed.

4   Why is due process important to grading?

Due process is the right that a student has to be heard and the assurance that university policies are followed. In public universities, students have won grade appeals when they were not give due process—when their side of the case was not allowed to be heard or the university policies were not followed. For example, if your school's policy is that students must pass a math test to progress to clinical courses, and you refuse to allow a student to take that test, thus leading to a failing grade, you would be liable.

5   What is contract theory?

This defense has been used by students in private universities, and it is applicable to public universities as well. Basically, this theory suggests that if students are admitted to a program and pay tuition and fees, they will receive a grade for each course and will eventually receive a diploma (assuming they maintain the prescribed level of academic performance and adhere to the university code of conduct). The basic premise is that the course syllabus is a contract (the student pays the university a fee, and the university provides a service, i.e., education). A prudent faculty member will consider the syllabus a contract and should adhere to the policies in the syllabus.

6   Why is contract theory important to grade disputes?

Sometimes you might be tempted to change something in the syllabus after it has been distributed to the students. Just as with any contract, once the syllabus has been distributed to the students, it should be followed carefully. The method for determining assignment of grades should be clear and followed judiciously. The contents of the syllabus should not be changed, if at all possible; however, if they are changed, a hard copy should be provided and honored for all students.

7   What is arbitrary or capricious conduct?

According to Kaplin and Lee (1997): "An arbitrary and capricious act is one that is willful and unreasonable and one without regard to the facts and circumstances of the case; an act without some basis which would lead a reasonable and honest person to the same conclusion . . ." (pp. 31–32). "Arbitrary and capricious" is allowing some students to do certain things but not others. It is giving exceptions only for some students. If you make an exception for one student, be prepared to do the same for all.

8   What does estoppel mean?

This means giving poor advice to a student. For example, if a student comes to you to clarify course requirements, and you give poor or misleading advice that leads the student to receive a failing grade, you may be liable for your actions. An example is *Olsson v. Board of Higher Education*, in which a student was told by a faculty member that he could take a comprehensive written examination instead of doing a master's thesis. When he failed the comprehensive examination, he sued because he said that the faculty member did not inform him about how much weight was being placed on the test for his graduation. While this argument did not hold up in court, giving students bad advice is always risky.

9 What should I do if a student complains to my dean/director about a grade I gave?

As the teacher, you should always encourage students to talk with you first if they are unhappy. If, however, they go to the dean/director first, that person should refer them back to you. If the student has already talked to you but is not satisfied, then he or she has the right to approach the dean/director, who would then follow the school's grade appeals process.

10 Do the courts ever require specific policies or procedures related to grading or evaluating clinical performance?

No. The courts will, however, look for evidence that the policies and procedures were followed and whether grades were assigned in an arbitrary, capricious, malicious, or prejudicial manner. Be as objective, consistent, and as fair as possible when assigning grades or evaluating students clinically. If you recognize unsatisfactory clinical performance, confront the student with specific examples of behavioral deficiencies, then give the student an opportunity to improve performance. Deliberately tell the student that a failing grade is pending if performance is not improved; then follow through.

11 What is a rubric, and how does it relate to grading?

A rubric is a detailed evaluation plan for grading a written assignment, such as a care plan, essay, or research paper. It utilizes verbs that are leveled like a taxonomy in order to give the student an objective sense of what is expected or considered unsatisfactory work. For example, in a four-level rubric, leveled wording may be "problems not identified," "problems partially identified," "problems identified adequately," and "problems thoroughly analyzed and completely identified." Leveled wording allows points or letter grades to be assigned more objectively.

12 Under what circumstances should I change a grade on an assignment or course grade?

Generally, a grade on an assignment or for a course should be changed only if it is clear that a mistake was made. Follow your school's policies for making such a change. Occasionally, however, a student may try to persuade you to add a few points to improve a grade. Take caution doing this; if you add points to one student's score, you must do so for all students. If you give points only to one student, you may be open to litigation for being arbitrary or capricious. A student does not have the right, however, to demand a detailed explanation of how you assigned your grades or what grades other students receive.

13 What is the Family Educational Rights and Privacy Act (FERPA), and how does it concern teachers?

The FERPA was passed in 1974 as a method of ensuring that student records be kept confidential. The law pertains to students who are of majority age (i.e., 18 years old) or the parents/guardians of students younger than 18 years. The FERPA states that university officials may not share educational records (grades or other academic records) with anyone who does not have a legitimate educational interest in those records without written authorization from the student. It also ensures that students have the right to view their educational records and to request that inaccurate or misleading records be corrected (if the request is denied, the student must be given a hearing). The law means that if parents call you to ask why you assigned a particular grade to their son or daughter, you are not allowed to discuss the grade with them without the student's permission. You are also not allowed to contact the student's parents for academic reasons without permission. Additionally, you must allow students to view all their academic records but no records of any other students. Records may be shared among faculty directly involved in the academic progress of the student but not with others within the university unless the individual has a direct need to see the records. For example, the school of nursing faculty may discuss the progress of an individual student among themselves, but they should not discuss such information at the lunch table with faculty outside the school of nursing. As another example, a faculty member would be in violation of the FERPA if she looked up the grades of her daughter's new boyfriend, just to be sure that he is a good student; but it might be appropriate to share that information with the athletic office to ensure athletic eligibility.

14 What should I do if a parent calls me about his or her child's grades/performance in school?

Remind the parent of the FERPA and that you are not allowed to discuss these grades unless you have permission from the student. The parent may protest being denied information, but the FERPA is very clear about maintaining confidentiality and allowing students who are of majority age to choose whether they want parental involvement.

15 Under FERPA rules, can I share an example of good or poor student work with other students?

Yes, but eliminate the student's name or any other identifying marks. It is prudent to show students examples of good and poor work, but keep the work anonymous. If possible, get the student's permission first before showing the work to other students.

16 How does the Americans With Disabilities Act affect grading/admission policies?

Students with disabilities should be held to the same standards as other students. However, universities must provide reasonable accommodations to facilitate student success. First, obtain documentation of the student's specific type of disability. Second, discuss with the student the type of accommodations requested. Consult with university administration if the accommodations are more than what you as faculty or the school believes is appropriate. In any case, allow the student the opportunity to be successful in the nursing program, but do not allow the student benefits that you would not give nondisabled students.

---

17 What legal obligation does a college or university have in "certifying" that a student is a capable practitioner, and how is this linked to grade disputes?

When a student graduates from a university, the institution is giving its approval that the student is capable and safe to practice nursing. If a student is not performing at the level of clinical course expectations, the student should receive a failing grade. This may mean that the student does not graduate on time and may have to pay for additional semesters of tuition. It may also mean that a student threatens to sue. However, institutions have an ethical obligation to patients and to the health-care facilities that employ their graduates to ensure the students are safe practitioners.

---

18 How should I handle a student who claims he/she turned in an assignment but I have no record of receiving it?

If you have no record or recollection of receiving the assignment, you have no obligation to accept an assignment after the due date or to give any credit for the assignment. If you do accept the assignment late, be willing to do so for other students. A good plan is to make a statement in your syllabus about grade penalties for late assignments (such as a 5% deduction per day for each day it is late). Encourage students to keep all returned assignments until final grades are posted as proof of having received a grade for a particular assignment.

---

19 Can I require a student to make up a clinical experience or a test?

Yes. Students sometimes have legitimate reasons for missing one or the other, but you may require them to make up the assignment or substitute a different assignment that meets the course objectives. If a student refuses, he or she can receive a failing grade or even fail the course. However, Kaplin and Lee (1997) suggest not assigning a failing course grade strictly for a missed assignment unless there are unusual circumstances and, especially, if the course failure would delay graduation for the student.

20 What should I do if a student misses an examination?

The mechanism for making up a test should be stated in the syllabus. If the student has a legitimate reason, such as illness or the death of a family member, you may allow the student to take the test later or take a substitute test. Make the substitute examination similar to the one given in class or at least of equal difficulty. The substitute test should not be so difficult that it appears to be punishing the student for the absence.

21 How do I recognize and document a pattern of unsatisfactory performance?

Faculty members must be diligent in observing student performance in clinical. Keeping anecdotal notes has been covered in other chapters. However, when a student is not performing satisfactorily, note it on the student record, and watch for a pattern. A failing course grade should be given, not for an isolated incident of poor performance, but for a pattern of unsatisfactory performance. This pattern may be evident over more than one semester. *Susan M. v. New York Law School* (1989) established that a student's performance in previous courses can influence grade decisions in subsequent courses.

22 Who has the right and/or responsibility to determine if a student's performance is unsatisfactory?

The primary right and responsibility belong to the faculty member who is assigned to teach the course or supervise the student in clinical. However, if a course is team-taught, all faculty assigned to the course should be consulted. It is prudent to consult with other faculty for advice and support, unless there is a clear reason to give an unsatisfactory score, evaluation, or grade.

---

23   If agency nurses and preceptors have a higher or lower opinion of a student's clinical performance than I do, but I am responsible for grading, how much weight should I give to the preceptor's opinion?

First, try to get to know both your students and the precepting nurses who are supervising your students. Make visits to the clinical facility, and be available for consultation with both the student and the preceptor. You can make better judgments about the situation if you know the parties involved. The bottom line, however, is that it is your call as to what grade to assign. Use your judgment.

---

24   What is a grade appeals process, or what should be in a grade appeals process/procedure?

Every university should have a grade appeals process that is published in a student handbook or other documents provided to students and faculty. The general chain of communication should be used — the student should first talk to the faculty member involved in providing the grade. If the student does not receive satisfaction, then the student should discuss the situation with the next person in the chain (course coordinator, lead teacher, department chair, or director of the program). If the student is still not satisfied, then the student must follow the published guidelines for appealing a grade. The courts have never specified what actions or steps universities should take to hear an appeal. However, most universities require that an appeal be submitted in writing and that students have the right to have their side of the story heard. The courts only say that the appeals process must allow for due process.

---

25   Should I keep notes about student behavior from clinical experiences?

Yes. Think about these notes like an incident report: stick to the facts. If you need to fail a student for unsatisfactory clinical performance (often based on your professional but subjective opinion), clearly state what the student did and why the student's performance was not satisfactory. Avoid using pejorative terms or other words that might be construed as biased.

26 How likely is it that clinical notes may be subpoenaed?

Very unlikely, but attorneys have been known to do so. Therefore, your clinical notes should be objective and descriptive of behavior. Do not insert disparaging remarks about the student as an individual or information that might lead a reasonable person to believe you are being arbitrary or vindictive. For example, it is appropriate to say that the student was unable to state the correct locations for an IM injection, but it is inappropriate to record, "The stupid student does not know where to give an IM."

27 How long should I keep records of grades?

Your university may have a policy regarding how long grades should be kept. As a general rule, in absence of a formal policy, keep all grades and notes until after the course grade has been recorded on the university records. Some faculty members keep records until after students graduate, but this is not necessary in all cases. Students may not sue for "educational malpractice" even if they fail the NCLEX examination, so keeping records until after graduation may not be necessary.

28 How can I avoid grade disputes?

Be fair, consistent, and kind. You may not feel like being kind, but often simply allowing the student to be heard is enough to defuse a situation. Additionally, students will often be able to accept bad news if they believe they have been treated fairly and in a manner consistent with their classmates. Be prepared to give specific reasons why you graded a paper in a specific manner or what your reasoning was for specific test questions, but do not get into an argument with a student. No matter what the student says, you are the professional, and the student is the novice.

References

Kaplin, W.A., & Lee, B.A. (1997). A legal guide for student affairs professionals. San Francisco: Jossey-Bass Publishers.

Weinberger, H., & Schepard, A. (1993). Judicial review of academic student evaluations: A comment on Susan M. v. New York Law School from those who litigated it. West Educational Law Reporter 77, 1089–1102.

Resources

Beezer, B. (1985). Using academic grades to discipline students: A legal caution. West Educational Law Reporter 21, 765–771.

Boley, P., & Whitney, A. (2003). Grade disputes: Considerations for nursing faculty. Journal of Nursing Education 42(5), 198–203.

Lallo, D. (1992). Student challenges to grades and academic dismissals: Are they losing battles? Journal of College and University Law 18, 577–593.

Miller, P. (1982). Student grade appeals: Procedure and process. Journal of Nursing Education 21, 34–38.

26

Using Standardized Achievement Tests

Julia Aucoin, DNS, RN-BC, CNE

1 Why do programs administer standardized achievement tests?

Achievement tests serve as an external measure to assess the progress of both individual students and the mastery of content in a nursing program. They can be used to demonstrate performance in comparison with national norms for both self-assessment and program improvement. Often these measures are integrated in a program's evaluation plan as a part of the accreditation process. Some programs use achievement tests to give faculty feedback on the effectiveness of teaching by providing student performance scores on content offered in the curriculum. The use of achievement tests is voluntary, adopted at the program level, and must have a clear purpose and application.

2 Why is there a surge in the achievement test business?

When the National Council Licensure Examination (NCLEX) format changed to Computerized Adaptive Testing (CAT), graduate performance dropped. Historically, each time the test plan has changed and the pass score is adjusted, graduate performance has dropped as well. Achievement tests become a formative method of evaluation to consistently measure performance throughout a program and offer feedback to students. Achievement test developers construct NCLEX-style questions written at the application and analysis level, making them more like the items that graduates would see on the NCLEX (the NCLEX refers to both the RN and PN versions of the test).

As nursing programs became increasingly concerned about substandard NCLEX performance, achievement test developers responded with tests to offer evaluation experiences authentic to the types of tasks and knowledge relevant for entry-level practice. Some end-of-course, comprehensive achievement tests are designed to predict the graduates' likelihood of passing the NCLEX. In doing so, the test vendors were able to promote comprehensive achievement test packages to help students learn how to be successful from the beginning of their nursing programs. These packages can provide content-specific tests associated with nursing content areas, testing for the end of program, and opportunities for retesting students who have performed poorly. Packages may also include remedial materials, NCLEX review course, and faculty development.

3　What factors should faculty consider when selecting content-specific achievement tests?

The tests have to be a match for the content as it is delivered in the program. For example, for Adult Health I and II achievement tests, all adult health content must be taught before the tests are administered, or the first semester's content must be a match for Adult Health I. The content of the questions must be current with practice; for example, questions concerning mixing a heparin drip would not be appropriate when heparin solutions are provided as pre-mixed with standard concentrations. Comprehensive assessment tools should reflect the curriculum in its entirety and thus be offered near the end of the program.

The questions have to be written at the application and analysis levels using Bloom's taxonomy. It is not useful to include the "all or none of the above" type of responses as these questions generally do not discriminate those who know from those who do not. Nor is it helpful to include pairs of opposites, for example, increased and decreased sodium levels. These items become essentially true/false responses or might be tricky, thus not providing quality opportunities for students to demonstrate what they know.

The faculty must be actively willing to review and use the results to improve student and faculty performance. Administering these tests without a plan to use the findings is not ethical, as test results are more than a label to attach to a student. Test results are an opportunity to identify content deficiencies as a road map for further study and reinforcement of material. A fee is charged for the tests, often paid by the students. Dissemination and explanation of the findings are the responsibility of faculty. Accessible, clear, and discernible score reporting is the responsibility of the test developer.

4   How can faculty determine content validity?

Reputable achievement test vendors will allow the faculty to view examinations before making a purchase. At the very least, faculty should be provided a list of the item descriptors. However, it is most helpful for faculty teaching in each specialty to take the test with the students. In doing so, the faculty becomes very aware of the content of the test and can judge if the test is current with practice (or if the faculty is current with practice). Many achievement test vendors have rigorous review processes and will share their content validity data with the programs. Construct validity is determined by alignment of the test with the NCLEX Practice Analysis findings.

5   How often should achievement tests be updated?

The NCLEX plan is updated every 3 years based on a practice analysis. The achievement test vendors should be making adjustments in their comprehensive predictive tests at least every 3 years to correlate with the practice analysis. Content examinations should undergo similar revisions. As items are kept in a test bank, the achievement test vendor should be able to have a flexible enough process that as practice changes, items can be pulled and not appear in print or electronic versions of the test. For example, the drug Propulsid is no longer available through U.S. pharmacies and therefore should not appear on tests.

When tests with norm-referenced scoring are updated, then test norming should be repeated reflecting these changes. Caution should be used in comparing groups that have actually taken two different tests.

---

6   What is the difference between secure and nonsecure versions of a test?

Secure versions are administered within standardized and proctored settings in order to protect the integrity of the scores, particularly percentile ranks. Both paper and electronic versions are scrambled and monitored by the test proctor to prevent cheating, note taking, copying, or downloading. Computer-based tests are accessed through a password issued to the faculty only. Nonsecure versions are often previous versions of the test or those designed with less rigor. Scores on these versions are often for personal improvement, not for incorporation into national norms. In some cases the nonsecure version can provide the test taker with the rationale for its still active items.

---

7   Which method of test giving is better: paper or computer?

For a while there was a hunch that practicing tests on the computer would lead to better performance on the NCLEX. However, that has not happened. Taking achievement tests as paper versions, especially early in the program, allows students to "think" with their pencils: underline important words, mark out incorrect replies, and make helpful notes as they create their pool of answers. As students mature in their test-taking skills, the computer version creates a more authentic testing environment to ready them for the NCLEX. By using computer-based tests throughout a program, students become familiar with the online testing format, develop the psychomotor skills for computer-based testing, and often gain confidence for taking the NCLEX on the computer.

Another advantage to the electronic version of the test is the ability to update the test immediately as items need to be changed in the question bank. Pulling or delivering items randomly can be accomplished easily in the electronic delivery system. Paper versions circulate more than a year without being updated. One such test had a typo in the correct response that remained in place for 3 years, and students typically will not select a response that is spelled incorrectly because they think it is a trick. When talking to a test developer, determine if the paper test is the same as the computer-based test for consistency in score interpretation.

---

8   Percentage or percentile: which is useful?

Percentage reflects raw score: how many right responses divided by how many questions. Students understand percentage because it is the way their examinations are graded. Percentile reflects a ranked performance within a larger pool of test candidates. It indicates what percentage of candidates did better and what percentage did worse than the individual test taker. Percentile is calculated from a large pool of candidates and can be used to compare the individual with the class, type of program, or all testers.

The important aspect of percentage or percentile is how the faculty and the tester use the information. Clearly, a student who performs at the 2nd percentile has not done well, no matter with which group the student is compared. Conversely, the student who performs at the 98th percentile is doing quite well. Someone has to perform at the top and someone at the bottom for the scoring to have meaning. What percentile will make your program happy? Is it the 50th, 60th, or a higher percentile? Many programs are happy to achieve the national mean or slightly higher. Perhaps a score of 40th percentile will be acceptable because the purpose of achievement tests is for performance improvement, so approaching the national mean may be acceptable.

9   Do achievement tests have predictive validity for the NCLEX?

Most teachers would be very eager for something that could accurately predict NCLEX performance. No one can predict anything with 100% certainty. However, the performance on predictive tests can correlate highly with performance on the NCLEX. Most teachers can predict fairly easily those who will pass. A low achievement test score could be a motivating factor for a graduate to study hard for the NCLEX. Many schools are relying on exit examinations to make decisions about graduation. However, there are many factors that contribute to NCLEX failure other than performance on the final predictive test. And predicting failure is harder than predicting success.

The information that is helpful from a predictive achievement test is how students performed in a testing situation similar to the NCLEX. The tests tend to be about 150 items, longer than the average NCLEX of 108 items. The predictive achievement tests cover the NCLEX categories, content areas, and nursing process in the same proportion as the NCLEX. The test can be administered from a computer station, just like the NCLEX.

What such tests do not measure are the affective factors that influence test performance. When is the test given in relation to the students' other examinations and graduation? How seriously do the students take the test? What distractions are influencing their performance on test day? What is the student stress or fatigue level? Most important, has the curriculum addressed everything it should to prepare students to take the NCLEX? There are still faculty members who are not familiar with NCLEX activities derived from the practice analyses, and thus needed content is not addressed. For example, performing a 12-lead EKG is an NCLEX activity.

10   How can the costs of achievement tests be managed?

Some schools assess a fee per semester, and others include the fees as a laboratory fee integrated with the tuition. The worst plan is to try to collect the money from students before the test is administered. Students resent the extra fee and may not perform well on the test as a result. This is the opposite of what might be expected: if they pay for the test, then they will do their best. The least intrusive method can promote the best student performance. Keep it simple so that no one is collecting money and checking off student payments on a list.

Consider the needs of your program. Are there a couple of key courses in which you would like to track student progress? Is the faculty dedicated enough to the process that it would consider buying a total testing package? A total package often includes many content mastery tests in both secure and nonsecure versions, a comprehensive predictor, study materials, and possibly a review course. The total package price is a discount from purchasing each test individually.

11   How does the achievement test help the individual student?

Students deserve an explanation how the achievement test can help them. They need to know the purpose of the testing program, how and when they will receive their results, and the consequences or benefits of their scores. They should be advised to do their best on the achievement test as it is practice for their final test, the NCLEX. The results can guide their study plans.

If a student performs poorly on the achievement test but satisfactorily on the teacher-made tests, then the faculty should examine the causes of that. Standardized tests can cause this student anxiety as can extraordinary pressure to perform or not graduate. This student may have become used to the faculty's style of writing test questions. Suppose a student fails the course yet scores very well on the achievement test. The explanation may then lie with the validity of the teacher made tests. Nevertheless, the student should receive specific feedback regarding individual performance and be guided to improve that performance with appropriate content and strategies.

12 How can you get students to do their best on the achievement test?

Achievement tests must be scheduled at logical times. Instructors often try to cram the achievement tests in the end of the semester during finals. If they are a mandatory part of the program, and the results are considered to be valuable, then time should be allotted for the tests.

Many teachers administer the achievement test before finals as an opportunity for students to self-identify content they do not know so they can study that and be successful on the teacher-made final. Other programs administer finals, then call the students in for the achievement test.

Generally, achievement tests do not have any bearing on the final grade for the course. Perhaps, like high school achievement test programs, 25% of the course grade should be based on the final, and 25% should be based on the achievement test. Grade-driven students often perform better when they know that points are attached to their assignments. Weighing achievement tests as little as 10% of the final grade may still give the student some impetus to perform better.

13 How does the achievement test help the program?

The intent is to get some validation that the students are being prepared throughout the curriculum for the NCLEX and that the courses present the concepts that all nursing students should know. Faculty can set target percentiles for all achievement test performance and implement strategies to improve performance until targets are reached. Whereas a target of 90th percentile or greater may not be reasonable, achieving the national norm would be desirable, given the 83% pass rate in recent years on the NCLEX.

14 How does the achievement test support accreditation?

Accrediting bodies have allowed programs to set their own measurement and evaluation strategies. Programs can define terms and how they will be measured. If a program has chosen measures such as achievement tests, then generating annual reports to document improvement is quite easily done for accreditation self-studies and visits. Using achievement test performance to document clinical judgment could be an easy application. When looking for a vendor, consider the Commission on Collegiate Nursing Education (CCNE) or the National League for Nursing Accreditation Commission (NLNAC) for indicators of success.

15 What are the responsibilities of faculty to provide feedback on achievement tests?

It is irresponsible of faculty to withhold achievement test results. The students have paid for the test; they deserve timely and easily understood results. As the achievement tests are often given at the end of the semester, it is only fair that results be mailed to the students for their review and consideration between semesters. A phased study plan can accompany the results so that those up to the 40th percentile know that they should practice taking NCLEX-style questions and review important course content before progressing. Those at the 70th and higher percentiles might be told to review all medications that were taught during the semester. Even though students think the time between semesters is a break, teachers know that in order to be prepared, students need to review content continuously. Some follow-up to online reporting of performance is required. Students need assistance in knowing what to do with the results.

16 What should faculty do about poor achievement test results?

Create study plans, and devote time to offering remediation. It is unreasonable to think that poor achievement test results are only the student's problem. As nursing programs continue to receive sanctions for poor NCLEX performance, faculty must come to agreement that NCLEX success is a shared responsibility. This is why tying achievement test performance to a grade is a good topic for discussion at a faculty meeting.

Instructors should examine course content in relation to the NCLEX activities to be sure that they are teaching relevant concepts. From the 2005 Registered Nurse Practice Analysis, only 8% of the NCLEX is related to obstetrics, yet there is increased emphasis on hemodynamic monitoring. Should a three- or four-credit maternity course with details about underwater births still be taught, or can some of that course credit be shifted into another course?

---

17 What should students do about poor achievement test results?

Students must devote themselves to a study plan and be offered a nonsecure version of the test to take again to demonstrate improvement. Tutoring or practicing taking NCLEX questions using one of the major publishers' NCLEX disks can be required. The achievement test results can be incorporated into the syllabus using a number of strategies, such that the students are held to the contract of the syllabus and thus perform those strategies.

---

18 What should faculty do about excellent achievement test results?

Instructors should continuously monitor their courses and update them to reflect NCLEX activities. They should continue to use peer evaluation to improve their teacher-made tests and watch for slight dips in performance to be sure they are not the beginning of a downward trend.

---

19 What should students do about excellent achievement test results?

They should continue to study and review important content. They should not sit back and wait for the NCLEX to arrive; practice NCLEX-style questions to achieve a rhythm and maintain a consistently high level of performance.

---

20 What about use of mobility tests for RN-to-BSN students?

RN completion programs need a defensible strategy to justify awarding credit for RN experience. Some programs choose to require a prescribed number of years' experience for admission to the program. Some require that experience to be current, and others state within the past few years. Others accept newly graduated RNs with no experience. The mobility tests allow for documentation to note a minimum performance level as the nurse progresses through the BSN curriculum. The decision to use mobility tests depends on the niche that school is trying to fulfill in the competitive RN-to-BSN marketplace.

---

21 Suppose a program does not use achievement tests?

There is no rule that a program must use an achievement test. However, it is risky to measure a program's success only against itself. In this era of benchmarking, using achievement tests provides a means of comparing a program with its peers. Relying only on self-evaluation could result in a program that is detached from the mainstream and that produces graduates who are not competitive in the national marketplace.

---

22 What are some achievement test companies?

Arnett Development Corporation: www.arnettdevcorp.com
Assessment Technologies Institute: www.atitesting.com
Center for Nursing Education and Testing: www.cnetnurse.com
Education Resources Inc.: www.eriworld.com
Health Education Systems Inc.: www.hesitest.com
National League for Nursing: www.nln.org

Resource

Smith, J., & Crawford, L. (2006). Report of findings from the 2005 RN practice analysis: Linking the NCLEX-RN examination to practice. Chicago: National Council of State Boards of Nursing.

27

Preparing Students for the NCLEX-RN®

Loretta Manning, MSN, RN, GNP

---

1   What is the purpose of the NCLEX-RN®?

The National Council of State Boards of Nursing (NCSBN) reports that "The NCLEX-RN® is developed to ensure public protection. The examination evaluates specific competencies needed by the newly licensed, entry-level registered nurse to perform safely and effectively. The National Council of State Boards of Nursing, Inc., develops the licensure exam, the National Council Licensure Examination for Registered Nurses (NCLEX-RN®), which is used by state, commonwealth and territorial boards of nursing to assist in making licensure decisions" (NCSBN, 2007).

---

2   How does the NCSBN determine what is appropriate information to include on the NCLEX-RN®?

As reported by the NCSBN, "There are several steps that occur in the development of the *NCLEX-RN® Test Plan*. The first step is conducting a practice analysis that is used to collect data on the current practice of the entry-level" (NCSBN, 2006a).

"In the study more than six thousand newly licensed nurses were asked about the frequency and priority of performing 150 nursing care activities. An analysis was completed of the nursing activities in relation to the frequency of performance, impact on maintaining client safety and the location of the client care settings where the activities are performed. This analysis directs the development of a framework for entry-level nursing practice incorporating specific client needs in addition to processes fundamental to nursing practice. The second step of development is the development of the *NCLEX-RN®* *Test Plan.* This becomes the guide for the selection of content and behaviors to be tested" (NCSBN, 2007).

---

3   What is the structure of the Test Plan?

The NCLEX-RN® Test Plan provides an abbreviated summary of the content and scope of the licensing examination. It provides a compass for examination development as well as the preparation of the nursing student. Each NCLEX-RN® examination reflects the test plan. Each examination assesses ASK (abilities, skills, and knowledge) that are essential for the nurse to assist with client needs requiring maintenance, promotion, or restoration of health. The framework of Client Needs was selected for the examination (NCSBN, 2007).

---

4   What is meant by Client Needs?

The NCSBN selected the framework Client Needs as a universal approach for defining nursing actions and competencies crossing all settings for all clients. See Box 27–1 for the distribution of Client Needs. The NCSBN Examination Committee reviews, revises, and approves the Test Plan information every 3 years based on research reflecting changes in practice. Each revision to the Test Plan is supported by resources supporting the rationale (this chapter uses the current percentages for Client Needs from April 2007 through April, 2010 [NCSBN, 2007]). Refer to the Web site (www.ncsbn.org) for full information about the Test Plan and ongoing communication regarding revisions.

BOX 27–1

Distribution of Client Needs on the NCLEX-RN®

Safe and Effective Care Environment

Management of Care	**13%–19%**
Safety and Infection Control	**8%–14%**
Health Promotion and Maintenance	**6%–12%**
Psychosocial Integrity	**6%–12%**
Physiological Integrity	
Basic Care and Comfort	**6%–12%**
Pharmacological and Parenteral Therapies	**13%–19%**
Reduction of Risk Potential	**13%–19%**
Physiological Adaptation	**11%–17%**

---

5 Are there any other processes included with these Client Needs?

Yes, there are integrated processes integrated throughout the Client Needs categories and subcategories. These processes have been identified as being fundamental to the practice of nursing. These are listed in Box 27–2. (The exact terminology used by NCSBN is in parenthesis [NCSBN, 2007].)

6 What content is included and evaluated in these Client Need categories?

In Boxes 27–3 through 27–6 are some examples from the 2007 NCLEX-RN® Test Plan.

BOX 27–2

Integrated Processes (The 4 Cs)

Clinical-oriented, scientific problem solving (Nursing Process)
Caring
Communication and documentation
Change in behavior (Teaching and Learning)

BOX 27–3

Safe and Effective Care Environment

Management of Care

Advance Directives
Advocacy
Case Management
Client Rights
Collaboration with Interdisciplinary Team*
Concepts of Management
Confidentiality/Information Security*
Consultation
Delegation
Establishing Priorities
Information Technology**

Safety and Infection Control

Accident Prevention
Disaster Planning
Emergency Response Plan
Ergonomic Principles**
Error Prevention
Handling Hazardous and Infectious Materials
Home Safety
Injury Prevention
Medical and Surgical Asepsis
Reporting of Incident/Event /Irregular Occurrence/Variance
Safe Use of Equipment
Standard/Transmission-Based/Other Precautions

*Revised on *2007 NCLEX-RN® Test Plan*
**New concepts on *2007 NCLEX-RN® Test Plan*

---

7   The NCLEX-RN® Test Plan was revised for April 2007; what were the specific changes to the Test Plan?

As noted in the boxes, three concepts were revised (Collaboration with Interdisciplinary Team, Confidentiality/Information Security, and Chemical and Other Dependencies), and two

---

BOX 27–4

Health Promotion and Maintenance

Aging Process
Ante/Intra/Postpartum and Newborn Care
Developmental Stages and Transitions
Disease Prevention
Expected Body Image Changes
Health and Wellness
Techniques of Physical Assessment

---

new concepts were added (Information Technology and Ergonomic Principles) (NCSBN, 2006b).

8   What do these Test Plan changes mean in terms of the current nursing curriculum?

The practice of nursing is an evolving discipline. Because the practice analyses are completed every 3 years and given the minor nature of revisions on the 2007 NCLEX-RN® Test Plan, it is probably not necessary to revise your curriculum completely. The Test Plan, however, is very useful to use as a guide for nursing programs when reviewing and revising curricula because it reflects the abilities, skills, and knowledge necessary for the student/new graduate to practice effective and safe nursing care (NCSBN, 2006b).

BOX 27–5

Psychosocial Integrity

Abuse/Neglect
Behavioral Interventions
Chemical and Other Dependencies*
Coping Mechanisms
Crisis Intervention
Cultural diversity
End-of-Life Care

---

*Revised on *2007 NCLEX-RN Test Plan*

BOX 27-6

Physiological Integrity

Basic Care and Comfort

Assistive Devices
Complementary and Alternative Therapies
Elimination
Mobility/Immobility
Nonpharmacological Comfort Interventions
Nutrition and Oral Hydration

Pharmacological and Parenteral Therapies

Adverse Effects/Contraindications
Blood and Blood Products
Central Venous Access Devices
Dosage Calculation
Expected Effects/Outcomes
Medication Administration
Parenteral/Intravenous Therapies
Pharmacological Agents/Actions
Pharmacological Interactions

Reduction of Risk Potential

Diagnostic Tests
Laboratory Values
Monitoring Conscious Sedation
Potential for Alterations in Body Systems
Potential for Complications of Diagnostic Tests/Treatments/Procedures
Potential for Complications from Surgical Procedures and Health Alterations
System-Specific Assessments
Therapeutic Procedures
Vital Signs

Physiological Adaptation

Alterations in Body Systems
Fluid and Electrolyte Imbalances
Hemodynamics
Illness Management
Infectious Diseases
Medical Emergencies
Pathophysiology
Radiation Therapy
Unexpected Response to Therapy

9   Are teacher-made examinations different from the NCLEX-RN®?

Generally speaking, every faculty member is at a different developmental level in test item writing, from novice to very experienced. Most tests contain predominantly "nice-to-know" versus "needs-to-know" information. In other words, they do not reflect the activities outlined on the NCLEX-RN® Test Plan.

Many teacher-made tests also do not reflect questions at the application or higher levels of cognitive ability using Bloom's taxonomy and revised taxonomy (Anderson & Krathwohl, 2001; Bloom, et al., 1956), as utilized by the NCLEX-RN®. The majority of the NCLEX-RN® items are written at the application and analysis levels because nursing practice mandates the application of ASK. These questions require more complex thought processing than recall of simple facts.

10   What are examples of "nice-to-know" versus "need-to-know" questions?

A nice-to-know question has no link to the Activity Statements as outlined in the NCSBN Practice Analysis and does not evaluate the nursing process and/or require decision making/problem solving. See Box 27–7.

A need-to-know question, for example, evaluates the NCLEX Activity Statement "Assess/triage client(s) to prioritize the order of care delivery." See Box 27–8. The question evaluates assessment in the nursing process. Each of the distracters is a possible answer; however, Option d is the best answer because this may be indicative of a ruptured appendix. The physician will need to be notified immediately for possible extensive abdominal surgery.

11   What is an example of a question evaluating the knowledge level in contrast to the application level of the cognitive domain?

The question in Box 27–7 evaluates knowledge. The learner has to memorize this information in order to answer this

---

BOX 27–7

A Nice-to-Know Question

What purpose is an appendectomy serving?

a. Ablative
b. Constructive
c. Diagnostic
d. Palliative

---

successfully. In contrast, the question in Box 27–8 requires the student to know the clinical assessment findings for a client with appendicitis; the student also needs to know the assessment findings for a potential emergency due to a ruptured appendix. All the options are correct statements, but they do not answer the question correctly. Clients with appendicitis do present with findings in options a, b, and c. Option d is the only one that indicates a potential emergency with this diagnosis. This is also different from the question, Which assessment finding would the nurse expect a client with appendicitis to exhibit? This question would require the reader to know only the signs and symptoms of appendicitis.

---

12 Should passing the NCLEX-RN® be an identified program outcome?

Yes. The Commission on Collegiate Nursing Education, the National League for Nursing Accreditation Commission, and

---

BOX 27–8

A Need-to-Know Question

After the nurse receives report, which of these client's assessment findings, for the diagnosis of appendicitis, is most important in determining an immediate need for intervention? A client who:

a. Complains of pain in the right lower abdominal quadrant.
b. Complains of anorexia, nausea, vomiting.
c. Assumes a characteristic position of side-lying with the knees flexed.
d. **Experiences a sudden relief from pain.**

---

state boards of nurse examiners use NCLEX pass rates as criteria for accreditation (AACN, 2003; NLNAC, 2003). There are also significant financial and emotional implications for nursing graduates who are unable to achieve successful outcomes on the licensure examination (Nibert & Young, 2005; Vance & Davidhizar, 1997). Employers who provide orientation programs for newly hired graduates may also lose their investments when their new employees are unable to achieve successful outcomes on the NCLEX-RN® (Messmer, Abelleira, & Erb, 1995).

Also, the question in Box 27–8 provides an additional rationale for why passing should be a program outcome. If the plan for the NCLEX-RN® is formulated from data collected about the safe practice of entry-level nurses, then it is imperative that nursing programs incorporate these Client Needs and integrated processes throughout their curricula. Achieving positive outcomes for the graduate is a ticket to success both on the NCLEX-RN® and in clinical practice.

13 Are commercial practice tests available?

Comprehensive, commercial exit examinations are being used by many schools to assess students' readiness for the NCLEX-RN® and as a benchmark for additional remediation. (Morrison, et al., 2005). In the early 1990s, identification of students at high risk for failure and the initiation of strategic interventions in the senior year were shown to be successful strategies for preparing students for the NCLEX examination (Ashley & O'Neil, 1991; Baradell, et al., 1990; Frierson, Malone, & Shelton, 1993; Wolahan & Wieczorek, 1991).

The annual NCLEX-RN® pass rate for first-time candidates educated in the United States dropped from 90.3% to 83.8% between 1994 and 2000 (NCSBN, 2005). Furthermore, the pass rate for similar candidates educated in the United States dropped to 80% during the first quarter of 2005, suggesting that this downward trend is continuing (Sifford & McDaniel, 2007). In light of these declining pass rates, few recent studies have examined the efficacy of these comprehensive tests.

Educators need to be cautioned about using exit examinations as the only predictors of NCLEX-RN® success. Rather, they should carefully evaluate all factors that contribute to NCLEX-RN® success. If graduates are progressing through the nursing programs successfully and then fail the test, these factors must be analyzed and addressed throughout the nursing curriculum. Poor test-taking skills, poor program preparation, inadequate study habits, employment, and anxiety have been identified as factors that contribute to graduates' unsuccessful outcomes on the NCLEX (Griffiths, et al., 2004).

Continued effort needs to be directed at analyzing course examinations so that critical thinking skills required to be successful on the NCLEX-RN® are also required on teachers' examination items. Examination items must be evaluated for adhering to the Test Plan format as well as for level of difficulty. As students are challenged both in the clinical setting and by their examination items to think critically and make clinical decisions, they will be better prepared to perform successfully on the NCLEX-RN®.

It is imperative that nursing faculty do not hand over the students' future to commercial testing. This displaces faculty accountability and responsibility for helping students achieve successful outcomes on the NCLEX. The NCLEX standards must be integrated throughout the students' entire education experience, and this needs to begin on the first day, both in the classroom and in clinical. NCLEX preparation is more than just preparing for a test. It is a way of thinking, studying, and practicing nursing care. If educators begin early preparing their students to think, this will become a lifelong habit and will last much longer than the NCLEX or the classroom.

---

14 Are NCLEX-RN® review courses recommended?

Yes. Some recent research examined requirements and interventions used by BSN programs nationally to promote and predict NCLEX-RN® success. The authors found that a few of the most frequently used interventions included academic referral, commercial reviews, social support referrals, and computerized reviews They concluded that the only significant intervention was the commercial review (Crowe, et al., 2004).

This question about recommending a review course is like asking, "Do you recommend a physician or nurse practitioner for a specific medical disease?" If the provider used by a client does not have appropriate skills for managing the illness, then the care will be ineffective. Perhaps the question to ask is "How do I know if I have an effective course?" Consider these basic questions:

- What is the framework for the course? Is it organized around the Test Plan, Activity Statements, Client Needs, and integrated processes?
- What is the educational and clinical background of the facilitators for the course?
- What do previous group participants report about the class?
- What is the passing percentage for the participants who take the class?
- Does the facilitator focus on how to answer questions evaluating clinical decision making, or does the course focus only on facts?
- What is the group's strategy for maintaining a high-quality NCLEX-RN® review?

A review course, however, is only as effective as the leader of the course. The individual must be knowledgeable about the Test Plan and have a strong clinical background. The course leader must be skillful in helping the graduate to understand the testing process, develop test-taking skills, increase knowledge of content, improve clinical decision-making abilities, and increase confidence. This plan also needs to begin during the student's first nursing courses and continue through graduation.

15 Does everyone need an NCLEX-RN® review course?

No. An excellent course will connect the nursing concepts and help students with their confidence in their ability to be successful. Graduates will know what concepts they need to continue to study upon completion of the course. Review courses are for graduates who experience a high degree of test anxiety, have achieved average grades in school, repeated any nursing course, or desire a formal approach to NCLEX-RN® preparation. However, many outstanding students who experience minimal test anxiety and have graduated with honors also appreciate the NLCEX-RN® review course. The majority of them report that the course assisted them in learning how to make clinical decisions and that they have a better understanding of how to answer questions evaluating the Activity Statements on the Test Plan. They report, "I feel so much more confident, and now I know I will be successful!"

16 How can I maximize student success on the NCLEX-RN®?

The first step is to initiate curriculum mapping by using the NCLEX-RN® Test Plan. List the content areas from the NCLEX-RN® Test Plan. The next step is to link each course objective to a content area. For example, consider a component of a medical-surgical course, such as Physiological Integrity: Pharmacological and Parenteral Therapies (13%–19%)

Example of Course Objectives:

1. Review the advantages and disadvantages of various routes of medication administration.
2. Accurately calculate doses of medications.
3. Review the factors influencing drug-drug interactions and incompatibilities.

In order to maximize the student's success, these objectives must be linked to the current NCLEX-RN® Activity Statements.

Examples of NCLEX Activity Statements for each course objective:

Objective 1: Evaluate appropriateness/accuracy of medication order for client.
Objective 2: Perform calculations needed for medication administration.

Objective 3: Review pertinent data prior to medication administration (e.g., vital signs, lab results, allergies, potential interactions).

After these two steps have been implemented, it is imperative that the teaching strategies focus on the nursing concepts in the Activity Statements. The SECRET to this process is as follows (Rayfield & Manning, 2006):

S   Start where the learner is; preparation ahead of time most likely will not happen.
E   Elicit the use of images to increase memory.
C   Connect a new concept to one the learner already knows.
R   Remember to simplify the concept.
E   Empower the learner with actions to increase clients' well being.
T   Teach concepts rather than disease processes.

"Making the simple complicated is commonplace; making the complicated simple, awesomely simple, that is creativity!" Charles Mingus (jazz musician)

See Figure 27–1 for an example of applying this SECRET in teaching NCLEX-RN® activities related to pharmacology above.

This figure and mnemonic will help students remember the activities for Objectives 1 and 3. The name will assist in remembering that most cephalosporins have a "Cef" or "Ceph" in their name. The goal is to actively engage the learner in the process of learning by making connections, thus resulting in an increase in memory.

The next step in this process is to help the learner make a connection with "need to know information." This has been determined through research the NCSBN has conducted. Focus on the activities regarding the "accuracy of the order and pertinent data prior to medication administration."

The mnemonic GIANT will assist the learner in remembering the major undesirable effects of these drugs. Of course, if the client has been hypersensitive or experienced an anaphylaxis response to penicillin, then more information needs to be assessed prior to administering these drugs. The NCLEX

CEF THE GIANT

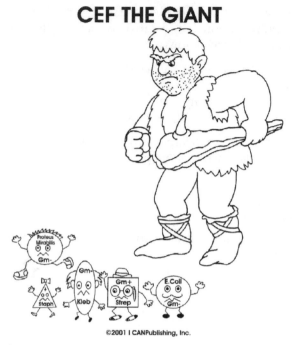

©2001 I CANPublishing, Inc.

GI: nausea, vomiting, diarrhea

I ncrease in glucose values

A naphylaxis may occur; alcohol may cause vomiting

N ephrotoxicity

T hrombocytopenia

Cef/Ceph, the "GIANT" is a powerful antibiotic that can destroy several types of bacteria and represents the 1st generation of cephalosporins. He can also produce "GIANT" undesirable effects.

Figure 27–1. CEF the giant. (Manning, L., & Rayfield, S. (2007). Pharmacology made insanely easy. Bossier City, La.: I CAN Publishing.) (Copyright 2008 I CAN Publishing, Inc. Used with permission.)

is all about client safety. If the client had a problem in the past with penicillin, the appropriate response would be to check the accuracy of the order. The learners are not *prescribing;* they are *managing* client safety. If the client who is taking these medications drinks any alcohol, there is a risk for an interaction resulting in vomiting. It is important to evaluate appropriate laboratory tests to determine if the client is experiencing any complications with nephrotoxicity or thrombocytopenia. Physical assessment findings are also pertinent with the complication of thrombocytopenia.

In review, this one teaching strategy has helped the learner remember the category of drugs (cephalosporins), the undesirable effects, potential interactions, and pertinent laboratory reports to monitor. The educator's job is to demonstrate the significance of this strategy through sample test questions, a case study, or a clinical experience.

---

17 Should I map clinical objectives to Activity Statements on the Test Plan?

Yes. Linking these activities to the clinical experience is a very powerful way to ensure that students have an appropriate clinical focus. For example, whether a student is in the pediatric, obstetrical, medical-surgical, intensive care, or community health clinical nursing curriculum, the clinical objectives should reflect the NCLEX Activity Statements. In order to demonstrate and simplify these, use the mnemonic PRIORITY (Manning & Rayfield, 2007) for the eight NCLEX-RN® (2006a) priority activities:

P   Proper client identification
R   Review pertinent data prior to medication administration
I   Infection control
O   Organize and prepare medication for administration
R   Review appropriateness/accuracy of medication order for client
I   Injury protection for client
T   Titrate/adjust dosage of medication based on assessment of physiological parameters
Y   Yes—perform emergency care procedures (e.g., CPR, Heimlich maneuver, respiratory support, automated electronic defibrillator)

The beginning nursing students (no matter what specialty they are in) should be accountable in clinical for identifying the client properly, infection control, and injury protection. When students begin to administer medications, then they will add the activities that relate to medications. Of course, this is only a small example of how to use the top activities. Review and adapt the activities as outlined in the Test Plan to your clinical objectives and evaluation tools.

---

18 How do test questions relate to mapping?

There are several approaches you may select. When matching the test items to the objectives/NCLEX-RN® activities, you may decide to link existing test questions or create new test questions. In addition to mapping the question to the activity, the item must also be constructed to measure the material at an appropriate cognitive level and within the framework of the nursing process. The cognitive levels were discussed in Question 9. Knowledge/comprehension may be used to evaluate basic nursing knowledge and the initial preparation in nursing school. Teachers need to move from these types of questions to the application/analysis level as the student progresses throughout the curriculum. The appropriate cognitive level alone without the designated activity reflected on the Test Plan cannot maximize the student's success. Both must be used together. See Box 27–9 for sample questions.

---

19 How can I remember how to prepare questions that evaluate higher-order thinking?

The word PATH can help instructors organize thoughts for developing these test items (Rayfield & Manning, 2006).

P   Plausible distracters
A   Application/Analysis
T   Thinking is multilogical
H   Has a focus on the NCLEX-RN® activities

BOX 27–9

Two Sample Questions

Question 1

Cognitive Domain: Knowledge

Nursing Process: Not present

NCLEX-RN® Activity Statement: Not present

What is the action of furosemide (Lasix)?

a. Inhibits sodium, chloride, and water reabsorption in the proximal portion of the ascending loop of Henle.
b. Promotes excretion of sodium and water but retains potassium in the distal renal tubule.
c. Increases osmotic pressure of glomerular filtrate, thus preventing reabsorption of water and increasing excretion of sodium and chloride.
d. Increases urine output by inhibiting reabsorption of sodium, chloride, and water in the distal portion of the ascending loop of Henle.

This question evaluates the memorizing of *knowledge,* which is the lowest level of cognition. The correct answer is Option a. Option b is a potassium-sparing diuretic, such as spironolactone (Aldactone). Option c is an osmotic diuretic, such as mannitol. Option d is a thiazide diuretic, such as chlorothiazide (Diuril).

Question 2

Cognitive Domain: Application

Nursing Process: Evaluation

NCLEX-RN® Activity Statement: Evaluate client's response to medications

The nurse administered furosemide (Lasix) to a client with congestive heart failure. Which of these clinical findings would be most important in determining the effectiveness of this medication?

a. Intake and output.
b. Skin turgor.
c. Urine specific gravity.
d. Weight of the client.

The question evaluates *application.* The reader must understand what the action of Lasix is and the pathophysiology of heart failure. The correct answer is Option d due to peripheral edema being a clinical finding with heart failure. When the heart is unable to pump effectively, the blood pools in the extremities, resulting in peripheral edema and a weight gain. Option a is incorrect because even if the client does void a large amount of urine, this does not quantify the client's physical response from the medication. Options b and c do not answer the question. They focus on the quality of hydration.

- **Plausible distracters:** Distracters should represent interventions or options (i.e., assessments, plans, etc.) that are appropriate for the client and/or condition described in the stem of the question. The reader must discriminate from similar options in order to identify the priority. This can be challenging for the novice, who is looking for one correct answer.
- **Application/Analysis:** The majority of the NCLEX items are written at the application or a higher cognitive level (Bloom's cognitive levels). These items require the learner to apply or analyze nursing knowledge.
- **Thinking is multilogical:** This means the question requires an understanding of application and knowledge of a minimum of two concepts to answer successfully.
- **Has a focus on the NCLEX-RN® activities:** Refer to the test plan (NCSBN, 2007).

20 Should all my questions be multiple-choice?

While the majority of items on the NCLEX® examination are multiple-choice questions, there also are alternate item formats. These questions may include fill-in-the-blank, hot spot, multiple-response, and drag-and-drop/ordered response items as well as chart/exhibit format. Refer to the NCSBN Web site at www.ncsbn.org for updated information. Examples of these questions are on the Web site.

21 What are your thoughts about writing true/false and matching questions?

Avoid these two formats because they evaluate basic knowledge. Including some alternate item formats in your tests will be beneficial for the student to begin experiencing this new format. The majority of your questions should be multiple-choice because this format evaluates the student's ability to think. This will continue to assist the student in experiencing how to successfully answer questions evaluating clinical decision making.

22 Are there any particular references for preparing students for the NCLEX-RN®?

In addition to those on the NCSBN Web site (www.ncsbn. org), consider the following:

Anderson, L.W., Krathwohl, D.R. (Eds.) (2001). A taxonomy for learning, teaching, and assessing: A revision of Bloom's taxonomy of educational objectives. New York: Addison Wesley Longman, Inc.

National Council of State Boards of Nursing, Inc. (April 2007). Test plan for the National Council Licensure Examination for Registered Nurses.

National Council of State Boards of Nursing, Inc. (March 2006). NCSBN research brief, vol. 21. Report of findings from the 2005 RN practice analysis: Linking the NCLEX-RN® examination to practice. Chicago: Author.

23 How can I contact the National Council of State Boards of Nursing for this information?

Web: www.ncsbn.org
Address: NCSBN, 111 E. Wacker Drive, Suite 2900, Chicago, Ill., 60601-4277
Phone: (312) 525-3660
Testing Services toll-free: (866) 293-9600

References

American Association of Colleges of Nursing. (2003). CCNE accreditation standards: AACN-CCNE (online). Available at www.aacn.nche.edu/Accreditation/standards.htm

Ashley, J., & O'Neil, J. (1991). The effectiveness of an intervention to promote successful performance on NCLEX-RN for baccalaureate students at risk for failure. Journal of Nursing Education 30(8), 360–365.

Baradell, J.G., et al. (1990). A comprehensive approach to preparation for NCLEX-RN. Journal of Nursing Education 29(3), 109–113.

Bloom, B.S., et al. (1956). Taxonomy of educational objectives: The classification of educational goals. Handbook I: Cognitive Domain. New York: David McKay.

Crowe, S.C., et al. (2004). Requirements and interventions used by BSN programs to promote and predict NCELX-RN success: A national study. Journal of Professional Nursing 20(3), 174–186.

Frierson, H.T., Malone B., & Shelton, P. (1993). Enhancing NCLEX-RN performance by assessing a three-pronged intervention approach. Journal of Professional Nursing 32(5), 222–224.

Griffiths, M.J., et al. (2004). The lived experience of NCLEX failure. Journal of Nursing Education 43(7), 322–325.

Manning, L., & Rayfield, S. (2007). Pharmacology made insanely easy. Bossier City, La.: I CAN Publishing.

Messmer, P., Abelleira, A., & Erb, P. (1995). Code 50: An orientation matrix to track orientation cost. Journal of Nursing Staff Development 11, 261–264.

Morrison, S., et al. (2005). HESI exams: An overview of reliability and validity. Nurse Educator 30(35), 395–455.

National Council of State Boards of Nursing. (2005). NCLEX statistics from NCSBN. Available at www.ncsbn.org/pdfs/NCLEX_fact_sheet.pdf.

National Council of State Boards of Nursing. (2006). Frequently asked questions about the 2007 NCLEX-RN® test plan. Available at www.ncsbn.org (NCSBN NCLEX Examinations Department).

National League for Nursing Accrediting Commission. (2003). Accreditation standards and criteria for academic quality for post-secondary and higher degree programs in nursing. New York: Author.

Nibert, A.T., & Young. A. (2005). A third study on predicting NCLEX success with the HESI exit exam. Nurse Educator 30(35), 521–527.

Rayfield, S., & Manning, L. (2006). Pathways of teaching nursing: Keeping it real! Bossier City, La.: I CAN Publishing, Inc.

Sifford, S., & McDaniel, D. (January and February 2007). Results of a remediation program for students at risk for failure on the NCLEX exam. Nursing Education Perspectives 28(1), 34.

Vance, A., & Davidhizar; R. (1997). Strategies to assist students to be successful the next time around on the NCLEX-RN. Journal of Nursing Education 36, 190–192.

Wolahan, C.G.H., & Wieczorek, R.R. (1991). Enrichment education: Key to NCLEX success. Nursing and Health Care 12(5), 234–239.

V

RECURRENT THEMES IN TEACHING NURSING

28

Facilitating Critical Thinking and Effective Reasoning

Pamela B. Webber, PhD, RN, CFNP

---

1 Where did the notion of critical thinking come from?

One of the most significant trends in nursing over the past 20 years has been the emphasis on more efficient and effective thinking in clinical situations. This trend emerged, in part, because of demands by health-care agencies that nurses be able to think and act more effectively and independently in a diverse and rapidly changing workplace. In response to this demand, the American Association of Colleges of Nursing (AACN) included critical thinking in its 1986 *Essentials of Baccalaureate Nursing* and subsequent essential documents. In addition, the National League for Nursing (NLN) (1992) included outcome criteria in its accreditation guidelines that placed emphasis on evaluation of students' ability to think critically. These and other nursing agencies continue to emphasize the importance of critical thinking in nursing. Unfortunately, while many people and organizations have talked and written about improving critical thinking over the last 20 years, there does not appear to be a significant corresponding improvement in clinical outcomes. There are many possible reasons for this, some of which are considered in this chapter.

---

2   Has the critical thinking movement universally been endorsed?

No. Some authors, such as Morin (1997), Tanner (1999), and Riddell (2007), urged caution in emphasizing critical thinking, given the lack of a clear definition, conceptual clarity, and reliable and valid methods of measuring it. Unfortunately, these and other words of caution were overwhelmed by the need to satisfy accreditation criteria and by nursing's willingness to jump first and investigate later.

---

3   Why are there so many synonyms for critical thinking?

Although the NLN and AACN were very effective in getting the phrase "critical thinking" disseminated, they failed to provide operational or even conceptual definitions (Scheffer and Rubenfeld, 2000; Scheffer, 2006; Riddell, 2007). As a result, schools of nursing and health-care facilities were encouraged to define critical thinking operationally within the context of their individual programs, goals, curricula, desired outcomes, and faculty beliefs. On one hand, this freedom was empowering to a nursing education system that had struggled in the past with rigid and prescriptive curriculum guidelines. On the other hand, however, this eclectic approach created a series of problems that the profession is still trying to address. Specifically, nursing collectively could not gain consensus on what critical thinking is and is not. Many schools defined critical thinking with descriptive words and phrases such as *critical analysis, clinical judgment, decision making, problem solving, evaluation, nursing process, reflection, concept mapping, logic mapping, and reasoning* (just to name a few). They then proceeded to use these same words and phrases as interchangeable synonyms for critical thinking. This blurring of meanings distorted understanding about what constitutes effective thinking in nursing and confused faculty, students, and nurses alike. Critical thinking is not one "monolithic thing" but has evolved into an "umbrella term" representing many diverse meanings and activities (Walsh & Seldomridge, 2006, p. 216). Unfortunately, the failure to clarify this essential skill has dramatically influenced the ability to teach and measure it in both education and practice.

---

4   What factors influenced how critical thinking is defined?

Since the movement of nursing education into university settings in the mid-20th century and the parallel movement toward developing nursing scholarship through the implementation and utilization of nursing research, nursing has had a strong scientific and quantitative slant. This is primarily because most early nursing research was modeled on quantitatively-based methodologies used in the traditional science disciplines. This predisposed nursing toward the belief that critical thinking is the resolution of clearly defined problems with easily identifiable solutions. Interesting, the more complex nursing and health care became, the less effective this scientifically rigid approach to thinking became. Strict association of critical thinking with scientific and quantitative methodologies was and is beneficial in the analysis of specific and empirically-based nursing phenomena; however, the more nursing scholars and expert practitioners learned, the more they realized that nursing included more than concrete and empirically based phenomena and began to question whether the phrase "critical thinking" really reflected the realities of practice. As a result, the use of other words, such as reasoning, which has broader meaning and application, began to emerge. While "critical thinking" is sometimes used synonymously with or in lieu of "reasoning," it is more of a foundational component of reasoning than a synonym. The scientific or quantitative aspects of phenomena can be understood without the complexity and significance of the qualitative and experiential aspects of the same phenomena also being understood. For example, physiological parameters such as vital signs and cardiac output in an intensive care patient can be quantified, but those numbers cannot explain the impact of the patient's faith on his recovery, nor can they explain the intuitive and experiential behaviors that an expert nurse might exhibit when providing care.

---

5   What is the language of thinking and reasoning?

The language of reasoning is one that is shared with theory and research and constitutes the basis of the knowledge typology. While there are many words and phrases in this typology, several are considered essential building blocks, such as *phenomena, ideas, concepts, variables,* and *propositions.* Words and meanings within the language are usually sequential and progressive in nature and provide order and structure when developing essential reasoning skill (Table 28–1). The following paragraphs review these building blocks, how they relate to one another, and how they influence reasoning in the clinical setting.

- **What are phenomena?**

Phenomena are observable connections or relationships between objects, events, ideas, or people. It is reasoning that enables you to recognize phenomena when they occur and make a determination about their significance. For example, observing that a postoperative surgical wound is red and swollen and observing that hospitalized children

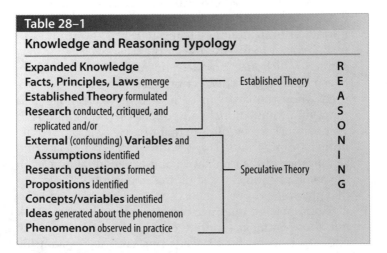

Table 28–1

Knowledge and Reasoning Typology

Expanded Knowledge		R
Facts, Principles, Laws emerge	Established Theory	E
Established Theory formulated		A
Research conducted, critiqued, and		S
replicated and/or		O
External (confounding) **Variables** and		N
Assumptions identified		I
Research questions formed	Speculative Theory	N
Propositions identified		G
Concepts/variables identified		
Ideas generated about the phenomenon		
Phenomenon observed in practice		

eat better when their mothers are present constitute recognition of the types of phenomena observed by nurses every day; however, they are seldom called phenomena. Instead, they are commonly called assessment data, problems, or simple observations.

A subtype of phenomena, called *noumena*, represents awareness of a connection or relationship between objects, events, ideas, or people, but the connection or relationship is a perception rather than an observation of things. For example, perceptions of intuitiveness, faith, feelings, and beliefs in patients and nurses influence their interactions and behaviors. For the sake of simplicity, "phenomena" is used for this chapter.

- **How do phenomena generate ideas, and why are ideas important?**

Once phenomena are observed, it is logical to generate thoughts or *ideas* about their origin, characteristics, and significance. As Example 1, if you observed a postoperative patient with a red and swollen surgical wound, you would use your established knowledge of microbiological theory to generate the idea that the wound is infected. As Example 2, if you observed that hospitalized children eat better when their mothers are present, you might generate the idea that having mothers present at mealtime is therapeutic and may shorten the child's hospital stay. In time, this idea may provide the basis of a clinical research study. Creative reasoning stimulates the formation of ideas that may become answers to questions, solutions to problems, and provide a way of exploring clinical phenomena further.

- **What are concepts, and how are they related to ideas?**

While phenomena are the source of ideas, *concepts* are the components of an idea. Concepts name and frame, or set boundaries for, an idea and usually consist of two or more descriptive words or phrases. Concepts included in the previous examples include:

- Example 1
  - Red, swollen surgical wound
  - Postoperative infection

- Example 2
  - Hospitalized child
  - Presence of mother
  - Amount of food being eaten by the child

Observable relationships among concepts are commonly described as *conceptual relationships*. Examples of conceptual relationships include:

- Example 1
  - Surgical wounds that are red and swollen may represent a postoperative infection.

- Example 2
  - The presence of mothers influence the amount of food eaten by hospitalized children.

The identification of concepts and conceptual relationships is not hard to do if students and faculty alike begin to look at clinical events in terms of observing and identifying phenomena and then naming and framing the components of the phenomena in terms of concepts and conceptual relationships. Clinical faculty frequently discuss diseases, signs, symptoms, and nursing interventions, but they seldom do so within the context of the common language of theory, research, reasoning, and practice, which further interferes with students' understanding of their essential interrelationships.

- **What are variables, and how are they related to concepts?**

Most concepts have the potential to vary in their characteristics; as a result, they are referred to as *variables*. The term *variables* is commonly used in research, but seldom used in the clinical setting, even though it applies. For example, the amount of redness and swelling associated with an infected surgical wound can vary, as can the amount of food that a child eats. Variables that are included within a proposition being examined are sometimes called *internal variables*.

- **Is there usually an element of cause and effect among internal variables?**

Whereas relationships among concepts are called *conceptual relationships,* relationships among variables that have direction are commonly called *propositions.* Direction means that one variable is influencing another variable. For example, infection causes postoperative wounds to be red and swollen, and mothers cause hospitalized children to eat better. In these propositions, there is a directional association, or a cause-and-effect relationship. In many cases, variables within propositions are measurable, which makes them potential research questions. Variables in a cause-and-effect relationship are considered to be either independent or dependent. *Independent variables* are those that influence or cause something to happen to a dependent variable. For example, infection is the independent variable that influences the dependent variables of redness and swelling, and mothers are the independent variable that influences the dependent variable of the amount of food that hospitalized children eat.

Effective reasoning in clinical situations involves determining the characteristics and boundaries of the variables involved and the nature and direction of their relationships. Teaching students to identify variables and to put them into directional relationships is a fundamental aspect of teaching them to reason effectively and establishes the basis for their understanding where and how their interventions are needed. In addition, it provides the basis by which students develop an understanding of the beginning stages of the research process. It all starts with the observation of phenomena, followed by naming and framing of involved variables, and then putting the variables into directional relationships.

- **What other types of variables influence reasoning?**

There are often variables outside the proposition created by the independent and dependent variables that have the potential to influence it. These variables are called *external* or *confounding variables.* Confounding variables have the ability to influence internal variables within propositions and ultimately the proposition itself. For example, your thinking about the redness and swelling in a surgical wound may be influenced by the fact that there is a methicillin-resistant *Staphylococcus aureus* (MRSA) outbreak on your unit. You think that now you have the possibility of an MRSA-infected wound. Instead of the independent variable being a simple infection, it is now an MRSA infection, which requires more complex treatment and nursing care. Another example of a confounding variable is the hospitalized child who snacks heavily on candy and, as a result, is not hungry when his mother comes in at mealtime. The confounding variable of snacking heavily influences the relationship of hospitalized children eating better when their mothers are present. The identification and analysis of independent, dependent, and confounding variables and their actual and potential relationships to a particular idea requires the ability to reason effectively.

- **What are assumptions, and how do they influence propositions?**

Assumptions are variables that are assumed to be true and are included as essential components of reasoning. For example, we assume the sun is going to come up tomorrow and plan our day accordingly. In nursing, we assume that everyone taking care of hospitalized patients wants the most positive outcome for that patient and plan our care accordingly. Somewhere during your education and practice you may have been told not to assume or make assumptions; the implication being that assumptions cause one to "jump to conclusions" and are therefore undesirable. In fact, we do want to identify them and determine how they might be influencing variables and propositions we are examining. Identifying and understanding assumptions that have the potential to significantly influence one or more of the variables and, thus, the proposition being examined is essential to effective reasoning. For example, you might assume that redness and swelling of a surgical wound is related to an MRSA and place the patient in isolation. However, if the wound is cultured, the culture comes back negative for MRSA, and the redness and swelling are determined to simply be an allergic response to the suture material, then your assumption is wrong, and you have put a patient through unnecessary treatment and expense. You could also assume that the relationship between a mother and hospitalized child is a nurturing one when in reality it may be an abusive one. Assumptions of this nature have the potential to influence reasoning and actual nursing care for patients and need to be identified and considered when making decisions about care. Whether you are caring for a patient or designing a research study, failure to identify assumptions and evaluate their potential impact could have a costly effect.

6   Why is this language not used more often?

The processes of observing and identifying phenomena; generating ideas; and naming and framing concepts, variables, propositions, and assumptions require an advanced level of reasoning and become particularly important when answering questions, solving problems, and exploring phenomena in nursing practice. Unfortunately, the profession assumes that everyone knows and understands these words, meanings, and relationships, when in fact many practicing nurses and nursing educators do not know, understand, or use these terms in a competent way. In a recent study on research language competency, Webber and Wanant demonstrated that some faculty teaching in baccalaureate and higher degree nursing programs could not adequately define essential words (phenomena, concept, variables, propositions, etc.) associated with theory, research, and reasoning, nor could they describe the inter-relationships among these terms; however, many of these same faculty members indicated that they used these terms frequently in class and clinical. Nursing education must assume a significant portion of the responsibility for this disconnection. Some nursing educators have written books or provided models on how to think or reason critically. However, few, if any, of these books and models include the language of theory, research, and reasoning. Failure to integrate this essential language has led to persistent gaps in understanding the sequential and progressive structure and order of theory, research, and reasoning and how they are operationalized in practice. This is not to say that nurses do not develop expert reasoning skills; they do; however, they more than likely develop this skill through the trial and error of experience and self-teaching, not because the nurses were taught. It is also apparent that at times even expert nurses are unable to analyze their thinking within the context of variables, propositions, assumptions, and so on. As a result, they struggle with implementing and utilizing research and other theoretical information into their practice. With the increasing emphasis on evidence-based practice, and evidence being defined largely as research outcomes, the lack of skill in recognizing and using this fundamental language will become more apparent. That is why it is critical for you to master the language and facilitate its correct use in students and peers.

---

7 How can effective reasoning be measured in students?

What does effective reasoning specifically allow teachers and students to do in the clinical and classroom setting? In nursing, effective reasoning provides the basis for the selection of nursing actions, and these nursing actions then constitute the outcomes of reasoning. Just as the language of reasoning develops progressively and sequentially, so do the outcomes of reasoning, as demonstrated in Table 28–2 (Johnson & Webber, 2005).

Table 28–2

Progressive and Sequential Outcomes of Reasoning

Control
    Influence
        Predict
            Explain
                Understand
                    Relate
                        Identify
                            Observe

8   Explain each step in the sequence.

Simply speaking, reasoning enables nurses to **identify** independent and dependent variables, confounding variables, and assumptions associated with a particular phenomenon observed in practice. They put these variables into relationship by **relating** them to one another in the form of propositions and work to **understand** the significance of those relationships to the health and well-being of the patients for whom they are caring. The nurses use their understanding to **explain** (interpret and translate) the significance and possible outcomes of these propositions to others, including patients, families, peer, and providers. They may also **predict** outcomes of similar propositions in future situations. Frequently, nurses make decisions and take actions designed to **influence** or **control** one or more variables within a clinical situation in order to bring about a desired outcome. The progressive nature of this type of reasoning is demonstrated in Table 28–3 (Johnson & Webber, 2005).

For example, a nurse may identify a potentially infected wound by noting redness and swelling (**identification of phenomena; naming and framing concepts and propositions**). Because the nurse realizes the significance of these findings to the well-being of the patient, the nurse notifies the physician, obtains appropriate orders

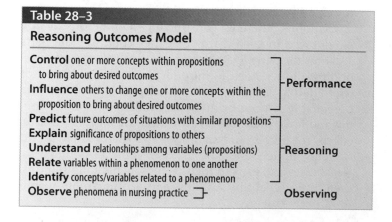

Table 28–3

Reasoning Outcomes Model

Control one or more concepts within propositions to bring about desired outcomes	**Performance**
Influence others to change one or more concepts within the proposition to bring about desired outcomes	
Predict future outcomes of situations with similar propositions	**Reasoning**
Explain significance of propositions to others	
Understand relationships among variables (propositions)	
Relate variables within a phenomenon to one another	
Identify concepts/variables related to a phenomenon	
Observe phenomena in nursing practice	**Observing**

for culturing the wound, places the patient on wound and skin precautions, determines patient allergies, and starts intravenous antibiotic therapy ordered by the physician. The nurse then discusses the situation with the patient and the family and explains in detail what is being done and why as well as what will happen if these procedures are not done (**the nurse understands, explains, predicts, and influences the situation**). Teaching this fundamental process will assist students in developing their ability to reason effectively in clinical situations.

---

9   How can I facilitate the development of this level of reasoning skill?

One of the best methods of teaching can be traced to ancient Greek philosophers and teachers, Socrates, his student Plato, and Plato's student, Aristotle. In studying the key topics of the day, such as justice and religion, Socrates encouraged his students to replace their vague, unsubstantiated thoughts and opinions with information founded in truth and reality. To accomplish this, he initiated, and Plato and Aristotle continued, a method of teaching and learning through inquiry known as the **Socratic method**. This method involves teaching students to study phenomena by exploring "who, what, when, where, why, and what if" types of questions and insisting that students define, describe, clarify, relate, explain, and justify their opinions. This approach encouraged Socrates' students to be specific in identifying concepts, variables, propositions, and assumptions, thereby constructing and deconstructing phenomena in such a way that they could see the parts and how the parts relate to one another. This type of questioning allowed for the introduction and exploration of confounding variables and assumptions that had the potential to change or influence students' original thinking and force them to look for multidimensional causes, effects, meanings, and significance. Socrates knew that if students understood the nature, context, boundaries, weaknesses and gaps in their own thoughts and opinions, then truth, reliability, validity, and accountability would most likely emerge.

10 How do teaching and learning through inquiry apply today?

Effective nursing educators use inquiry to explore and deconstruct nursing phenomena and, in so doing, they teach students to analyze independent and dependent variables within propositions, confounding variables, and assumptions, and then determine the significance of these elements within specific clinical situations. In addition, students are taught how to influence or control one or more of the involved variables in order to bring about a desired outcome. As a teacher of nurses, it is important that you train your students to use this basic method of learning through inquiry in order to ensure structure and thoroughness of thought, reliability, and validity in their reasoning that can be used throughout their careers.

11 What is patterning, and how does it influence reasoning?

An effective method of facilitating the development of reasoning skills in students is to teach them to identify patterns. Patterns are recurring variables, propositions, or assumptions within similar situations. Knowledge used in nursing, such as nursing and biological theory, has unique embedded patterns that students can be taught to discern. Once a pattern is identified, students can begin to determine, through reasoning, the significance of the pattern to patient care. Analyzing variables in patterns and using that analysis to guide nursing actions and predict future outcomes is called *trending*. For example, as a clinical exercise, ask your students to trend the following variables concerning a postoperative patient who is not deep-breathing and is refusing to ambulate. The patient is a heavy smoker with a history of chronic bronchitis.

Using teaching through inquiry, ask the students to identify essential independent and dependent variables, propositions, confounding variables, and assumptions involved by posing the following questions:

• What are the variables involved?
• Which variables are independent, dependent, and confounding?

Data	Baseline on Admission	Prior to Surgery	12 Hours Postoperative	24 Hours Postoperative	36 Hours Postoperative	What Is the Pattern?
Blood pressure	150/92	144/88	140/82	122/82	118/74	↓
Heart rate	88	90	96	108	120	↑
Ventilatory rate	24	22	26	28	30	↑
Temperature	98	98	99	99	99	Normal to ↑
Breath sounds	Normal	Normal	Diminished at bases	Diminished at bases	Diminished throughout	↓
Pain scale	0	0	9	8	7	↓

- What patterns can they identify?
- What is the significance of the patient's history and postoperative activity?
- What is the significance of the trend in the pattern?
- What assumptions are being made?
- What are the possible consequences if one or more of the variables in this situation are not changed?

Junior and senior nursing students would most likely determine that, in the absence of bleeding and other postoperative complications, the trended data are most likely the result of the patient's reluctance to deep-breathe and ambulate because of the pain combined with the patient's history of smoking and chronic bronchitis. They could further determine the significance of these patterns to the patient's current health status. For example, students should be able to identify that the patient is most likely hypoventilating, which is decreasing the oxygen level and resulting in a compensatory increase in the ventilatory rate and tachycardia. The tachycardia, in turn, results in decreased cardiac output and a lower blood pressure over time. Once the student has put all these propositions together and determined the significance of these patterns to the patient, the student should be able to predict what could happen to the patient if these trends are allowed to continue. In addition, the student should be able to identify specific nursing interventions to influence or control one or more of the variables in this situation in an attempt to improve this patient's outcomes, such as initiating the following patient care measures:

- Create a turning and coughing schedule every 2 hours
- Assess breath sounds every 2 hours and as needed
- Develop a deep-breathing schedule with use of an incentive spirometer ten times every waking hour
- Monitor for possible development of pneumonia
- Ambulate the patient every 4 hours or more often
- Talk with the physician or nurse practitioner about obtaining a chest x-ray and arterial blood gases or using an oxygen saturation monitor and subsequent use of aerosol therapy, supplemental oxygen, and so on

Learning to trend patterns helps students reason in an organized manner and be specific about the design of their nursing interventions. Perhaps most important, it focuses the students on prevention. Students who trend patterns similar to this case would probably never have to be reminded again about the need to turn, cough, deep-breathe, and ambulate postoperative patients, especially those who smoke and have a problematic history.

12 Are there different types of reasoning; if so, which is best for students to use?

There are several types of reasoning. The two most common types are deductive and inductive and, although they are different, they are often used in combination. With **deductive reasoning**, students use established knowledge (facts, principles, and laws) when analyzing and explaining phenomena, concepts, propositions, and so forth. With deductive reasoning, outcomes are presumed to be true because the facts, principles, and laws used to explain them are considered to be true. For example, a student who sees a red and swollen surgical wound may deduce that these are signs of infection. Students primarily use deductive reasoning while in school because it is a safe way to make clinical decisions, and because most nursing faculty teach that way.

The second most common type of reasoning is called **inductive reasoning.** Students make observations about a particular phenomenon and begin to identify variables and propositions that lead to new and creative answers and solutions. For example, a student may observe that visitors going in and out of a child's room are sneaking candy into the child. The student may work with the child to set up a system by which every time the child refuses candy, the nurse will allow 15 more minutes of television at night, an extra trip to the toy room, or a ride in a wheelchair around the hospital. There is also an amount of uncertainty with inductive reasoning because of its speculative nature. However, inductive reasoning encourages creativity and use of imagination within nursing practice. While there are other types of reasoning, deductive and inductive provide the basic foundation and are easy to teach and evaluate in nursing students.

13 How quickly should students develop the ability to reason effectively?

Reasoning skill may develop slowly or quickly depending on students' cognitive level, their ability to operationalize the language and meanings in practice, and their ability to learn through formal inquiry. The more they practice using the language and formal inquiry in classroom and clinical discussions, written assignments, and evaluation tools, the better their reasoning skills will become.

14 What factors influence students' ability to reason effectively?

There are several factors that provide direction and structure for reasoning in nursing. These factors include nursing knowledge, skills, values, meanings, and experiences (KSVME) and personal KSVME (Webber, 2002; Johnson & Webber, 2005; Webber, et al., 2007).

- **Knowledge.** While it may seem repetitive to have knowledge as a factor that influences reasoning, the fact remains that students have to have some knowledge before they can apply it even at an elementary level, and it is anticipated that the level of students' knowledge will continually grow and develop. Students have to have at least fundamental knowledge about nursing to be able to identify basic concepts or variables relevant in clinical situations. As students read, study, and take more classes, their knowledge grows, and the more variables and assumptions they will be able to identify and relate in clinical situations. For example, students take a course in microbiology and apply what they learn when studying the difference between aseptic and sterile technique, changing sterile dressings on a burn victim, and administering antibiotics to a patient who is in septic shock. Knowledge is not static; it is dynamic and constantly evolving. As a result, reasoning that utilizes knowledge is also constantly evolving.

- **Skills.** It is commonly assumed that the word *skill* means how well something is done and implies action more than thought. However, the term originated from an Old Norse word that means demonstration of knowledge, which shows the intricate relationship between action and thought. Nowhere is this more important than in health care. Knowledge is operationalized through skill, and skill must be rooted in knowledge. Nursing skills are intentional acts or activities implemented for, with, or on behalf of patients. The application of skills requires reasoning that reflects nursing knowledge, values, meanings, and experiences. Nursing skills have historically been viewed as technical acts, such as bed baths and bed making. Now, nursing skills have both an intellectual and technical dimension and are dependent on effective reasoning. What constitutes nursing skills has evolved and become more sophisticated over time to include not just the traditional psychomotor activities, but also more intellectually complex activities such as the effective application of theory and knowledge in meeting diverse patient care needs;

utilization of research findings in practice; communication with other health-care professionals, patients, and families; management of patient care; and financial stewardship. Even reasoning is considered a skill that is to be continually developed.

A concept often associated with skill development is that of **competency,** or level of ability in implementing skills. In nursing, competency is defined as the ability to think and act effectively and safely and is not synonymous with experience. Competency requires continual development of nursing knowledge, skills, values, meaning, and experiences, and the application of these when identifying, relating, understanding, explaining, predicting, influencing, and/or controlling nursing phenomena. It is assumed that when students pass the National Council for Licensure Examination–RN®, they are competent enough to protect the safety of the public. However, competency in basic patient safety does not equate to the level of competency associated with expert practice that takes years of experience and active learning to develop.

In nurturing the development of competency in students, you must first realize that competency is not instantaneous. Teaching the theoretical basis of a skill is a relatively quick process. Perfecting the performance of that skill takes time and experience. When working with students, remember that developing competency may not be measured in the perfect performance of each and every skill but in the fact that students recognize what they do not know about implementing a particular skill and seek appropriate resources such as their clinical faculty and policy and procedure manuals to fill in the gaps in their knowledge.

- **Values** are enduring beliefs that establish the moral and ethical boundaries of what is right and wrong. These beliefs establish guidelines for value-based reasoning. Values develop over time based on individual, family, social, cultural, and religious influences. In addition, they provide a sense of individuality as well as a sense of community with those who share the same or similar values. Values shared by individuals within a particular profession, such as nursing, reflect important beliefs of that profession and are usually stated in the form of professional standards. Nursing values include concern for others; truth and honesty; integrity; ethical thought and behavior; personal choice; dignity; and justice. Nursing values guide behavior and influence reasoning in nursing situations and have become a significant part of nursing's professional identity. Nursing faculty should model these values and facilitate their development in students.

Nursing values also include the concept of **care** and **caring**, which means to have concern for, protect, and accept responsibility for others. Nurses care through the intentional application of nursing knowledge, skills, values, meanings, and experiences. The intent to care guides all reasoning in nursing. Caring motivates nurses to want to identify, relate, understand, explain, influence, and control nursing phenomena. Unfortunately, you cannot assume that students have the ability to care in a way that is meaningful to nursing. Their ability to care must be assessed and nurtured as with any other nursing skill.

- **Meanings.** Meanings define the purpose and intent of language, the study of which is called hermeneutics. Hermeneutics is named for the Greek god Hermes, who in Greek mythology delivered and interpreted messages from the gods for people on Earth. Hermeneutics allows for the selection, adaptation, and organization of verbal and nonverbal language and meanings into a subset within existing language, such as nursing language and meanings. These unique subsets convey what is epistemologically important to a particular discipline. For example, nursing, medicine, and law each have a specific language to meet their particular needs. All professions, including nursing, medicine, and law, have unique words and meanings, acronyms, abbreviations, and symbols that have significance to them. For example, Florence Nightingale, the mother of modern nursing, was known as the "lady with the lamp" because of her diligent and dedicated nursing of wounded and dying soldiers during the Crimean War (Bostridge, 2007); therefore, the lamp has special meaning and significance to nurses.

Nursing language is derived from its knowledge, skills, values, and experiences and is shared among all nurses. It characteristically includes acronyms, abbreviations, symbols, and unique meanings that are used in nursing texts, journals, and in daily conversations among nurses. For example, what does it mean when nurses say they care or when they describe themselves as professional? How does this differ from physicians who describe themselves as professionals who care? Nurses assign meaning and significance to nursing situations through the utilization of nursing knowledge, skills, values, and experiences. Once meaning is assigned, it becomes the basis for nursing action. Students are constantly learning and internalizing what it means to be a nurse, and they will look to you to interpret meanings they do not understand. Faculty awareness that students do not always know the meanings of words, events, and actions encountered in nursing practice and making sure that they receive an adequate introduction to new and specialized meanings is essential to student development. For example, nursing uses a tremendous number of acronyms that students simply may not know.

- **Experience** usually refers to the length of time in a particular position. However, the role experience plays in learning is much more complex than this definition represents. Nursing experience refers to the process of continually developing knowledge, skills, values, and meanings used in clinical reasoning as a result of actively engaging in nursing situations over time. It is the change that occurs that defines experience, not only the passage of time. Experience is filled with successes and failures, and it is how students and faculty cope with experience that is crucial to learning. Students usually compensate for the lack of experience by relying on established knowledge and maintaining a certain amount of rigidity in their thinking. As they gain more confidence and move toward a higher level of competency, they begin to integrate experiential understanding into their practice. Experience, as defined by change, cannot be provided by faculty. Each clinical experience has the potential to teach students something if they are paying attention. As a faculty member, you can plan classroom experiences and schedule clinical time, but the student has to become actively and intellectually involved in the experience if growth is going to occur.

15   What role does nursing process play in reasoning?

Reasoning allows students and nurses to use their personal and professional KSVME to identify, relate, understand, explain, predict, influence, and/or control phenomena in nursing. The question many people ask at this point is where does the nursing process fit into all of this? The answer lies in the identification of propositions among variables. However, to understand this connection, the nursing process must be reviewed. The nursing process (and its components of assessment, planning, implementing, and evaluating) has been used for decades as a means of introducing nursing students to basic problem solving. The key word in this phrase is *process*, which usually means ordered activities or steps. When using the nursing process, students learn to identify and build ordered and directional relationships among variables. For example, students collect patient assessment data and then put that data into relationship with specific patient and nursing problems. They then plan, implement, and evaluate care designed to address these problems. However, although these steps help students develop focused and logical thinking, the nursing process is not without limitations. The most obvious limitation is that it predisposes students to basic problem-oriented thinking or the resolution of isolated problems with clearly defined solutions, which is not reflective of actual nursing practice. Nursing process is valuable when helping students identify significant variables and relationships; however, it does not support more complex, multidimensional reasoning necessary for nursing practice today, which is the most likely reason why nurses practice without it.

16 Where does nursing diagnosis come into play?

Nursing diagnosis was added to the original steps of the nursing process in the 1970s, which paralleled the onset of widespread use of computers in health care. The decision to add nursing diagnosis was influenced by the need for nursing to have a common language that could be stored as computer data. Nursing diagnoses categorize common patient problems according to prescribed categories. The validity of nursing diagnosis has come under serious question over the past two decades because of its rigid, esoteric language, its "canned" approach to thinking, and the fact that practicing nurses simply do not use it at the bedside. Having students match and copy nursing diagnosis phrases directly out of textbooks or from a computer drastically limits thinking and is inconsistent with facilitating upper-level reasoning skills. The unfortunate reality is that nursing diagnosis language is embedded in textbooks and in the computerized documentation systems of health-care agencies, which means that practicing nurses do what they must do with nursing diagnosis in computerized documentation systems and then proceed to actually practice without it.

So what do you do when teaching students? Until the profession can successfully remove nursing diagnosis from textbooks and patient care documentation systems, educators should ensure that students know the minimum nursing diagnosis language that they may see in the NCLEX-RN® and current patient care documentation systems. Most important, educators should also teach students to reason independently and effectively by using the strategies presented here as well as other creative strategies designed to stimulate their intellectual development.

17 How will reasoning be taught in the future?

Expert nurses use actual, potential, and perceived variables in quantitative and qualitative domains to make clinical decisions. In its simplest form, expert reasoning is about influencing and controlling relationships among complex and multidimensional variables, propositions, and assumptions; however, when asked, most expert nurses will tell you nursing process never entered their mind. It is likely that the ability of the expert nurse to look for relationships among variables was originated with the nursing process; however, most students and nurses very quickly and subconsciously move on to a higher level of reasoning and let the traditionally defined nursing process go. Whereas the nursing process serves a purpose at the introductory level, students and practicing nurses quickly move past it as their reasoning abilities develop. Various methods of facilitating advanced reasoning, such as integrative concept mapping and logic models (Ellerman, Kataoka-Yahiro, & Wong, 2006), are providing ways of promoting effective reasoning; however, the profession has yet to develop a comprehensive model that shows a clear way of developing advanced reasoning in students that integrates the common language of theory, research, and reasoning.

18 **How can I learn to incorporate all of this information when teaching students?**

Tanner (2006) indicated that there are five factors that influence clinical judgments made by nurses. These factors include (1) what nurses bring to the situation: KSVME; (2) awareness of patients' unique responses (the patient's KSVME) and the integration of these responses into nursing reasoning; (3) awareness of the context and culture of clinical situations and practice settings and integration of these into nursing reasoning; (4) specific reasoning patterns or combinations of patterns used in practice; and (5) analysis (through inquiry) of practice situations where reasoning breaks down. This chapter has introduced some of the essential language, meanings, processes, and tools necessary to facilitate the development of these five areas in students. As you continue to prepare for the important task of teaching future nurses, it is important to keep in mind that your job is not to teach students everything you know and it is not to teach them about the latest trend or newest technology. These trends and technologies will be obsolete before they graduate. Your job is to teach them how to reason effectively within the context of nursing KSVME and within a diverse and ever-changing health-care environment. If you do this, then your students will be able to answer questions, solve problems, and explore nursing phenomena on their own.

References

American Association of Nursing (1986). Essentials of baccalaureate nursing. Washington DC: Author.

Ellerman, C.R., Kataoka-Yahiro, M.R., & Wong, L. C. (2006). Logical models used to enhance critical thinking. Journal of Nursing Education 45(6), 220–227.

Johnson, B., & Webber, P. (2005) Introduction to theory and reasoning in nursing, 2nd ed. Philadelphia: Lippincott Williams & Wilkins.

Morin, K. (1997). Critical thinking—say what? Journal of Nursing Education 36, 450–451.

National League for Nursing. (1992). Criteria and guidelines for the evaluation of baccalaureate and higher degree programs in nursing. New York: NLN.

Riddell, T. (2007). Critical assumptions: Thinking critically about critical thinking. Journal of Nursing Education 46(3), 121–126.

Scheffer, B.K. (2006). Critical thinking: A tool in search of a job. Journal of Nursing Education 45(6).

Scheffer, B.K., & Rubenfeld, M.G. (2000). A consensus statement on critical thinking in nursing. Journal of Nursing Education 39, 352–360.

Tanner, C. (1999). Evidence-based practice: Research and critical thinking. Journal of Nursing Education 38, 99.

Tanner, C.A. (2006). Thinking like a nurse: A research-based model of clinical judgment in nursing. Journal of Nursing Education 45(6), 204–211.

Walsh, C.M., & Seldomridge, L.A. (2006). Critical thinking: Back to square two. Journal of Nursing Education 45(6), 212–219

Webber, P., & Wanant, W. Linguistic competence in nursing faculty: A missing piece in theory and research. Unpublished raw data.

Webber, P.B. (2002). A curriculum framework for nursing. Journal of Nursing Education 41(1), 15–24.

29

Teaching Evidence-Based Practice

Lisa Sams, MSN, RNC,
and Donna G. Knauth, PhD, RN, FACCE

---

1 What is evidence-based practice (EBP)?

EBP is the implementation of patient care that is derived from:

1. Valid and reliable research evidence
2. Expert clinical knowledge
3. Patient preferences and values

It requires that clinical decision making about patient care be based on the integrative result of these three components. The expected outcome of EBP is the highest quality patient care.

---

2 Does EBP differ from the usual care patients receive?

Yes. Usual care refers to the most common approach to care, which relies on clinical decision making based on both pathophysiological principles and clinical experience. This often means we are relying more on habits and opinions than evidence. The systematic approach to evidence-based care includes the pathophysiologic principles but relies on the inclusion of relevant research findings along with clinician expertise to focus on outcomes and the measurement of outcomes. Here clinical decision making is based on critical thinking rather than rote learning and routines.

Two primary reasons account for our laggardly adoption of EBP. These are: (1) the majority of clinicians today have not been trained in the evidence methodology, and (2) the infrastructure of most organizations is not configured to support EBP.

---

3   Is there a specific series of events in evidence-based practice?

Yes. There are five systematic steps of EBP that provide transparency in critical analysis and improve patient outcomes. These steps are:

1. Define and ask the specific clinical question based on the patient population, the intervention of interest, comparison interventions, and outcome.
2. Collect the best evidence by identifying, appraising, and synthesizing studies to answer the specific clinical question.
3. Critically evaluate the evidence for validity and whether benefits outweigh risks for patient care.
4. Integrate the evidence with the provider's clinical expertise, the health-care status and preferences of the patient, and the health-care resources available in making a clinical practice decision.
5. Evaluate the practice decision (Sackett, et al., 1997).

With the rapid evolution of health-care knowledge, health-care professionals must take the responsibility to deliver evidence-based care to ensure the best outcomes for their patients. The systematic steps of EBP provide the necessary framework for health-care providers to translate research findings into practice to achieve the best possible clinical outcomes. Thus, it is up to the educators to teach students how to find and use this evidence.

---

4   How does EBP differ from research utilization?

Research utilization is the use of research findings in clinical practice, a movement that began in the late 1970s. Its purpose was to increase nurses' awareness of research results and to assist them to incorporate these results into their practice. Many models of research utilization have been developed, including models for individual clinicians and those for organizations or groups of clinicians. Research utilization models all involve several steps as follows:

1. Select a topic.
2. Retrieve and critique relevant literature.
3. Assess the implementation potential of an intervention.
4. Develop the intervention protocol.
5. Evaluate the outcomes.
6. Make decisions about adoption of the intervention.

Research utilization is a forerunner of EBP, which is more complex and includes additional components. One major difference is that the research knowledge in research utilization is typically based on a single study, whereas EBP involves knowledge from a thorough search and critical appraisal of all relevant studies. Additionally, EBP takes into consideration the practitioners' expert knowledge, the individual patient's health-care status, preferences, and values, and the available health-care resources. EBP differs also in the methods for defining and asking the specific clinical question that guides the search and appraising the research findings to aid in clinical decision making (Melnyk & Fineout-Overholt, 2005).

---

5   Is there a consensus on how to define EBP?

Not entirely. There are several working definitions, however, all of which involve the following:

• Appraising and applying the current best evidence from research
• Using clinical expertise
• Applying the patient's history, health status, preferences, and values
• Using shared clinical decision making between the patient and practitioner to achieve quality patient care and to improve patient outcomes.

These components are depicted in Figure 29–1.

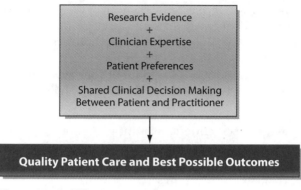

Figure 29–1. EBP components.

---

6 Why is EBP important?

The quality of health care depends on health-care providers knowing:

- What questions to ask.
- How to search for and evaluate relevant research evidence.
- How to integrate this knowledge with their own expert clinical knowledge and the patient's health status and preferences.
- Available health resources that can aid in making clinical practice decisions that lead to the best quality patient care.

Over the past three decades, three major issues facing health care have been poorly addressed. These issues are:

1. **The gap between research and practice.** Research findings that could benefit patients take up to 17 years before clinicians apply them in their practices. [Institute of Medicine 2003]
2. **Health-care knowledge volume and speed.** Clinicians who graduate today can expect to see their knowledge turn over completely four times during an average career.
3. **Variations in care.** Clinician preferences continue to drive many aspects of daily care; not always are these preferences based on sound evidence.

---

7   How much attention are these issues receiving nationally?

There are a number of agencies and organizations press-ing for improvements in the health-care delivery models that exist today, and they have identified the lack of EBP as a major detriment to improving outcomes and patient safety. As recently as 2006, the director of the Agency for Health Research and Quality (AHRQ) described the trans-lation of evidence into care as "cumbersome" with a con-tinued lag time into practice of 17 years (Clancy, 2006). The AHRQ Web site is an important resource for EBP: http://www.ahrq.gov

---

8   Is there national guidance for education on this issue?

The Institute of Medicine (IOM) report, *Health Professions Education: A Bridge to Quality* (2003, p. 46), listed EBP as one of the five core competencies needed in all health professions education, thus challenging health-care pro-fessionals to provide care based on the best available sci-entific evidence. The report identified the lack of training in this area and called for schools to redesign their curric-ula to include this competency.

---

9   If I would like to include EBP in my course, how do I get started?

Convey to students that it is a systematic way to approach clinical decision making using five important sequential steps:

1. Ask the clinical question.
2. Search the literature for the most relevant and best evidence.
3. Appraise the evidence for its application to patient care.
4. Integrate all research evidence with one's clinical exper-tise and patient preferences and make a practice deci-sion or change when indicated.
5. Evaluate the results of the decision or change.

EBP is a process of "patient problem-centered lifelong learn-ing," as described by one of the early leaders, David Sackett and colleagues (1997, p. 2). There are a number of resources on the Web:

> http://www.jr2.ox.ac.uk/bandolier/
> http://www.mdx.ac.uk/www/rctsh/ebp/main.htm
> http://www.mclibrary.duke.edu/training/cinahlovid/ebp

Once you accept the notion that mastering EBP is part of a "lifelong learning" process, you will feel less intimidated and find your knowledge base growing every year. There are three strategies that will help you bring an evidence-based approach into your course:

1. Develop a sense of competency in structuring clinical questions, both background and foreground questions, and their role in clinical decision making.
2. Become familiar with the principle of an evidence hierarchy as a way to quickly grasp the concept of "evidence strength."
3. Locate evidence-based guidelines and systematic reviews that will be useful in your course, and compare those findings with current course content.

---

10 What are background questions, and how can I use them in my classes?

Background questions are aptly named because they help determine what lies behind a problem or how a process occurs. For example:

- What are the most common bacteria found in lower urinary tract infections (UTIs)?
- How does cellulitis develop?
- Why is labor divided into stages?
- Where is the impact of age-related macular degeneration?

This information provides the "skeleton" around which the clinician continues to build knowledge. Sackett et al. (1997, 2000) describe these as answering the *how, what, when,* and *where* questions about patient issues. Answers to background questions can typically be found in current texts (no more than 2 years old) or valid Web resources for basic knowledge, such as academic centers or online versions of texts. Your students may find the National Library of Medicine resource called Medline Plus a useful resource for answers to background questions: http://www.nlm.nih.gov

Experienced clinicians may have more trouble than students formulating background questions because the background knowledge has been integrated into their thinking. The experienced clinician can practice structuring these questions with colleagues who are outside of their area of expertise.

11 What are clinical foreground questions, and how can they be included in classroom presentations?

Clinical foreground questions are the driving force for evidence-based clinical decision making. Foreground questions build on the background knowledge and seek specific information about managing a patient problem. To answer the foreground question one uses "scientific evidence about diagnosing, treating, or assisting patients with understanding their diagnosis" (Melnyk & Fineout-Overholt, 2005, p. 28). Formulating clinical foreground questions is the process of "asking the answerable question" (Sackett, et al., 1997, p.3), and is the first of the five steps of EBP as described above.

To yield the most relevant and best evidence, clinical foreground questions should be formulated using the PICO format. This mnemonic indicates the structure of the question:

- P: Patient-specific statement
- I: Intervention under consideration
- C: Comparison with another intervention (if relevant)
- O: Outcome desired (Sackett, et al., 1997)

Guyatt and Rennie (2002) add a fifth element, time frame (PICOT), but this is not always necessary. Using the UTI example, practical questions about care can be developed. For example: *In a healthy middle-aged woman with occasional episodes of lower UTI, will self-treatment with Macrobid for 3 days, as compared with usual care, effectively eliminate the infection?*

Patient (be specific)	A healthy middle-age women with occasional episodes of lower UTI
Intervention of interest	Does self-treatment with Macrobid × 3 days
Comparison	Compared with "usual care"
Outcome	Effectively eliminate the UTI

In class, you can incorporate many examples of the PICO question as you present content related to various aspects of patient care. For example, using the age-related macular degeneration (AMD) as a background question, "What is AMD? "How do you differentiate dry from wet AMD? Now you can structure a foreground question: *In patients diagnosed with the dry form of AMD, does use of a vitamin supplement, compared with no supplement, slow the advance of AMD?* You can expand on the research related to the supplement in course discussion as well as show students how they engage the individual patient in their own decision making regarding the use of supplements.

12　What is meant by an evidence hierarchy?

An evidence hierarchy is a rating system that identifies the level of strength of the evidence. It is a way to visualize evidence or the findings from research from simple opinion in a textbook all the way through high-level, systematic reviews. A systematic review includes a meta-analysis of all relevant randomized controlled trials (RCTs) or evidence-based clinical practice guidelines that are based on systematic reviews of RCTs. These are identified as the highest level (level I) in a hierarchy of evidence. As you progress from lower to higher levels, there is increasingly more strength in the evidence. There is a graphic that the University of Washington Library modified from University of Virginia. The graphic is a colorful pyramid depicting the evidence chain from textbooks and opinions to the most rigorous form of systematic reviews such as those prepared by the Cochrane Collaborative. See http://healthlinks.washington.edu/ebp/ebptools.html

13 How should I help my students differentiate the evidence hierarchy from the concept of "grading the evidence"?

Grading the evidence is a way for a group that has conducted an appraisal of research on a specific topic to convey the complexity of its appraisal process and the basis of its recommendations. There are many different grading schemes in use. A professional organization or a government agency may choose to develop its own grading criteria rather than use a method developed elsewhere. The AHRQ, in collaboration with the American Medical Association and the American Association of Health Plans, provides a public resource for clinical practice guidelines, the National Guideline Clearinghouse. These practice guidelines, produced by professional organizations and others, are specific practice recommendations that are based on review of the best evidence on the topic. The clearinghouse presents all guidelines in a standardized format. One component in the format is an explanation of the grading criteria that were used to produce the recommendations within the guideline. The Web site is http://www .guideline.gov

Another resource can be found on the Registered Nurses of Ontario Web site http://www.rnao.org. These guidelines are produced via a systematic method, and all address nursing care issues, such as assessment and management of pain. The evidence is graded and clearly defined, so it is easy to show students how any one recommendation fits into the evidence hierarchy. For example, in the guideline, *Subcutaneous administration of insulin for people with Type II Diabetes*, there are 15 recommendations for practice, each with an evidence "grade" that reflects the strength of the evidence on which the recommendation is based. The second recommendation states: "Education and administration of insulin should be tailored in collaboration with the individual to address current knowledge ability and needs." Clearly noted next to the recommendation is the level of evidence, 1A, which in the rating scheme means the evidence is drawn from a meta-analysis or systematic review of RCTs.

14 What is a systematic review, and is it a good source of information for students?

Simply stated, this is a study of studies, and this secondary source is often a good first step in the search process. In the glossary of *Bandolier* (2007), an online journal about evidence-based health care, a systematic review is defined as "a summary of the medical literature that uses explicit methods to perform a thorough literature search and critical appraisal of individual studies and that uses appropriate statistical techniques to combine these valid studies. Systematic reviews are not all equal, and quality issues are important" (http://www.jr2.ox.ac.uk/bandolier/learnzone.html). Although full access to this journal is by subscription, you can learn more about systematic reviews at this Web site. What differentiates systematic reviews from traditional reviews is their design. A systematic review typically:

1. Defines a specific question for investigation, which is usually a foreground question; hence, these reviews are conducted to be clinically useful.
2. The search methods are delineated.
3. Inclusion and exclusion criteria for study selection are delineated.
4. Methods of evaluation of the study are defined.

Some systematic reviews include a meta-analysis, a technique for quantitatively combining and integrating the results of multiple studies on a given topic, but this is not a requirement. For examples of systematic reviews, go to Cochrane Library at http://www.cochrane.org where you can access the abstracts online without a fee. Full text of the review is by subscription. Ask your university librarian to access the full text for you. It is a good teaching tool for understanding systematic methods. These reviews are conducted by review groups, and these are listed on the Web site. The groups are designated by their clinical focus, such as Pregnancy and Childbirth or Musculo-Skeletal. The reviews are contained in those review groupings. For example, look at the abstract that is located under the Pain, Palliative Care, and Support group: *Epidural analgesia for pain relief following hip or knee replacement.*

15   How can I evaluate the quality of practice guidelines?

As previously stated, practice guidelines are another source of evidence designed to guide clinical decision making. There are many guidelines; they are not all evidence-based or constructed with systematic rigor. To evaluate the strengths and weaknesses of a guideline, you can teach students to use these four questions (Guyatt & Rennie, 2002, p. 185):

1. Did the recommendations consider all relevant patient groups, management options, and possible outcomes?
2. Is there a systematic review of evidence linking options to outcomes for each relevant question?
3. Is there an appropriate specification of values or preferences associated with outcomes?
4. Do the authors indicate the strength of their recommendations?

Here is a guideline example where the methodology is explained and the recommendations are graded by the strength of the evidence:

- Evidence-based guidelines for weaning and discontinuation of ventilatory support. Chest (2001). 120(6 Supp), 375–484S (224 references) http://www.guideline.gov

16   How should students search the literature?

- Begin with a well-constructed clinical foreground question, and have the key words already identified.
- Search first for the systematic reviews or evidence-based guidelines. These secondary sources are excellent for busy clinicians: other groups have already conducted the search and appraisal work. But you may have many questions that are not answered by one of these resources.
- Set a time limit for searching. Remember, a key member of the EBP clinical team should be the health sciences librarian. A librarian has an advanced degree in the science of researching. If you have limited or no workable findings when you have met your time limit for searching, consult with your librarian colleague.
- Invite a librarian to provide an overview to searching specific clinical foreground questions in one of your classes.

Ask the students to generate the foreground questions, and provide them to the librarian beforehand. Many classrooms can show real-time Web access on a screen so students can follow along.

Ann McKibbon (1999), one of the leaders in EBP and a health science librarian, has several publications that will help you learn effective search strategies. With over 25,000 journals in print and only 4,000 of those in MEDLINE and fewer still in CINAHL, it is easy to see how literature can be missed without a librarian's aid.

---

17 Is there a recommended way to review the literature in the context of EBP?

This is called critical appraisal of the literature. This is the systematic analysis of research to arrive at the clearest understanding possible of risks and benefits of a particular intervention on patient outcomes. Learning to appraise the literature critically is a lifelong skill. The two references cited previously, Melnyk and Fineout-Overholt (2005) and Guyatt and Rennie (2002) will guide you through the basic elements of appraising various forms of the literature. Many academic libraries have links to tutorials such as:

> http://www.hshsl.umaryland.edu/corporate/resources /evidence.html#TUTORIALS
> http://www.cche.net/usersguides/decision.asp

---

18 Are synthesis publications also a good resource?

Yes, because these are intended to be quick evidence-based resources for busy clinicians. Two examples that follow evidence-based methods and offer synthesis information in a one-page format are *Evidence-Based Nursing*, a British Medical Journal, and *ACP Journal Club*, published by the American College of Physicians. Both offer online subscriptions as well so their databases can be searched:

> http://ebn.bmj.com/
> http://www.acponline.org

19 How can I integrate the evidence-based approach into the students' clinical education?

Establish the expectation that background and clinical fore-ground questions (PICO) will be used in clinical rotations. This can be accomplished in many ways; for example:

- Students generate one background question for their patient every day. If they keep a log, the answers to the background questions become a resource for them.
- Use the questions in pre- and post-conference time.
- Build post-conferences around PICO questions. As students discuss patients, have the group generate questions for which they will bring answers to the next post-conference.
- Ask students to identify resources for background and foreground questions that are available to clinicians on the clinical unit where they are assigned.
- Use the unit policy/procedure manual or any clinical pathway, order set, or protocol. These are valuable teaching tools. Select one that is appropriate for the students' level, and ask them to review it for its congruence with current evidence.

20 How can I include an assignment that walks students through the critical thinking in EBP?

Figure 29–2 shows an excerpt from an assignment developed to foster evidence-based thinking. Students were guided through evidence-based thinking with questions that helped them answer the background and foreground questions, all based on selected cases from their clinical educational experience.

21 How was this assignment graded?

Figure 29–3 gives the grading criteria that were used.

22 Are there suggested references for learning more about EBP?

1. DiCenso, S., Guyatt, G., & Ciliska, D. (Eds.). (2005). Evidence-based nursing: A guide to clinical practice. St Louis: Elsevier Mosby.

Purpose:
This paper is designed to support your use of best evidence in clinical practice. In an average career, clinicians face a four-fold turnover in the knowledge necessary to practice. The problem-based learning principles within the systematic methods of evidence-based practice are the only way clinicians can be assured they will be offering their patients the most effective care.

Objectives:
You will have the opportunity to question a specific practice in common use today. Because this assignment is constructed around a background question, you will delve into the current knowledge to better understand the common practice, then compare what you have learned with what you observe in your clinical time.

The second question within each practice is called a foreground question. Here you will be guided to specific evidence reviews to help you compare what you have learned in exploring the background of a clinical question with direct clinical application that foreground answers provide.

The Cochrane Library of Systematic Reviews (SR) is where you will find answers to each foreground question with the exception of Question #4, where you are directed to the National Guideline Clearinghouse.

www.cochrane.org
www.guideline.gov

You can access the Cochrane abstracts free on-line. This paper, however, requires you to use the entire SR., which in some cases may be more than 40 pages. You will need to work with the Health Science Librarian to access the full review with tables when applicable.

Select one of the questions below and complete the following objectives to prepare a paper that critically analyzes what you have learned in your review of key literature and what you have observed in clinical practice.

Questions:
Background Question#1
What methods are available to evaluate fetal well-being during the process of labor?

Develop a comparative table to: (1) name the method, (2) describe how this method gains information about fetal heart rate, (3) describe the benefits and the risks with each.

What national-level policies or guidelines offer guidance on assessment of fetal well-being during labor? (check the Guideline Clearinghouse, AWHONN, and ACOG)

- How were these documents developed? Is a methodology for development clearly explained within the document?

- Is there a policy on the clinical unit where you work that governs this practice?

- Discuss the nursing role with each of these methods.

- Explain the risks and benefits to both patients (mother and fetus) in the context of the national documents.

Foreground Question #1
In pregnant women undergoing normal term labor (spontaneous or induced) does auscultation of fetal heart rate compared to electronic fetal monitoring provide for equivalent or improved neonatal outcomes?

- Review the Cochrane Systematic Review (SR) on Continuous EFM
  - Discuss your reaction to this SR and provide a thoughtful analysis of the background evidence and the foreground evidence in this topic compared to your clinical observations of the practice during this term.

Figure 29–2. EBP assignment.

109

NURS 172: Health Care of Women
Evidence-Based Practice Paper Assignment: Grading Criteria

This small group project (two students per group) has been designed to assist students in 1) searching for the best evidence to answer a clinical question, and 2) critiquing the evidence so that the best-quality, up-to-date care can be provided for children and families. This paper assignment constitutes 15% of your course grade. Each group of two students will select one of the eight clinical questions provided and will conduct an in-depth search for the best scientific evidence regarding that question. The final paper should clearly describe the methods used to identify and retrieve the evidence. Also, recommendations for practice based on research evidence should be articulated. This assignment will provide you with experience in how to turn a clinical issue into a searchable, answerable question. It will provide you the opportunity to discuss basic knowledge, to conduct time-efficient retrieval of the best evidence, and to analyze, in detail, your clinical experience related to the topic and the findings from the evidence for its relevance to practice.

The paper should be written in APA format, should not exceed 10 pages in length, and the reference list should cite all included studies.

*Please submit this grade sheet with your paper, along with all studies included.

Content Area	Possible Points	Your Points
Background Questions 30%	**30**	
All questions addressed	10	
Thoroughly described the following: Background to the problem. Clinical significance of the problem. Methods used to search for knowledge about the background question.	20	
Foreground Questions 60%	**60**	
Evidence of thorough review and discussion of the SR or guideline: Methods used to identify and retrieve the evidence to answer the foreground question.	30	
Analysis of the findings from both background knowledge and foreground best evidence and your clinical experience. Recommendations for practice	30	
Format (APA, clarity of writing, organization of ideas, grammar, and spelling) 10%	**10**	
TOTAL		

Figure 29–3. Grading criteria.

2. Guyatt, G., & Rennie, D. (Eds.). (2002). Users' guide to the medical literature: A manual for evidence-based clinical practice. American Medical Association Press. NOTE: This book presents the process of critical appraisal in an easily digestible format.

3. Melnyk, B.M., & Fineout-Overholt, E. (Eds.). (2005). Evidence-based practice in nursing and healthcare. Philadelphia: Lippincott–Williams & Wilkins.

References

Bandolier. (2007). Accessed May 8, 2007, at http://www.jr2.ox.ac.uk/Bandolier/

Clancy, C. (2006). AHRQ action in Health Policy Newsletter, Thomas Jefferson University 19(4). Accessed May 8, 2007, at http://www.jefferson.edu/dhp/newsletter.cfm

Institute of Medicine of the National Academies. (2003). Health professions education: A bridge to quality. Washington, DC: Author.

McKibbon, A., Eady, A., & Marks, S. (1999). PDQ evidence-based principles and practice. Hamilton, Ontario, Canada: B.C. Decker.

Sackett, D.L., et al. (1997). Evidence-based medicine: How to practice and teach EBM. New York: Churchill Livingstone.

Sackett, D.L., et al. (2000). Evidence-based medicine: How to practice and teach EBM (2nd ed.). Edinburgh: Churchill Livingstone.

30

Ethical Issues in Teaching Nursing

Esther H. Condon, PhD, RN

1   What are my obligations to myself as an educator?

Your obligations to yourself as an educator include finding an environment that supports the nursing profession and that supports your teaching, research, practice, and community service efforts. Other obligations to yourself include finding a cadre of supportive colleagues with whom to share ideas, issues, and collaborative ventures. Should you find yourself in an environment that does not support your efforts and progress, you are obliged to withdraw from it and find another environment that is supportive. You have an obligation to yourself to continue to study and learn, to maintain competence in your areas of expertise, and to find mentors who will assist you with this.

2   What are my obligations to my students as an educator?

Having faith in students is a primary obligation because it sets the stage for a relationship that will allow students to reveal strengths and weaknesses that the educator can help them to utilize or minimize. Being open to the student as a whole person is where the educator can begin to work as a guide with the student, always mindful that the student will move on with what has been learned from having known the educator. Realizing that the educator occupies a position of privilege in relation to the student is important, and being receptive to students is of great importance. Educators are obliged to see students as they are and to envision what they will become. It is of the utmost importance to pay attention to what concerns students, even if it is difficult to do so.

3   What are my obligations to my colleagues as an educator?

Your obligations to your colleagues are to be respectful and helpful. Colleagues are very influential to one's development as an educator. Some will have a positive influence, whereas others will have a negative influence. Civility and helpfulness are qualities that should be developed in oneself and in others. Being civil and helpful helps others to do likewise and often leads to rich and satisfying collegial relationships. Being kind and bringing about benefits for colleagues can bring satisfaction and acknowledgement. People practice what they know, and when they know better, they practice better. Mentoring colleagues as well as students is critical to successful collegial relationships.

4   What is most important for a teacher to remember?

It is important to remember that teachers are powerful and influential and that teachers will be remembered long after the lesson has been forgotten. Therefore, it is critical that teachers exemplify positive role behaviors as well as authentic human behavior because students and colleagues will use this as a guide for their own development.

5   How do my ethics affect my teaching?

One's ethics have a profound impact on one's teaching. There can be no separation of one's ethics and what one does as a teacher. One's ethics provides the grounds for every action taken or not taken in relation to students and faculty colleagues. Teachers accept an obligation to lead a morally defensible life and do not restrict ethical thinking to the professional role domain. Teachers must exemplify ethics in action and help students and faculty colleagues to understand all ethical dimensions of life and of practice.

6   What if I am unable to reach my moral ideal as an educator?

It is important to understand that a moral ideal is something that is not static or something that can be reached once and for all. Achieving one's moral ideal is a daily project that demands being reflective and acting on one's values and principles. One significant moral ideal is to be in relationship with those around us and to examine often the extent to which students, self, and colleagues benefit or do not benefit from the relationship. Understanding one's own moral point of view and that of students and colleagues can bring one closer to understanding one's moral ideal and judging its worth.

7   When colleagues are difficult, how should I respond?

How conflicts are resolved is at the heart of collegial relationships. The values at stake will determine if and what action is to be taken. Being honest and willing to listen to all points of view is a good beginning with difficult colleagues. Knowing what central values are supported or compromised in the conflict will point the way to resolving it. Sometimes people must "agree to disagree without being disagreeable" when there is no harm in doing so, and this can be done with integrity. Displaying faith and trust in colleagues lets them know that the relationship will not be destroyed as a result of the conflict.

8   What is the most important moral advice for a new teacher?

New teachers are typically focused on their own shortcomings, feelings of discomfort, and the use of teaching techniques. This is an early stage in the acquisition of competence as a teacher. When levels of comfort and proficiency have developed, the new teacher must focus on the relationship with students. It is critical that the new teacher connect with students in ways that will allow students to benefit from contact with the teacher. It is important to constantly remind oneself that the entire teaching-learning process exists within a relationship. That relationship will profoundly affect the teaching-learning process and its outcomes. New teachers who are able to insightfully navigate their development as a teacher will be able to develop authentic and helpful relationships with students. The teaching-learning moment is created by teachers and students together, so building caring coalitions with students is an agenda to be pursued daily so that both students and teachers will become better human beings. Understanding that having the intention to emancipate self and students is an important moral position.

---

9 Should I use a nursing theory to guide my teaching practice? Where does moral theory fit into this?

It would be questionable to say that nursing theory is not suitable for teaching practice. However, just as there may be more than one theoretical approach to a nursing situation, so it is in the teaching-learning situation. Knowing who the students are—their backgrounds, knowledge, and culture—and experience with teaching and learning can provide important context for the educator to select a theoretical approach. Developmental approaches are useful, and these are represented in many nursing theories and frameworks. Moral theory in teaching-learning must include consideration of the learner as having uniqueness and dignity above all else. Cultural context should be examined to assess the appropriateness of theory and principles. When using theory, the educator should reflect on what is "good" and "right" within the theory and ask "for whom, and when?" In this way, a theoretical approach is critically appraised for its benefits and shortcomings. The educator should reflect often on the idea that what is taught and how it is taught will become the practice of the student.

---

10 How can I be fair to students?

Fairness involves giving to students according to their needs. Fairness is a minimal standard and can be greatly enhanced by being caring, especially when being fair results in failure for a student.

11   How do I maintain appropriate relationships with students?

Accepting the relationship of trust that the teacher engages in with students is an important concept. Acknowledging the asymmetry of power inherent in relationships involving inequality of knowledge and status is critical to establishing appropriate relationships with students. Students are held in trust by teachers, and their good and well-being must be the deciding factor in all aspects of the relationship. Where conflicts of interest arise, the educator must act in the student's best interest or withdraw from the situation.

12   How should I handle dishonesty and cheating with students?

Students bring a wealth of experience to the teaching-learning process. This includes values and patterns of previous behavior that may or may not have been challenged or even evaluated by others. Informing students of expectations with regard to dishonesty and cheating is of primary importance and must be done early in the relationship. Education is about changing behavior, values, and beliefs and as such provides students and faculty opportunities to adopt or relinquish behavior, values, and beliefs. Involving students early on in determining how the teaching-learning process will be conducted promotes their investment in the process and outcome. Making them responsible for upholding academic integrity and expressing trust in their ability to do so can set students on the right path. However, faculty are obliged to take steps to make cheating and dishonesty difficult to engage in and also to respond appropriately when they occur. Students should be exposed to the impact that dishonest behavior has on their credibility and on relationships of trust with teachers and other students. They must understand that the professional life requires integrity.

13   What should I do when parents ask me about students' grades?

At the present time, grades are considered private information that cannot be shared with parents. The teacher can encourage students to discuss grades with their parents and convey the idea that parents have a natural concern for the student's progress. Discussion of grades must be between the student and the parent. The teacher is obliged to maintain confidentiality regarding the student's grades.

14 What should I do when students come to me with personal rather than academic problems?

Often students arrive in a teacher's office burdened by personal issues. It is important to listen to what the student has to say and offer appropriate guidance in the short term while encouraging students to use campus resources such as the counseling center or student health services. If a student is in immediate danger, the teacher should activate services that would protect the student. Teachers must recognize that maintaining appropriate boundaries is required but that expressing human concern is never inappropriate.

15 What should I do when students betray my trust in them?

When students betray a teacher's trust, the teacher must openly discuss this with them. They may not realize that this has occurred or understand the effect on the teacher. Being honest with students is one important way to earn and maintain their trust. A frank discussion of what it means to trust and be trusted may move students to another level of integrity. It is also likely to reveal something that the teacher needs to know about his or her teaching practice that should be changed. Discussion with a trusted colleague can help to sort out the process and feelings that accompany this.

16 How do I handle situations in which students arrive without the requisite skills and knowledge from previous classes?

This can be a difficult issue with a variety of underlying causes. One's first reaction is to ask how this situation occurred. This must be asked so that formative evaluation processes can be used to correct the problem over the long term. Students are on the threshold of new experiences for which they are not prepared and must be made aware of this. Early assessment of student knowledge is a wise practice. Rates of learning vary among students, and the teaching-learning environment can have a strong impact on what is learned and when. Developmental phenomena are also influential and transitions from one level of the curriculum to another may affect how students perceive their knowledge and competence. It is important for the educator to make it known to students when they lack the requisite skills or knowledge and its likely effect on their continued learning. Doing this in an interested and supportive manner is crucial to gaining the students' cooperation to resolve the problem. Offering additional support and tutoring can make a major difference in how students receive this information. Asking students to generate possible solutions to the problem involves them directly. Students need to know that faculty can be depended on to assist them and that the students must be held accountable for standards of performance. Guidelines and timelines should be set for students to acquire the skills and knowledge so that they can progress. Gaining the assistance of colleagues and students who already possess the skills and knowledge can help to turn the situation into a positive outcome. Being proactive is much better than being reactive and judgmental.

17 How can I maintain academic standards and be empathetic to students experiencing academic difficulties?

Academic standards must be met because they represent the trust placed in academic institutions that competent nurses will graduate from them. Students experience academic difficulties for a variety of reasons. They may have difficulty learning or may be experiencing illness or other situational factors that make it difficult to maintain academic standards. Regular and thorough advisement of students is important for discovering trends in student performance. Students should be made aware of the required standards and what action to take should they have academic difficulties. Students should be encouraged to seek the counsel and advice of their instructors early and to perform self-appraisal at each evaluation point in a course or curriculum sequence. Faculty must be open to the fact that students face new challenges that are academic and developmental and that these can easily be overwhelming when unexpected events such as illness or family crisis occur. The faculty member should be willing to accept expressions of anger and disappointment when students face academic difficulties. Allowing students to express feelings is an appropriate empathetic response. Helping the student to mobilize campus resources is an appropriate academic response. Realizing that violence can and does occur in these circumstances should prompt the faculty member to assess any potential for harm to self or others and to act accordingly.

18 What effect can I have as an educator on nursing knowledge and its transmission to students?

Educators constantly appraise the state of knowledge in nursing. Faculty members have the responsibility to create and to test the worth of knowledge developed for practice. By critically appraising theory and research findings, educators are in a position to judge their value for practice. When there is evidence to suggest that knowledge is not valid, reliable, or applicable in the manner intended, nursing faculty contribute to the construction of new knowledge. Research and theorizing are the bedrock of knowledge development for any discipline. They must evolve continuously if the discipline is to be of service to society. When students are presented with the knowledge of the discipline, they must be socialized to the fact that knowledge is ever-changing. Students and faculty must appreciate the evolutionary character of knowledge and practice and be constantly engaged in the critical appraisal of their effectiveness. Therefore, students and faculty must think innovatively and creatively about a variety of issues in knowledge generation and application. Each must know that knowledge is never exhausted, nor is it ever complete.

19 How can I maintain my enthusiasm for teaching?

It is important for new teachers to understand that it is daily practice that sustains teaching and that, consequently, teachers must plan for periods of renewal and rest. Time should be set aside for rest and reflection and enjoyment of life. Without this, it is difficult to be enthusiastic. Teaching should not be an all-consuming endeavor. Rather, balanced with a rich and interesting life, teaching can become an expression of great enthusiasm for life. The practice of seeing the lighter side of situations can refresh students and colleagues when things take a dull turn. By surprising students with innovation and creativity, it is possible to help the fires of enthusiasm burn brighter. A good sense of humor and willingness to laugh at oneself is essential.

20 If I am asked to do something unethical such as falsify a grade for a student, how do I handle this?

When asked to violate the standards of ethical practice in teaching, the answer must always be no. The teacher who is willing to do something unethical can never recover credibility; the student knows this, and the teacher knows this. Considerable damage is done to all parties in such a situation because all lose faith in their ability to trust themselves and others. Reputations are built on trust, and a teacher who has a poor reputation with respect to integrity will not succeed. Administrative solutions can be invoked to handle issues of grading after the teacher has submitted what is believed to be the appropriate grade. Schools also have advisory or judiciary committees that can be helpful in resolving such issues. The teacher must always be sure that the grade given was accurate and reflective of the student's performance.

An author once said, "We must first see our students if we are to believe in them." This we should never forget.

Resources

American Nurses Association. (2001) Code of ethics for nurses with interpretive statements. Author: Washington, DC.

Baxter, P.E., & Boblin, S.E. (2007). The moral development of bac-
    calaureate nursing students: Understanding ethical and unethi-
    cal behavior in classroom and clinical settings [electronic
    version]. Journal of Nursing Education 46(1), 20–26.
Begley, A.M. (2005). Practising virtue: A challenge to the view that
    a virtue-centered approach to ethics lacks practical content
    [electronic version]. Nursing Ethics 12(6), 622–637.
Noddings, N. (2003). Caring: A feminine approach to ethics and
    moral education, 2nd ed. Berkeley: University of California
    Press.
Noddings, N. (2002). Starting at home: Caring and social policy.
    Berkeley: University of California Press.
Polifroni, C.E. (2007). Ethical knowing and nursing education.
    Journal of Nursing Education 46(1), 3.
Watson, J. (1999). Postmodern nursing and beyond. Edinburgh:
    Churchill Livingston.

31

Legal Issues in Teaching Nursing

Susan Sweat Gunby, PhD, RN

1 It seems there are more legal issues involved in higher education at this time compared with several years ago. What are some reasons for these challenges?

The advent of the Internet has allowed most of the world to be more aware of and more knowledgeable about challenges in higher education and the legal recourses to address some of those challenges. In past years, it would have been attorneys or skilled users of library resources who had access to knowledge and information that can now be discovered by anyone with Internet access.

As tuition and related expenses have continued to increase, many students feel entitled to more from academic institutions. Utilizing multiple types of Web-based sites, students may disclose their perceptions about adverse decisions rendered by a college or university and its faculty and administrators. Many of the legal implications of this current trend have yet to be identified.

A final reason centers on the increased demands for accountability for outcomes of higher education. Colleges and universities must account to multiple constituencies about how student learning is being measured, the number of students who graduate, and how many graduates are able to get a job in their chosen field of study. These external regulations may generate pressure to make tough decisions about what constitutes success in courses and in many nursing courses, faculty must decide about clinical competency of students.

---

2 Have the demographic changes in students over the years affected the way colleges and universities respond to legal issues?

In past years, the doctrine of *in loco parentis* permitted the educational institution and its administrators and staff to act in place of the parents of students. This doctrine tended to shield the institution from challenges about decisions related to multiple types of disciplinary actions. Colleges and universities enforced the rules, and students had few legal rights.

Through the years, students, attorneys, faculty, and higher education administrators began to understand that there are differences between disciplining a student for academically related infractions as compared with, for example, breaches of rules related to living in a dormitory. Additionally, the evolution of higher education led to the establishment of more community-based institutions, and the demographics of college and university students changed. The average age of undergraduate students increased from the previously traditional range of 18–22 years. Many students commuted instead of living on campus. Many of these types of challenges led to the decreased emphasis on the *in loco parentis* doctrine.

---

3 What type of faculty behavior is particularly troublesome from a legal standpoint?

In general, the courts have viewed faculty actions and decisions legally troublesome if the actions or decisions appear to be arbitrary, capricious, adversarial, or in bad faith. An arbitrary and capricious action or decision could be characterized by a faculty member acting by impulse, whim, or randomly toward a student rather than based on facts or principles. An example of an arbitrary and capricious decision would be if faculty decided to not follow the course syllabus about grading students and, at the end of the semester, made changes in the expectations for a successful grade for a particular experience. If a faculty member acted in a hostile manner toward a student, the teacher could be charged with acting in an adversarial manner, in bad faith, or displaying ill will against that student.

---

4   I have noticed that some educators post students' grades on their office doors and leave graded papers outside their offices for students to pick up. Do these actions have legal implications?

Yes. Institutions that receive federal funding are required to comply with the Family Educational Rights and Privacy Act of 1974, commonly known as FERPA or the Buckley Amendment. Faculty in those institutions need to understand and apply the FERPA regulations. In particular, faculty members should be aware of the legal protections provided to certain types of educational records and the release of information in those records as defined by FERPA.

Most teachers know that a student's grades, transcripts, and records about allegations of academic dishonesty should not be released to another person or institution without that student's written consent unless there is a legitimate educational interest. However, some educators do not realize that posting grades by social security or student identification numbers without the student's consent violates FERPA regulations. With the permission of students, grades can be posted by code names or random numbers provided these are not in the alphabetical order of the names of students in that class.

Leaving graded papers in locations where other persons can see those papers is a FERPA violation. Schools of nursing can designate a secretary or receptionist who may distribute graded papers to students with appropriate identification, or papers can be placed in locked mailboxes. Grades for papers can be disseminated through course Web sites that allow individual students to access their grade only with the use of a correct password or identification number.

---

5 Negligence is an important legal concept in the clinical practice of nursing. What defines a "negligent" educator?

Negligence in clinical practice means that a person fails to act in an ordinary, reasonable, and prudent manner and this subsequently becomes the direct cause of a foreseeable injury. The person's behavior or actions are not consistent with the standard of the ordinary, reasonable, and prudent person.

An educator may be found professionally negligent if professional conduct is below the standard of due care rendered by reasonably well-qualified professionals in the same or similar circumstance. A major aspect of the concept of professional negligence is that faculty members have a specific duty or responsibility to foresee or anticipate the possible adverse outcomes of their actions.

---

6 Are my actions judged against those of similar nurse educators in my region of the state/country or against other standards?

Years ago the standard of "locality rule" was the predominant method by which the standard of care was framed. This local standard meant that professionals would be judged against what a reasonably well-qualified professional would do under similar circumstances in that same or similar region. Some states still utilize elements of the locality rule.

However, emphasis has shifted toward a national standard. Some reasons for this change include increased access to Internet resources, increased use of various forms of communication (such as cell phones equipped with instant messaging capability, photographic capabilities, and international accessibility), increased attendance at national conferences, availability of online resources and materials from national or international conferences (e.g., PowerPoint presentations and full lectures), national certification of nurses, national standards for licensure, national standards for advanced practice nurses, nationally accepted standards of professional care and behavior, state standards of care, and national accreditation standards.

7 Nurse educators should protect students from harm. What does this mean?

In addition to the more obvious methods of protecting nursing students from harm, such as ensuring that students have the knowledge and skills about universal blood-borne pathogen precautions before caring for clients with acquired immune deficiency syndrome, faculty must be aware of safety concerns inside and outside the sites used for clinical experiences.

Incidents of violence on college campuses will most likely reshape the responses to the question of what constitutes the limits of educators' and administrators' legal duty to care for students in terms of campus safety issues.

Faculty should become sensitive to a new safety issue confronting nurse educators. In one situation, a student was found by her former husband through clinical assignments listed on a course Web site that was believed to be secure. This man contacted the faculty member who was teaching this student through the home phone number listed on the course Web site for students to use in case of an emergency. The man also sent e-mails to other faculty, staff, and administrators listed on course and college Web sites, pleading with them to contact his former wife and their child on his behalf.

8 I have heard that students practice under my nursing license when they are in the clinical areas. Is this true?

No. Vickie Sheets (2005, p.2), a nurse attorney who is Director of Practice and Regulation with the National Council of State Boards of Nursing, explains, "the only person who works on a nurse's license is the person named on the license." She further states, "The nursing student is accountable for nursing actions and behaviors to patients, the instructor, the clinical facility, and the nursing program" and that "the instructor must intervene if necessary for the protection of patients when situations are beyond the abilities of students."

Nancy J. Brent, a nurse attorney, used information from the University Hospital Consortium (2001) to further illustrate this important point: "When professional negligence is alleged against a student nurse, the standard of the graduate professional nurse in the same or similar situation applies" (p. 482).

---

9 What are some legal implications for nurse educators in addressing a student's unsafe clinical performance?

First, the concept of due process is pivotal. Due process of law requires that deprivation of education (whether that results from a classroom or clinical failure or both) by an institution must involve adequate notice and some type of hearing for the student involved.

Second, when a student has failed due to unsafe clinical performance, educators must ensure that the student is treated in a fair and equitable manner while also adhering to the specific policies and procedures concerning the clinical evaluation of students. Scanlon, Care, and Gessler (2001, p.7) noted that novice nurse educators may be reluctant to fail students in clinical practice "because they are unsure about the legitimacy of their judgments and their ultimate decision about the student's abilities."

---

10 What types of policies do faculty need to have in place to deal with students who are failing in class or unsafe in clinical?

Nursing faculties need to address clearly and thoughtfully such issues as:

- Do faculty adhere to the course syllabus? If it was necessary to correct a course syllabus, have all students been notified?
- Are grievance or appeal procedures clearly delineated? Can faculty articulate these procedures to students?
- What constitutes unsafe versus safe clinical practice?
- What factors would be involved in a situation in which a student's clinical practice is deemed safe for the entire semester but the student receives a failing grade for clinical experience?

- What documentation is needed to support a failing grade?
- How and when should students be removed from the clinical area when unsafe performance has occurred?
- How will faculty teach other students in the clinical area while evaluating a student who may have exhibited previous unsafe performance?
- How will the student's due process rights be respected?
- Will a student's lack of compliance with certain professional behaviors or expectations (such as incivility, tardiness, inconsistent class attendance, bullying, or inappropriate language) affect grades in class, clinical experience, or learning resource center experience?
- What will be done if a student's behavioral response to a failing grade is excessively emotional, harassing, or violent in nature?
- How will novice educators be supported in the challenging process of evaluating a student who is failing a course or is evidencing unsafe clinical practice?

---

11 How should faculty approach developing these types of policies and procedures?

It is critical that faculty realize that all course expectations, policies, and procedures must be consistent with the mission, philosophy, and expected outcomes of both the school of nursing and the college or university at large. Faculty must adhere to proper institutional procedures for securing approval of policies associated with admission testing, progression testing and evaluation, graduation testing, academic progression criteria, academic dismissal, misconduct leading to disciplinary actions, and students being denied access to clinical sites due to results from criminal background checks or drug and alcohol screening tests. Faculty may wish to collaborate with colleagues in clinical practice to craft some portions of the above policies and procedures and then submit the draft policies through the appropriate school of nursing committees and college or university approval process. Students need complete information about these policies and procedures, including students' clearly identified rights and responsibilities.

12 I must provide "reasonable accommodations" to students with disabilities. What is a reasonable accommodation according to the law?

Reasonable educational accommodations may be defined as any reasonable adjustment required for a student to fully participate in the college or university community. This may mean that accommodations be implemented inside and outside classrooms. However, in order to provide reasonable accommodations to a student with a disability, institutions are not required to fundamentally alter their programs of instruction, lower academic standards, or be placed in a situation that will produce an undue burden on the college or university.

Students seeking reasonable accommodations will be expected to provide sufficient evidence of the specific disability as well as documentation of the proposed accommodation. It is usual that institutions will require the student to provide updates on expectations for accommodations. Clinical educators must be aware that students with disabilities may have accessibility and other accommodation needs in the agencies where students have clinical experiences.

13 What are two of the most common types of academic misconduct?

Cheating and plagiarism. In essence, academic misconduct is composed of both academic and disciplinary elements and has both ethical and legal implications. For this reason, many differences of opinion exist about what disciplinary sanctions should be imposed on a student who has engaged in cheating or plagiarism. Some faculty believe these forms of academic misconduct have more ethical than legal implications.

Cheating and plagiarism are forms of stealing. Students who cheat are stealing from the academic institution, from other students who have worked hard to achieve their success, from faculty, from the nursing profession, and actual knowledge and understanding from themselves. These individuals are possibly stealing life or health from a future patient or client by not gaining the requisite knowledge to care for a vulnerable person.

Faculty and colleagues in an academic institution must engage in conversations about what constitutes academic misconduct, how a student's due process rights will be ensured, and what disciplinary sanctions will occur if allegations are found to be true. Additionally, students should be actively involved in the process of ensuring academic integrity.

---

14 What should I understand about Health Insurance Portability and Accountability Act (HIPAA) regulations and possible legal implications for nursing education?

The HIPAA affects everyone in a health-care setting and in a nursing education program. Nursing educators are legally and ethically obligated to protect the personal health information about students in the same manner as for patients and clients. The privacy portions of HIPAA regulations limit who may have access to health information and how that health information may be utilized. Confidentiality standards protect basic information that may identify a person's past, present, and future physical and mental health conditions.

Protecting the personal health information of students may pose ethical and legal challenges to nurse educators and administrators. For instance, if an instructor believes that a student's health status could create an unsafe situation in the clinical area, the instructor may be faced with how much information to share with a clinical preceptor or how much supervision may be required to ensure safe practice. Educators must work with colleagues in practice to address these evolving issues. It is extremely important that university legal counsel be involved in these decisions and policy development.

HIPAA standards have been established for electronic transmission of certain health-related information. When making clinical assignments, faculty must be very diligent about maintaining privacy and confidentiality of patient health information. Full names of patients should never be conveyed via fax, e-mails, clinical assignment sheets posted on online course pages, personal digital assistants, cell phone text messaging, and other forms of communication.

In addition, students need to be taught the importance of protecting all nursing care plan documents, which should not contain full names of patients. Students must understand that they cannot share information about patients or clients with individuals who do not have a need to know that protected information.

---

15 Is there any further information to help me address some of these legal challenges?

Focus on the majority of students who are committed to doing well as nursing students and who are passionate about their chosen profession. Often, nurse educators focus so much on the few students who are failing; are unsafe in the clinical area; who cheat, plagiarize, or engage in other forms of unprofessional behaviors. As a result, these faculty deprive the majority of students of a wonderful learning experience.

Dorothy E. Reilly (1996), the late nurse educator and scholar, asked "How did I become a master teacher?" (p. 131) and in her response she noted that "Significant incidents in teaching, like those in nursing practice, should not remain ends in themselves, but rather they must be subjected to analysis of their meaning and their contribution to the achievement of professional mastery" (p. 133).

References

Brent, N.J. (2001). Nursing and the law: A guide to principles and applications. Philadelphia: Saunders.

Reilly, D.E. (1996). A teacher looks back. The route to mastery. Journal of Nursing Education 35, 131–133.

Scanlon, J.M., Care, W.D., & Gessler, S. (2001). Dealing with an unsafe student in clinical practice. Nurse Educator 26, 23–27 [electronic version]. Accessed November 19, 2006, at http://gateway.ut.ovid.com/gw1/ovidweb.cgi

Sheets, V. (2005). Ask NCSBN. Leader to leader: Nursing regulation and education together [electronic version]. Retrieved from www.ncsbn.org/LDR_LDR_March_05.pdf

Resources

Alley, N.M., Marrs, J.A., & Schreiner, B. (2005). Nurses' promise to safeguard the public: Is it time for nationally mandated background checks? JONA's Healthcare Law, Ethics, and Regulation 7, 119–124.

Bellack, J.P. (2004). Why plagiarism matters. Journal of Nursing Education 43, 527–528.

Boley, P., & Whitney, K. (2003). Grade disputes: Considerations for nursing faculty. Journal of Nursing Education 42, 198–203.

Chasens, E.R., et al. (2000). Legal aspects of grading and student progression. Journal of Professional Nursing 16, 267–272.

Ehrmann, G. (2005). Managing the aggressive nursing student. Nurse Educator 30, 98–100.

Evans, B.C. (2005). Nursing education for students with disabilities: Our students, our teachers. In M.A. Oermann & K.T. Heinrich (Eds.) Annual Review of Nursing Education 3, 3–22. New York: Springer.

Farnsworth, J., & Springer, P. J. (2006). Background checks for nursing students: What are nursing schools doing? Nursing Education Perspectives 27, 148–153.

Goudreau, K.A., & Chasens, E.R. (2002). Negligence in nursing education. Nurse Educator 27, 42–46.

Helms, L., Jorgensen, J., & Anderson, M.A. (2006). Disability law and nursing education: An update. Journal of Professional Nursing 22, 190–196.

Hutton, S.A. (2006). Workplace incivility: State of the science. JONA 36, 22–28.

Kolanko, K.M., et al. (2006). Academic dishonesty, bullying, incivility, and violence: Difficult challenges facing nurse educators. Nursing Education Perspectives 27, 34–43.

Lashley, F.R., & deMeneses, M. (2001). Student civility in nursing programs: A national survey. Journal of Professional Nursing 17, 81–86.

Spurlock, D. (2006). Do no harm: Progression policies and high-stakes testing in nursing education. Journal of Nursing Education 45, 297–302.

Tate, E.T., & Moody, K. (2005). The public good: Regulation of nursing students. JONA's Healthcare Law, Ethics, and Regulation 7, 47–53.

32

Encouraging Professional Awareness and Activism

Rebecca Bowers-Lanier, EdD, RN,
and Karin Beecroft, MSN, RN

---

1 What are professional awareness and activism?

Professional awareness is an understanding of one's personal behaviors as behaviors related to the precepts of the profession. Nurses who are professionally aware know that their behaviors reflect the profession of nursing with its historical traditions of caring, advocacy, and promotion of health and wellness; they also have an awareness of current issues affecting nursing and health care.

One dictionary defines activism as "a vigorous and sometimes aggressive action in pursuing a political or social end" (2001). Activism is on a continuum—from delivering the very best nursing care to advocating for the profession through leadership in professional and specialty organizations and influencing legislative and regulatory policies that affect nursing and health care.

2   Why are professional awareness and activism important to the role of the faculty member?

Because faculty members are role models, they should demonstrate the skills and competencies central to professional awareness and activism. Students should see their faculty members advocate for them and for their patients. They should see faculty members as leaders in professional associations and specialty nursing organizations. Students learn by watching and trying on new behaviors.

3   Does the faculty member have a role in promoting professional awareness as an intrinsic value to nursing?

Yes, from the standpoint that professional awareness means being an active, aware, engaged nurse. Nursing is a profession that values caring, advocacy, and health promotion. Nurses who are professionally aware have a sense of their responsibility to nursing. Therefore, professional awareness does have intrinsic value. This can and should be woven throughout the curriculum.

4   If I value professional awareness and activism, should I evaluate the school's philosophy for its stated beliefs about them before I accept a position?

Sometimes faculty positions are taken because of convenience, such as geographic proximity or schedule flexibility. Consideration of such abstractions as the philosophy of the nursing program may not be at the top of the list. Nevertheless, most schools' philosophies include statements about what the faculty believe characterizes a member of the profession, and the faculty member may glean from those written words how the school will promote professional awareness and activism within their faculty members and students.

5   How can I assess a school's capacity for promoting professional awareness and activism to its students?

First, ask questions:

- Does the school have a nursing students' association and, if so, how active is it? How are faculty members involved in the students' association? Who is the association's advisor, and is the advisor active in his or her own professional associations?

- Do faculty members give clinical "time" for students to participate in such activities as the nursing students' association's annual conference, legislative days, or trips to volunteer at health fairs?

- Are nursing students involved in college activities, such as the student government association? Are students actively encouraged to become involved in college activities?

- How do faculty members describe nursing students they consider to be "outstanding"? Are these students who get good grades? Are they students who are involved in student activities? Are these students who have planned and implemented projects aimed at the greater good?

Second, evaluate student posters and other wall art:

- What types of posters line the walls of the school?
- What projects have students showcased?

Third, talk to the students. Do students believe they are an integral part of the college? Do they believe that their opinions and contributions are genuinely sought and appreciated? Younger people have their own unique perspectives; are these encouraged and supported by the college? Is there an atmosphere of open-mindedness and a willingness to consider different viewpoints?

6   How can I determine whether a school values professional awareness and activism among its faculty members?

Look first at the leadership. Is the dean/program head actively involved in the profession? Does the program head hold a leadership position in the professional association or a specialty organization? Is that person involved in the university at large? How does that individual answer questions aimed at finding out the level of commitment to the profession and to activism?

Are faculty members actively involved in the professional association and/or specialty organizations? How do they answer questions about activism for themselves and for their students? From your assessment of the program head and the faculty, how would you assess their willingness to assist you in honing your activist competencies and skills?

---

7   As a new faculty member, how active should I be in the profession?

An absolute for a faculty member is professional awareness. A teacher of nurses should have a broad understanding of the past and the future of the profession; the environment in which nurses work; what factors promote good nursing care and which do not; who are the profession's current and past leaders; and what personal attributes can be ascribed to leaders of nurses. Minimally, a faculty member should belong to the professional organization and to a specialty organization. If time permits, a young faculty member should participate in the organizations' activities or take on a leadership role.

---

8   What is essential for professional awareness for the faculty member?

The faculty member should demonstrate skills and competencies that reflect professional awareness and activism (see Questions 10 and 11). The overt expression of these skills and competencies may look different at various stages of the life of the faculty member. All faculty members should demonstrate activist skills, and these are on a continuum (see Question 11). Above all, a faculty member is a role model for students. As students take on behaviors of the professional, they learn from the interactions with their faculty members and other nurses. If they see activist behaviors in their role models, they will learn that those behaviors are valued components of the professional persona to which they are aspiring.

9 If I am an activist and a leader in my professional association, does it make me a better teacher?

Not necessarily. Some of the skills and competencies that reflect professional awareness and activism cut across roles. These include good communication abilities, critical thinking, and risk taking. Because faculty members serve as role models, to the extent that students take on these competencies from faculty members, they will learn how to assume activist behaviors. Those skills may make them better patient advocates.

However, a good teacher must be more than an activist and professionally aware. The good teacher is one who not only demonstrates the skills and competencies but also encourages these in students, helping students hone these skills while stepping back to allow the students to practice them. There are more skills and competencies to nursing education than those evidenced by professional awareness and activism.

10 What competencies reflect professional awareness and should be promoted in students?

These are the competencies that demonstrate professional awareness:

- **Critical thinking** (evidence of analytic skills, weighing options, synthesis of concepts, and so on)
- **Inquiry** (willingness to ask questions to gain better understanding and to guide actions)
- **Excellent communication skills** within a therapeutic context and as part of membership on an interdisciplinary team
- **Accountability and responsibility** for one's own actions

11 What competencies reflect activism?

Activism is dynamic; it can be conceived as on a continuum of behaviors that reflect concern for self, client, and society. An activist is one who is willing to express a set of beliefs about something of importance.

Activist nurses may limit their activism to the role of nurse-client interaction; that activism is called "advocacy." These nurses speak out for their patients and sometimes take risks that may jeopardize their own livelihoods. Other activist nurses become leaders within their professional organizations, and they speak out for other nurses and patients; again, sometimes at their own peril. It is an unfortunate reality of the nursing profession that chief nursing officers have been known to lose their jobs because of their advocacy for their nurses and the patients with whom they work.

The skills and competencies that make good activist nurses with their patients are the same skills that are used at a more global level: good communication including listening, speaking, and writing; risk taking; critical thinking; and willingness to take personal responsibility for one's actions.

---

12 What teaching/learning strategies help students develop professional awareness?

In a well-integrated curriculum, students will be exposed early to professional awareness. They learn professional awareness by:

- Studying past and present nursing leaders' accomplishments and personal attributes
- Meeting nursing leaders and hearing their personal stories
- Participating in and reflecting on professional activities, such as association meetings
- Engaging in discussions and debates about professional issues, such as regulation, the politics of health-care financing, reimbursement, quality and safety, and so on.

This pedagogy should take place throughout the curriculum and not be reserved for the final semester's trends and leadership courses.

---

13 What teaching/learning strategies help students develop activism?

Activism connotes taking on behaviors that reflect assertiveness and beliefs. That may be asserting beliefs that a patient needs a better understanding of his condition or another treatment. It may mean that the student believes classmates should receive clinical time for attending a political rally. It could mean that a student is nominated for a leadership position in the nursing students' organization. It could mean that the graduate student desires to critique the curriculum constructively.

Whatever the cause, the student must be guided constructively in an encouraging environment to take on activist behaviors. Faculty members have a critical role to play in this developmental process by offering suggestions for improved communication skills, encouraging risk-taking behaviors while providing a psychological safety net, and assisting students in debriefing episodes that involve activist behaviors.

---

14 How do professional awareness and activism affect patient care?

Activism, like advocacy, requires the same skills and competencies; educators want students to learn and practice those skills. By graduation, students should know how to advocate for their patients—students will not be experts, but they should know the essential components of advocacy. Faculty members should have provided them with opportunities to extend those skills to sample activism in the larger healthcare community.

---

15 Is there a connection between professional awareness/activism and clinical proficiency?

Probably not. Faculty members want undergraduate pre-licensure students to be able to deliver care that is safe, not harmful, and to know the difference between safety and harm. These students are, at best, novices at graduation. How does that relate to professional awareness and activism? Ideally, they possess some understanding of the profession and their current and potential contributions to the profession. If they possess the core competencies for activism, that is sufficient. First and foremost, they must be safe novice nurses.

16 How do you promote student involvement in activities that reflect professional awareness and activism?

As such, activities usually involve meetings, conferences, or community-based events, such as wellness fairs. Students respond very well to getting extra credit or clinical time-off for participating in these events. Some schools even provide registration fees for students to attend. Often, faculty cannot resist the temptation to require written reports about field experiences. Faculty members should avoid making the written report onerous; otherwise, students will resent the ties that go along with the privilege of missing a day's clinical or getting the extra credit. If the faculty member requires a written report, it should be short and concise as to the behaviors that are being promoted, such as activism or professional awareness.

An alternative might be for a faculty member to personally invite small numbers of students to attend a professional meeting with him or her (making sure that all students have an equal opportunity to spend time with the faculty member before the end of the semester). Having small numbers of students spend time with their faculty away from an academic setting may be just as valuable for student learning as getting credit for attending a larger meeting.

17 What about teaching professional awareness and activism for graduate students?

Working with graduate students is very different. They should be more than novices in the profession when they graduate. Graduate students tend to be older and more experienced. Graduate school should be about seeing the big picture and developing leadership skills. The curriculum should provide for honing their skills in professional activism. There should be exposure to current leaders in the field and discussions of leaders' professional development. An introduction to politics and how the graduate students can become involved is critical. Graduate students should be encouraged to become change agents in their jobs or communities. The importance of their role in the profession should be an ongoing theme in the curriculum. Emphasizing a sense of responsibility to advancing and improving the profession of nursing should be an integral part of the curriculum.

18 Can the nurse educator encourage activism throughout the curriculum?

Yes. In the curriculum in which professional awareness and activism are integrated throughout, the nurse educator will seek experiences and learning for the students that match the course content. For example, in a beginning course in medical-surgical nursing, students can hear a personal story from a medical-surgical nurse in the community who is in a leadership position. The nurse leader should talk about personal views on being a professional and how that individual demonstrates activist behaviors, in the immediate work setting or within in the profession. Similarly, the clinical faculty member should use vignettes of clinical stories that demonstrate professional awareness and/or activism.

In the curriculum where there is no overt emphasis throughout on activism and/or professional awareness, the responsibility for enhancing student learning is that of the individual faculty member to ensure that students are exposed to professional awareness and activism.

19 How can I incorporate electronic media and communication into activism?

The Internet is a powerful communication tool. Undergraduate students, especially those in the demographic group of 18–25-year-olds, rely on the Internet for communication. Social networking sites are popular forums for disseminating information about themselves to others. This can include political interests. Political action committees have been formed from these online groups, a sort of electronic grassroots activism. Younger voters do not use traditional media to the extent that older voters do. By encouraging students to use blogs, podcasts, and other forms of electronic media, a faculty member should be able to engage students in a comfortable, familiar forum.

Students could be encouraged to post their ideas about their views on various health policies, political leaders, and health-care issues. Other students could post responses to these blogs, and this could serve as an ongoing seminar for a class. This format could be expanded to traditional components of the curriculum as well. The benefit of using electronic media for discussion is that it shows a willingness to move beyond traditional communication and appeal to students at another level.

20 Suppose I am computer-illiterate?

If you are unfamiliar with any of these formats, help can usually be found at the college's computer center. Sometimes there are graduate student assistants who can help with electronic media. Other faculty members can also engage the students in a discussion of the various forms of electronic communication and how they can be used. An interactive group discussion in which student knowledge is being sought could generate some creative thinking and would also show the willingness of the faculty to try new things, keep current in the field, and speak the students' language through inquiry and engagement.

References

Microsoft Encarta College Dictionary. (2001). New York: St. Martin's Press.

Resources

American Nurses Association—Government Affairs. http://nursing-world.org/gova/

Black, L. (2006). From needlestick statistic to nurse advocate. American Journal of Nursing 106(3), 64–66.

Boswell, C., Cannon, S., & Miller, J. (2005). Nurses' political involvement: Responsibility vs. privilege. Journal of Professional Nursing 21(1), 5–8.

Edmunds, L. (2003). Opening the door to care. Accessed March 7, 2007, at http://www.son.jhmi.edu/JHNmagazine/archive/fall2003/index.htm

Gebbie, K., Wakefield, M., & Kerfoot, K. (2000). Nursing and
    health policy. Journal of Nursing Scholarship, 32(3), 307–315.
International Knowledge Network of Women in Politics. Available
    at http://www.iknowpolitics.org
Lumpkin, B.A. (2007). Lobbying: Not a bad word, but a core com-
    petency. Imprint: The Professional Magazine for Nursing
    Students 54(2), 40–43.
Mason, D., Chaffee, M., & Leavitt, J. (Eds.) (2006). Policy and poli-
    tics in nursing and health care, 5th ed. Philadelphia: Saunders.
National Nurse. Available at http://nationalnurse.blogspot.com
Peters, R. (2002). RN nurse administrators' role in health policy:
    Teaching the elephant to dance. Nursing Administration
    Quarterly 26(4), 1–8.
Underwood, P. (2000). Professionalism and activism. Imprint: The
    Professional Magazine for Nursing Students 47(4), 31.

33

Developing Students Into Leaders

Lydia R. Zager, MSN, RN, CNAA-BC

1 Is every nurse, regardless of educational level, a leader?

Yes. Every nurse is a leader; not just as a chief nurse, a supervisor, or a charge nurse. The nurse is a leader whether on the night shift with six to eight patients or in the intensive care unit with one patient: nurses are the leaders of their patients' care.

2 Why is vision an important leadership characteristic for nurses to have?

A vision statement takes thinking beyond the immediate outcomes to a belief that nurses are capable of giving extraordinary care for all patients. A vision propels achievement of personal and professional goals.

- **All nurses need to have a vision of their individual practice:** Students are taught to ask about the mission and vision of the organization where they want to work. The students need to be able to decide if that organization supports the philosophy they have about how they want to practice nursing. It is equally important for every nurse to have a vision of how they want to practice nursing. One opportunity for developing a shared vision was an intensive year-long program in which nurses from across the country met five times for executive leadership development. During the program, a group of nurses developed a vision statement that every individual student and nurse can adopt to guide their practice.

- **Individual Nurse Vision Statement**: "Nurses will unite to transform care-giving through excellent practice that empowers those we serve." It is a simple statement, but the context of the words say so much:
  - "Nurses": Refers to every nurse, regardless of education of specialty.
  - "Transform care-giving": Nurses need to not only care for their patients but also care for each other and to transform the work environment into a supportive place that promotes job satisfaction, increases retention, and ultimately improves patient care.
  - "Excellent practice": This refers to the standards that guide nursing practice. Excellent practice is what allows this vision statement to transcend time, as nurses use evidence-based practice to achieve excellent patient outcomes. Excellent practice also requires nurses to have a guiding belief that education, formal and informal, is a career-long, ongoing process that is necessary in order to provide the best care possible to patients.
  - "Empower those we serve": Care cannot just be provided; it is a partnership with patients and their families and other health-care team members, with the ultimate goal for patients and/or families to be able to care for themselves and to have choices in their care.

If every nurse, on every shift, in every kind of work environment believed that "I transform care by giving excellent practice that empowers my patients," excellence would be the standard.

---

3 Are leadership and management necessary in nursing, and what is the difference?

Both leadership and management are important in nursing. Nurses are managers of care when they follow physicians' orders, give medications, complete treatments, or make arrangements for care to be given by others. Nurses become leaders when they use clinical reasoning skills to make decisions about the priority of care given based on the needs of the patients. Nurses then follow up with necessary interventions, such as calling a physician to report abnormal laboratory values or critical changes in a patient's condition. As leaders, nurses take responsibilities for their actions and make necessary revisions to move patient care forward toward desired mutual outcomes for patients and their families.

---

4   What do students need to know about their own leadership style?

Students who are aware of their own leadership style, both their strengths and weaknesses, take the first step in understanding how others respond to them. Students who understand their own behaviors, their traits, and how they react and handle different and difficult situations will become more effective leaders. There are numerous tools, such as the Keirsey Temperament Sorter, to help students identify their style and their temperament and gain an insight into the temperament of others. This broad awareness will guide them as leaders and prepare them for challenges they may encounter in working with others.

Faculty play a very important role in helping nursing students become leaders. It begins with students taking the role of leader in the care of their patients. When you ask students questions in clinical, begin every question with, "As the nurse leader of your patient's care . . ." For example, "As the nurse leader of your patient's care, what is your priority intervention for this patient?" Leadership is an expectation of nurse graduates now and in the future.

---

5   What are the leadership characteristics that nurses need to demonstrate every day in the care of their patients?

Leadership characteristics include honesty, competence, fairness, open-mindedness, dependability, loyalty, ambition, caring, and cooperativeness. These characteristics are descriptive of all nurses. Nurses are expected to be honest, dependable, and caring. After all, the Gallup poll has shown for several years that nurses are the most trusted profession in the United States. Fairness and open-mindedness are often characteristics that must be developed through ethical, cultural, and leadership training. Instructors need to recognize leadership qualities in students and to encourage them to strive for leadership positions in student nurse organizations as well as membership in Sigma Theta Tau and other honor organizations.

6 Why is courage an important leadership characteristic for nurses to have?

Nurses can be excellent critical thinkers and make the right decisions, but if they lack the courage to implement the decisions, all the critical thinking will not help the patient. Consider the nurse who hesitates to call a physician with important information because the nurse is afraid the physician will not want to be bothered or is afraid of the physician's manner of responding. It takes courage to make decisions other nurses do not agree with. It takes courage when others tell you that you are wrong and you believe you are right, or they tell you to "let it go" because "it is the way we always do it." It takes courage to know you could be wrong but you are willing to go with your best judgment because it is in the best interest of the patient. It takes courage to make the transition from critical thinking and decision making to action. Courage is a vital leadership quality in nursing.

7 What are some of the responsibilities students need to know about as they become nurse leaders and managers who support nursing personnel in providing excellent care to patients?

Students may think that learning about management and leadership is not necessary because they are just new graduates and are not in a leadership role. The charge nurse position, however, often comes quickly to new graduates because of the current shortage of nurses. The role of the charge nurse still carries manager/leadership responsibilities and can be a challenge to new graduate nurses if they are not prepared. Some of these responsibilities, like delegation, patient room assignments, communication, and conflict management, are important to consider. Leadership is essential to help ensure the safe administration of medications. Certainly hospitals are trying to improve the ways medications are given, but it is the responsibility of all nurses to use the "five rights" and question if a medication is appropriate for the patient. New graduates, who become charge nurses or nurse managers, may be required to assess and take action if there are personnel issues or systems issues interfering with safe medication delivery.

The role of the manager/leader is diverse, but students can remember and learn from teachers as they model the leadership behaviors they want students to emulate. It is also important to stress that nurses should constantly model the behaviors they want to see in those they work with. The power of one can be an influential catalyst for positive changes in others.

---

8   What do nursing students need to know about how to delegate?

The most important thing anyone needs to know about delegation is that it does not relieve the delegator of responsibility. The second thing is that you must know what you can legally delegate to another, particularly in nursing, where the nurse practice acts vary from state to state. Good, positive communications skills go a long way in conveying what you want the other person to do. One way to help students practice delegation in the clinical area is to have them delegate to other nursing students, pretending their classmates are a nursing assistant, practical nurse, or another professional nurse. This allows you to review with the students (particularly the "manager") guidelines in delegating:

- Does the individual know how to do what you are requesting?
- Is the person legally able to do it? Is it within the scope of practice?
- Are you delegating a task that is more appropriately done yourself or by another registered nurse? (For example, is this a patient who needs to be taught how to

self-administer insulin for the first time, and should be taught by the RN and not delegated to a practical nurse?)

---

9 How can students be taught to prioritize their nursing care, including delegating appropriately to others?

A good time for faculty to do this is when the students are busy with their clinical assignments and need some help. Guide the students how to prioritize their care for the patients and decide what they could delegate by asking them these questions:

- What are the potential outcomes if something is not done immediately? (This will help them get started.)
- What needs to be done first? (Does a patient need your immediate attention? Is there a stat order that needs to be followed?)
- What could be safely delegated to another nurse, nursing assistant, or practical nurse that would be within their scope of practice?
- What can wait until later?

Initial assessments and patient teaching are the responsibility of the registered nurse. Praise students in their leadership ability to make good nursing decisions about their patients' care.

---

10 What should nursing students be taught about following-through?

It is critical for students to follow up with the individual to whom they delegated. They need to remember that responsibility and accountability remain with the delegator. Teach them to ask the staff or student to whom they delegated:

- Was the task done?
- What were the results, assessment, and/or evaluation?
- What still needs to be done?
- Was the care documented?

Delegation is a powerful leadership tool for others' development and motivation. Emphasize and role-model with students how important feedback is to the person to whom they delegated. Praise and genuine appreciation help build others' self-confidence, and strengthen teamwork.

11 How should students be taught to make patient room assignments?

Teaching how to make room assignments is an important leadership skill but can be difficult because students do not get many opportunities to do this. Even if they do not make the room assignments for their patients, you can have discussion with the students about what they would have done. Remind them that clinical judgment is a characteristic of leadership, and help them work through issues such as:

- Is the patient immunocompromised? Does the patient have an infection and need isolation?
- Are there safety issues, risks of falls, suicide precautions, risks of injury? Does the patient need to be near the nurses' station for observation?
- What is the age and gender of the patient? If the patient is a child, growth and development needs as well as gender must be considered.
- Does the patient have internal radiation and need a private room?

12 What communication skills do students need to be effective leaders?

Nursing students take classes in how to communicate effectively with their patients, and these same communication skills can work well for them as team members and as leaders. Nursing faculty can help guide the students to use vocabulary that is suitable and direct and is communicated with enthusiasm and confidence. Precise speech is always important but particularly when it relates to what needs to be done for patients. Teach students to evaluate if what they said and meant was what the other person heard and thought. This communication is necessary to prevent conflicts, misunderstandings and more importantly is essential for patient safety. It is important that students receive this same kind of feedback when they are in clinical and are communicating with other health-care providers. Create a role-playing exercise for students using scenarios, and videotape the interactions. Videotaping provides valuable feedback to students about what they said, how they said it, and what message their body language is communicating.

13 What do students need to know about conflict?

Conflict is unavoidable. Conflict needs to be approached with an open mind; the other's point of view needs to be heard. In health care, the best interest of the patient is always the common concern between parties. Conflict can have the following positive results:

- Be a catalyst for change
- Facilitate group cohesiveness
- Help improve organizational effectiveness

When conflicts are resolved, the result can be a tremendous source of personal and organizational growth. Personal insight into how we handle conflict is an important skill for nurse leaders.

14 How can students learn more about resolving conflict?

The Thomas-Kilmann Conflict Mode Index (2002) is a quick and easy tool for nursing instructors to order and use in the classroom. It determines which method of conflict resolution is preferable and when it is appropriate to use that method: According to Thomas and Kilmann, the five ways people deal with conflict are:

- **"Avoidance—I lose/you win"**—Appropriate if the issue is not worth the trouble
- **"Accommodation—I lose/you win"**—Appropriate when you know you are wrong, and the issue is more important to the other party
- **"Compromise—I lose/you lose"**—Appropriate as a quick fix for a temporary settlement or inconsequential issues

- **"Collaboration—I win/you win"**—Appropriate for complex issues; gains commitment for change and spreads responsibilities
- **"Competition—I win/you lose"**—Appropriate when quick decisions are needed and the issue is vital to the organization

None of the approaches is all right or all wrong. What is important to know is when to use which approach based on the situation. Nurses as a group tend to compromise or accommodate; they need to work toward collaboration whenever it is appropriate. Developing skills in conflict resolution is not easy and is developed over time. It is very important that this training be included in the nursing curriculum.

15 How should work environments be discussed with students?

Share the research by Kramer and Schmalenburg (2004) that found that 80% of the nurses they surveyed who perceived they had a supportive work environment, were satisfied in their jobs and their ability to provide quality patient care. Satisfied nurses are a positive factor in quality patient care. Students need to be guided to select places of employment where the nurse leaders/managers provide the mentoring needed for new nurses to advance in their careers. Students need to seek places of employment where middle managers have the leadership skills, knowledge, and abilities to ensure there is a supportive work environment. Those managers and leaders can serve as strong role models for the nursing graduates.

16 What should students seek in a work environment that will give them job satisfaction and utilize their leadership skills?

Students need to look for a work environment that will give them the best opportunity to develop as nurses and as leaders. This kind of work environment is essential in order to stop the revolving door of graduate nurses leaving the workplace in less than a year, or even more critically, leaving nursing altogether. The American Association of Colleges of Nursing has an excellent publication called *Hallmarks of the Professional Nursing Practice Environment* (2002). In the companion pamphlet for students, called *What Every Nursing School Graduate Should Consider When Seeking Employment*, there are sample questions to help identify a preferred work environment. These documents are free on the AACN Web site and are excellent resources for helping students identify strengths and weaknesses of a potential employing agency. Some of the considerations include a preceptorship or residency program; a collaborative, interdisciplinary team; encouragement of continuing education; clinical advancement programs; clinical and organizational decision-making characteristics; philosophy of patient care; and how the nurse's knowledge and contributions will be recognized.

It is important to teach students to visit the units where they are seeking employment. A positive work environment and being supported is more important to job satisfaction, particularly in the first year of employment, than the specialty of nursing chosen. More than ever, nurses are shopping for a facility with a positive atmosphere and teamwork, as much as they are looking at pay (Ferrie & Scott, 2004). It is essential that students not only seek positions with a supportive environment but that they model that behavior when they are in leadership positions. As Gladwell (2000) states, this can be the "tipping point" for change. If nursing students expect and choose to work only where there is a supportive work environment, support becomes the rule, not the exception.

---

17 What about the importance of having and being a mentor?

There are different types of mentoring roles. The first type of mentoring students will encounter will be their preceptor, who will help them refine their nursing skills and abilities needed for the position they are in. It is important to discuss with them about how finding the right mentor can help them achieve their goals and work in areas that are professionally challenging. Ask them to identify nurses whom they admire or who are in positions the student aspires to some day. Encourage students to ask these nurses how they achieved their goals. Share stories about your mentors. Tell students how someone special guided you, gave you insight and feedback about your career. Sharing personal stories about how a mentor encouraged and influenced you in the decisions you made about your education and career gives realistic examples of the important role of mentors.

18 What should students be taught about planning their careers?

Perhaps most important is goal setting. Writing out goals increases the chances they will be achieved. If all nurses write a career plan, update it each year, and share it with their nurse leader, they will be prepared to assume roles of increasing responsibilities and leadership in the future. This planning needs to begin with students. Before they graduate, have nursing students write their 3-year career plan to take with them to job interviews. With a written plan, new graduates will be able to make better decisions about which place of employment will help them achieve their career goals. This type of pre-planning will increase the chances of a good relationship between the new nurse and the health-care facility.

References

American Association of Colleges of Nursing. (2002). Hallmarks of the professional nursing practice environment. Washington, DC: Author. Accessed April 28, 2007, at http://www.aacn.nche.edu/Publications/positions/hallmarks.htm

Ferrie, B., & Scott, A. (2004). Seeking satisfaction. Advance for Nurses 6(4), 9–10.

Gladwell, M. (2000). The tipping point. New York: Little Brown.

Kramer, M., & Schmalenburg, C. (2004). Development and evaluation of essentials of magnetism tool. Journal of Nursing Administration 34(7–8), 365–378.

Thomas, K.W., & Kilmann, R.H. (2002), Thomas-Kilmann conflict mode instrument. Available at www.cpp.com

Resources

Aiken, L.H., et al. (2003). Educational levels of hospital nurses and surgical patient mortality. Journal of American Medical Association 290(12), 1617–1623.

Keirsey, D. (1998). Leadership, temperament, and talent. Del Mar, Calif.: Prometheus Nemesis Book.

Keirsey, D. (1998). The sixteen types. Del Mar, Calif.: Prometheus Nemesis Book.

Kerfoot, K.M. (2006). Leadership/management and the workplace. Nursing Administration Quarterly 30(4), 373–374.

Kramer, M. & Schmalenburg, C. (2004) Essentials of a magnetic work environment. Nursing 34(6), 50–54.

Nanus, B. (1992). Visionary leadership. San Francisco, Calif.: Jossey-Bass.

Pinkerton, S.E. (2003). Mentoring new graduates. Nursing Economics 21(4), 202.

Sherman, R.O. (2005). Growing our future nursing leaders. Nursing Administration Quarterly 29(2), 125–132.

Sleutel, M.R. (2000). Climate, culture, context or work environment? Journal of Nursing Administration 30(2), 53–58.

Thompson, P.A., Navarra, M.B., & Antonson, N. (2005). Patient safety: The four domains of nursing leadership. Nursing Economic$ 23(6): 331–333.

Zager, L.R., & Walker, E. (2005). One vision, one voice: Transforming caregiving in nursing. Orthopedic Nursing 24(2).

34

Considering Emerging Curriculum Issues

Joan M. Stanley, PhD, RN, CRNP, FAAN

---

1 What external forces are affecting nursing education and practice?

- **Global nature of health care.** Health care can no longer be perceived as national; it is global. Advances in communication and transportation have opened many avenues for world travel and commerce, leading to increased exposure to infectious diseases, access to new technologies and treatments, and changes in health-care policies and economics.
- **Changing demographics.** A growing aging population and increased percentages of underrepresented minorities will continue to have an increasing impact on health-care needs and health professionals' practice. In 2002, 12% of the U.S. population (more than 35 million people) was older than 65 years of age. By 2030, approximately 70 million persons, or 20% of the U.S. population, will be older than 65 years (Administration on Aging, U.S. Department of Health and Human Services, 2004). The Institute of Medicine (IOM) (2003b) report, *Unequal Treatment*, confirmed that racial and ethnic disparities in health care include differences in access, clinical appropriateness, and patient preferences.
- **Increasing prevalence of chronic diseases.** A rising prevalence of chronic health problems, primarily due to

lifestyle, increasing rates of obesity, and increases in the number of older adults, will place significant demands on the health-care system and affect the types and quantity of health-care services needed. The predominant health problems of older adults are chronic rather than acute and are exacerbated by normal changes of aging.

- **Health professional workforce shortages.** Current and projected workforce shortages in other health professions, including pharmacy and medicine, will affect the numbers of professional nurses needed, areas of specialization, and scope of practice. Physician shortages in primary care and gerontology are projected to be particularly dramatic.
- **Demands for changes in health profession education.** Over the past 10 years, reports, including those from the IOM (2000, 2001, 2003), the American Hospital Association (2002), the Joint Commission (2002), and the Robert Wood Johnson Foundation (2002) have exhorted health professions to change the way future practitioners are educated.
- **Complexity of health-care system.** The health-care system is growing increasingly complex. Patients, both inside and outside the acute care facility, are at the center of an increasingly intertwined web of specialists, practitioners, administrative personnel, information resources, government requirements, and so on.

---

2 What internal forces are affecting nursing education and practice?

- **Nursing shortage.** Current shortages of nurses are projected to continue in certain geographic areas, specific health-care settings, and particular practice areas (Biviano, et al., 2004).
- **Dissatisfaction with work environment.** Many nurses (41%) are dissatisfied in their work environments and plan to leave their current positions. Nurses younger than 30 years are particularly vulnerable to becoming dissatisfied and burning out quickly; one report indicated that 33% planned to leave their job within the year (Aiken, et al., 2001).

- **Increased demand for nursing services and specialization.** With the growing shortages of other health professionals, nurses increasingly are providing access to care in medically underserved areas, to diverse populations, and in growing areas of specialization, e.g., palliative care, chronic disease management, oncology, critical care, and school health.
- **Faculty shortage.** Shortages of nursing faculty limit the ability of schools of nursing to expand enrollments: 71% of generic baccalaureate nursing programs and 70% of master's degree programs reported an insufficient number of faculty as the primary reason for not admitting all qualified applicants (Fang, Wisniewski, & Bednash, 2007a). In addition, nursing faculty have continued to age. For doctoral faculty, the mean age is 55.3 years (Fang, Wisniewski, & Bednash, 2007b), up from 49.7 in 1993 and 54.3 in 2004 (American Association of Colleges of Nursing, 2005).
- **Limited clinical sites.** Competition among health professions for available clinical or training sites also limits the ability of schools to expand enrollments to address the nursing workforce shortages. For baccalaureate and master's programs, respectively, insufficient clinical sites (56% and 45%) and insufficient clinical preceptors (30% and 46%) were cited as limiting a school's ability to accept qualified applicants (Fang, Wisniewski, & Bednash, 2007a).

---

3 In light of these changes and pressures within the health-care system, how should nursing education respond?

- All nurses need new knowledge and skills through expanded and different educational experiences. With growing evidence of improved patient care outcomes, increasing numbers of national nursing organizations and foundations, the military, federal agencies, and state nursing associations are recognizing the need for nurses to be educated at the baccalaureate and master's level.

    The American Association of Colleges of Nursing (AACN) has crafted a new vision for nursing education, which includes evolving all advanced specialty nursing practice to the practice doctorate (DNP) and a new advanced generalist role, the clinical nurse leader (CNL), prepared at the master's level. These parallel initiatives have evolved after many years of dialogue, both within and outside nursing. The minimum level of education required for entry into professional generalist nursing practice would continue to be the baccalaureate degree, which provides a significant resource for patient care in all settings.

4 What is a generalist nurse?

The generalist nurse is a registered professional nurse currently prepared at the entry level through a variety of education models, e.g., associate degree, baccalaureate degree, second-degree baccalaureate, or master's generic nursing program. Graduates have broad preparation in the professional nursing role across the continuum of health care. Generalist preparation enables nursing care for a variety of patients and in most health-care settings.

5 What is an advanced generalist nurse?

The advanced generalist nurse is a new concept in nursing education and practice. This nurse is prepared at the master's level. Master's preparation can be post-baccalaureate in nursing or generic master's education. The generic master's advanced generalist education would provide the graduate with the entry-level or baccalaureate competencies in addition to the more advanced generalist competencies that include knowledge and skills over and above those expected of a graduate of a generalist nursing program. One advanced generalist nursing role that is currently being implemented by more than 90 nursing schools is the CNL.

6 What is a CNL?

The CNL is a new nursing role currently being implemented by over 90 schools of nursing. The CNL practices across the continuum of care and in all types of health-care settings, including acute care hospitals, long-term care, outpatient settings, public health, school health , and home health care. Graduate preparation is in a master's advanced generalist nursing education program. As an advanced generalist, although the graduate may have practice experiences that provide additional knowledge and skills in a specialty, the education program prepares the individual with knowledge and skills applicable to all practice settings and patient populations. The CNL is not an administrative role but is expected to provide and manage clinical care at the point of care for a cohort of patients within a health-care setting. Some of the key components of the CNL role include an emphasis on the lateral coordination of care; risk anticipation and the design or redesign of plans of care; quality improvement strategies; implementation of evidence-based practice; and the development and leveraging of human, environmental, and material resources (American Association of Colleges of Nursing, 2007).

7 What is the DNP degree? How is this degree different from a research-focused degree (PhD, DNS, DNSc)?

The DNP degree is the designation for practice doctorate programs in nursing. Practice-focused doctoral programs prepare experts in any area of specialized advanced nursing practice. DNP programs focus on nursing practice and build on the baccalaureate and master's nursing competencies. The AACN, in a position statement approved by the membership in 2004, proposed that the practice doctorate be the graduate degree for advanced nursing practice preparation, including the four advanced practice registered nurse (APRN) roles: clinical nurse specialist, nurse practitioner, nurse midwife, and nurse anesthetist (American Association of Colleges of Nursing, 2004). Other areas of specialty nursing practice that will be prepared at the DNP level include community health, informatics, and leadership/nursing administration.

Research-focused doctoral nursing programs primarily grant the Doctor of Philosophy degree (PhD); however, some offer the Doctor of Nursing Science degree (DNS, DSN

or DNSc). The research-focused program is designed to prepare nurse scientists and scholars with a heavy emphasis on
scientific content and research methodologies to conduct
original research and generation of new knowledge in the
discipline of nursing (American Association of Colleges of
Nursing, 2006).

---

8   How can schools of nursing maximize clinical experiences?

One limiting factor in expanding enrollments in schools of
nursing is the dearth of clinical sites. Also, calls for graduates
to have increased opportunities to integrate didactic learning into clinical practice are mounting. New models of clinical education to expand enrollments and maximize clinical
experiences are being implemented in all types and sizes of
nursing schools across the country. One model that is receiving increased attention is community-based education.
Community-based education is not the same as community
health nursing, which is a specialized area of nursing practice. Rather, community-based education provides the
opportunity to use different teaching strategies and diverse
settings. It exposes the student to patient needs from a variety of perspectives, provides opportunities to provide care
along a continuum, work more readily with interdisciplinary teams, work within and across diverse health-care delivery environments and communities, and provide care for
diverse populations (American Association of Colleges of
Nursing, 2000). A critical feature of community-based education is the development of true, innovative academic and
community partnerships that are unlimited. Innovative
health-care experiences may include such diverse settings as
senior day-care centers, school health clinics, churches,
migrant clinics, occupational health-care settings, or even
the local laundromat.

The use of simulation and other technologies provides
a growing array of teaching/learning methodologies. As
schools seek ways to expand student enrollments and
address growing faculty shortages and insufficient clinical
practice sites, the increased use of simulation is being

considered and evaluated. Simulation and other forms of technology cannot totally replace the more traditional clinical experiences and face-to-face encounters. However, increasing evidence highlights the positive learning outcomes and innovative uses of technology, including assuring students have the opportunity to practice specific skills, receive adequate feedback, obtain experiences that may be limited in a given time period, and develop sufficient skills prior to performing in a real patient environment. (For additional information, see Chapter 19 on the use of simulation.)

---

9   What emerging areas of knowledge and skills will all nurses need to practice in the future health-care system?

- Evidence-based practice
- Patient safety
- Quality improvement
- Health-care and information technologies
- Gerontology (care of older adults across the continuum from well to the frail elderly)
- Population health, health promotion
- Cultural competence or cultural awareness
- Spirituality
- Globalization of health care
- Genetics and genomics
- Emerging infectious diseases
- Management of chronic illnesses
- Environmental health
- Disaster or emergency preparedness
- Interprofessional practice, including team building, communications, dynamics and team leadership
- Complex systems, microsystems

This list is not prioritized and is not meant to be exhaustive. Rather, it indicates the array of increasingly important issues. The depth of content will be different for the generalist, advanced generalist, and advanced nursing specialist. For many of these areas, a few select resources are listed in Figure 34–1 to get you started.

322

Selected Resources for Areas of Emerging Nursing Curricula

PATIENT SAFETY & QUALITY IMPROVEMENT:
- Quality and Safety Education for Nurses (QSEN) initiative website
  http://www. qsen. org
- Series of 5 articles on the QSEN competencies in *Nursing Outlook*
  May/June 2007.
- American Association of Colleges of Nursing. (2006). Hallmarks of Quality and Patient
  Safety. Accessed at
  http://www.aacn.nche.edu/publications/WhitePapers/Qual&PatientSafety.htm

GERONTOLOGY: CARING FOR OLDER ADULTS ACROSS THE CARE CONTINUUM FROM WELL TO THE FRAIL ELDERLY
- American Association of Colleges of Nursing. (2004). Nurse Practitioner and Clinical
  Nurse Specialist Competencies for Older Adult Care. Can be accessed at
  http://www.aacn.nche.edu/
- American Association of Colleges of Nursing. (2000). Older Adults: Recommended
  baccalaureate competencies and curricular guidelines for geriatric nursing care. Can
  be accessed at http://www.aacn.nche.edu/
- Thomlow D, Latimer D, Kingsborough J, Arietti L. (2006). Caring for an Aging America:
  A Guide for Nursing Faculty. Washington, DC: American Association of Colleges of
  Nursing.
- The John A. Hartford Institute for Geriatric Nursing website
  http://www.hartfordign.org/resources/education/bsnPartners.html. Provides access
  to several excellent geriatric curriculum resources.
- NICHE Program: Nurses Improving Care for HealthSystem Elders. Can be accessed at
  http://www.nicheprogram.org/programs
- American Journal of Nursing (2007). How to Try This: Assessments and Best Practices
  in Care of Older Adult. Accessed at http://www.NursingsCenter.com/AJN olderadults

END-OF-LIFE CARE
- American Association of Colleges of Nursing. (1998). Peaceful death: Recommended
  competencies & curricular guidelines for end-of-life nursing care. Access at
  http://www.aacn.nche.edu/Education/deathfin.htm
- American Association of Colleges of Nursing & City of Hope. ELNEC, End-of-Life
  Nursing Education Consortium Advancing End-of-Life Nursing
  Care Training Program.

POPULATION HEALTH, HEALTH PROMOTION
- Association for Prevention Teaching and Research. Prevention Education Resource
  Center (PERC). Online interprofessional exhange of teaching resources and
  education activities for prevention and population health education. Access at
  http://www.teachprevention.org
- US Preventive Services Task Force (2006). Guide to clinical preventive services, 2006:
  Recommendations of US Preventive Services task force. Access at
  http://www.ahrq.gov/clinic/pocketgd.htm
- Allan J., Barwick T., Cashman S., Cawley, J., Day C., Chester D., Evans C., Garr D.,
  Maeshiro R., McCarthy R., Meyer S., Riegelman R., Seifer S., Stanley J., Swenson M.,
  Teitelbaum H., Timothe P., Wemer K., Wood D. (2004). Clinical prevention and
  population health curriculum framework for health professions. *American Journal of
  Preventive Medicine 27(5)* Elsevier Inc.
- Allan J., Stanley J., Crabtree M.K., Wemer K., Swenson M. (2005). Clinical prevention
  and population health curriculum framework: The nursing perspective. *Journal of
  Professional Nursing 21(5)* Elsevier Inc.

Figure 34–1. Resources.

323

Selected Resources for Areas of Emerging Nursing Curricula

CULTURAL COMPETENCE

- American Association of Colleges of Nursing (in draft). Competencies for Cultural Competency in Baccalaureate Nursing Education. After May 2008 can be accessed at http://www.aacn.nche.edu
- Purnell LD, Paulanka BJ. (2003). *Transcultural Health Care: A Culturally Competent Approach, 2nd edition.* Philadelphia: F.A. Davis.
- Purnell LD, Paulanka BJ. (2005). *Guide to Culturally Competent Health Care.* Philadelphia: F.A. Davis.

GENETICS AND GENOMICS

- Consensus Panel. (2006). Essential Nursing Competencies and Curricula Guidelines for Genetics and Genomics. Silver Spring, MD: American Nurses Association. Available at http://www.aacn.nche.edu/Education/pdf/Genetics%20%20Genomics%20Nursing%20Competencies%2009-22-06.pdf or http://www.genome.gov/17517037
- Jenkins J, Calzone K. (2007). Establishing the essential nursing competencies for genetics and genomics. *Journal of Nursing Scholarship, 39 (1)* 10-16.

ENVIRONMENTAL HEALTH

- Commission for Environmental Cooperation. (2006). *Children's Health and the Environment in North America.* Montreal, Canada: Author.
- National Environmental Education & Training Foundation. (2005). *Environmental Management of Pediatric Asthma, Guidelines for Health Care Providers.* Washington, DC: Author.
- National Environmental Education & Training Foundation. (2003). *National Pesticide Competency Guidelines for Medical & Nursing Education.* Washington, DC: Author. http://www.neetf.org/health/providers/index.shtm
- National Environmental Education & Training Foundation. (2003). *National Pesticide Practice Skills Guidelines for Medical & Nursing Practice.* Washington, DC: Author. http://www.neetf.org/health/providers/index.shtm

DISASTER OR EMERGENCY PREPAREDNESS

- Nursing Emergency Preparedness Education Coalition (NEPEC) website can be accessed at http://www.mc.vanderbilt.edu/nursing/incmce.
- International Nursing Coalition for Mass Casualty Education (2003). Educational competencies for registered nurses responding to mass casualty incidents. Access at http://www.aacn.nche.edu/Education/pdf/INCMCECompetencies.pdf
- Veenema T.G. (2006). Ready RN: Disaster Nursing and Emergency Preparedness. Elsevier/MCStrategies. Accessed at http://www.webinservice.com/
- George Washington University. National Nurse Emergency Preparedness Initiative. Includes six online learning modules for nurses. Information can be accessed at http://www.gwumc.nnepi.org
- Veenema, TG. *Disaster Nursing and Emergency Preparedness for Chemical, Biological and Radiological Terrorism and Other Hazards, 2nd edition.* New York, NY: Springer Publishing Company.

COMPLEX SYSTEMS & MICROSYSTEMS

- The Plexus Institute website can be accessed at http://www.plexusinstitute.org/About/New to Complexity.cfm
- Series of 9 articles. Microsystems in Health Care, published September 2002-November 2003 in *The Journal on Quality Improvement* by The Joint Commission. Authors are Nelson EC, Batalden PB, Huber TP, Mohr JJ, Godfrey MM, Headrick LA, and Wasson JH.
- The Dartmouth Institute for Health Policy and Clinical Practice. http://www.clinical microsystem.org

Figure 34–1. *Continued*

10 How can all this new content be added to an already full curriculum?

Nursing faculty continuously ask how can they possibly fit any additional content or experiences into an already over-loaded curriculum. In many situations, the maximum number of credits allowed by the institution for a degree are already required, the maximum number of clinical and didactic hours are already built into the curriculum, and the expectations/learning assignments for each course credit have ballooned. As health-care knowledge and com-plexity of the health-care system increase, nursing cannot continue to prepare new practitioners in the same tradi-tional ways. Content and learning experiences, including general and professional education components, must be integrated, build on previous learning, and not be duplica-tive or isolated.

One practical approach to integrating new content is to refocus what is currently taught within any given learning session, section, or course. Case studies can be used to inte-grate multiple principles or content areas. For example, a geriatric patient in a critical care setting provides an oppor-tunity to focus on principles and differences in aging, spiri-tuality, cultural variations/beliefs, interprofessional team communications, as well as critical care. Other examples are a mass casualty scenario that involves biological or infec-tious agents and working in an interprofessional team to develop quality improvement strategies. Through refocusing strategies, newer content and learning can be integrated into existing courses. Response to disasters may be integrated into health assessment, health policy, critical care, infection control, mental health experiences, and interprofessional communication content. Environmental health content and learning experiences may be integrated into more traditional pediatric, community health, health policy, health educa-tion, and health promotion content and experiences.

Due to time constraints, limited opportunities, and expectations of graduates to provide care in an increasingly complex health-care system and to diverse populations, nursing educators do not have the luxury of providing uni-focal learning experiences that do not integrate and build on previous learning experiences and opportunities.

---

11 When might this "new future" for nursing education exist?

Nursing education has consistently been in an evolving state, at times more rapidly than others. For example, nurse practitioner education began in certificate programs and, gradually through the 1970s and 1980s, increased in number and transitioned to master's degree education programs. This transition occurred primarily in response to changes within schools of nursing and in response to the community's demand for an increasing number of APRNs prepared to provide accessible, high-quality care to diverse populations. The current changes in nursing education will not occur at any one point in time. The proposals that have been made by the AACN and others have developed over 5–10 years. In 2004, the AACN membership set 2015 as the target date for all specialty advanced nursing education, which includes all APRN education, to move to the practice doctorate. Whether this target will be reached remains to be seen. Schools of nursing are developing new advanced generalist master's degree and DNP programs. In 2006, 93 schools were at some stage of developing a CNL track within the master's degree program. Also in 2006, 20 schools indicated they were admitting students to a DNP program, with an additional 63 schools indicating they were in the planning phase (Fang, Wisniewski, Bednash, 2007a). In June 2007, at least 49 schools had indicated they were admitting students to a DNP program and the list continues to grow (AACN, 2007). At what point these numbers reach a critical mass or tipping point is not known. The amount of energy invested in the dialogue surrounding these initiatives has been tremendous and continues to grow, indicating a high level of focus and interest in making these transitions.

The influences and changes described here are just a few out of many that we must consider as we design and (continuously) redesign nursing curricula. We cannot continue to teach the way we have in the past without being left in the wake of a rapidly changing health-care system.

References

Administration on Aging, U.S. Department of Health and Human services. (2004). Statistics. Available at http://www.aoa.dhhs.gov/prof/Statistics/statistics.asp

Aiken, L.H., et al. (2001). Nurses' reports on hospital care in five countries. Health Affairs May/June 2001, 43–53.

American Association of Colleges of Nursing. (2007). Doctor of Nursing Practice (DNP) Programs. Accessed October 2007 at http://www.aacn.nche.edu/DNP/DNPProgramList.htm.

American Association of Colleges of Nursing. (2005). Faculty shortages in baccalaureate and graduate nursing programs: Scope of the problem and strategies for expanding the supply. Accessed April 27, 2007, at http://www.aacn.nche.edu/Publications/pdf/05FacShortage.pdf

American Association of Colleges of Nursing. (2000). Implementing community-based education in the undergraduate nursing curriculum. Washington, DC: Author.

American Association of Colleges of Nursing. (2004). Position statement on the practice doctorate in nursing. Washington, DC: Author. Accessed April 27, 2007, at http://www.aacn.nche.edu/DNP/DNPPositionStatement.htm

American Association of Colleges of Nursing. (2006). The essentials of doctoral education for advanced nursing practice. Washington, DC: Author. Accessed April 27, 2007, at http://www.aacn.nche.edu/DNP/pdf/Essentials.pdf

American Association of Colleges of Nursing. (2007). White paper on the education and role of the clinical nurse leader. Washington, DC : Author. Accessed April 27, 2007, at http://www.aacn.nche.edu/Publications/WhitePapers/CNL2-07.pdf

American Hospital Association Commission on Workforce for Hospitals and Health Systems. (2002). In our hands: How hospital leaders can build a thriving workforce. Chicago, Ill.: Author.

Biviano, M., et al. (2004). What is behind HRSA's projected supply, demand, and shortages of registered nurses. Washington, DC: Health Resources and Services Administration.

Fang, D., Wisniewski, S.W., & Bednash, G.D. (2007a). 2006–2007 Enrollment and graduations in baccalaureate and graduate programs in nursing. Washington, DC: American Association of Colleges of Nursing.

Fang, D., Wisniewski, S.W., & Bednash, G.D. (2007b). 2006–2007 Salaries of instructional and administrative nursing faculty in baccalaureate and graduate programs in nursing. Washington, DC: American Association of Colleges of Nursing.

Institute of Medicine. (2001). Crossing the quality chasm. Washington, DC: National Academies Press.

Institute of Medicine. (2003a). Health professions education: A bridge to quality. Washington, DC: National Academies Press.

Institute of Medicine. (2000). To err is human: Building a safer health system. Washington, DC: National Academies Press.

Institute of Medicine. (2003b). Unequal treatment. Washington, DC: National Academies of Science.

Joint Commission on Accreditation of Healthcare Organizations. (2002). Healthcare at the crossroads: Strategies for addressing the evolving nursing crisis. Chicago: Author.

Robert Wood Johnson Foundation. (2002). Health care's human crisis. Princeton, NJ: Author.

VI

FLOURISHING IN THE FACULTY ROLE

35

Understanding the Nursing Faculty Shortage

Linda E. Berlin, DrPH, RNC,
and Karen R. Sechrist, PhD, RN, FAAN

1 How serious is the nursing shortage problem?

The problem of inadequate numbers of faculty in all nursing programs is extremely serious. The objective of this chapter is to quantify the extent and severity of the problem based on factual information.

2 What is the extent of the problem?

For academic year 2006–2007, there was a 7.9% vacancy rate for full-time faculty positions in schools with baccalaureate and graduate programs, according to the American Association of Colleges of Nursing (AACN) (2006). In addition, 55 (16.7%) of the 329 responding schools had no vacant positions but needed additional faculty. Vacancies per school ranged from 1 to 18. The National League for Nursing (2006) also found a 7.9% vacancy rate in baccalaureate and graduate programs and a 5.6% vacancy rate in associate degree programs. Vacancy rates of less than 10% may not seem like much, but even one or two vacant positions can have a significant impact on the workload demands of the remaining faculty.

3 Why is the faculty vacancy rate significant?

The vacancy rate is significant because it restricts the number of students that schools can admit. In academic year 2005–2006, 41,683 qualified applications were not accepted to baccalaureate, master's, and doctoral programs. As the most important reason for not accepting all qualified applications, 44% of schools reported insufficient numbers of faculty (Fang, Wilsey-Wisniewski, & Bednash, 2006a). The result is not only will fewer people become nurses but the pool of future faculty will also be further diminished.

4 What is the primary reason for the shortage of faculty?

The important reason is related to demographics—the aging of the faculty. There are large numbers of faculty at or approaching retirement and not enough younger faculty to take their place. This is a serious situation that will not improve in the foreseeable future.

5 What about current faculty?

In academic year 2005–2006, there were data on 11,635 full-time nurse faculty teaching in 575 schools with baccalaureate and/or graduate degree programs (82% response rate). Of these, 47% held doctoral degrees (in nursing or other fields), and 53% had master's degrees (Fang, Wilsey-Wisniewski, & Bednash, 2006b).

6 What is the average age?

Like the overall nursing workforce, the average age for doctoral degree faculty has increased steadily, going from 50.7 years in 1995 to 54.7 years in academic year 2005. Faculty members with master's degrees are 5.6 years younger, going from 46.6 in 1995 to 49.2 in 2004, with a slight dip to 49.1 in 2005 (Fig. 35–1).

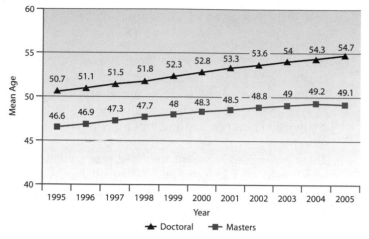

Figure 35–1. Average age of full-time nurse faculty, 1995–2005 (AACN, 1995–2005a).

---

7 Why the slight dip the age?

The most likely reason is due to the increased recruitment of individuals who are primarily engaged in precepting students at clinical sites. These individuals are given the faculty rank of clinical or faculty associate, clinical instructor, specialist, and adjunct faculty. These individuals are often younger than faculty with the rank of instructor, assistant, and associate professor. Faculty members in these categories increased by 1.2% from 2004 to 2005 (Berlin, Wilsey, & Bednash, 2005; Fang, et al., 2006b).

---

8 How fast are teachers aging, and have any studies been done to determine how many faculty will be eligible to retire over the next several years?

In 2002, we calculated that full-time nurse faculty members who were teaching in 2001 and were age 62 or younger were aging almost half a year each subsequent year for doctoral faculty and a third of a year each year for master's faculty. We also did retirement projections for the group by creating statistical models for doctoral and master's-level faculty.

9 What were the findings related to retirement over the next several years?

- From 2004 to 2012, anywhere from 200 to 300 doctoral faculty members will be eligible to retire each year.
- Because master's-level teachers are generally younger, the peak years for retirement eligibility will be 2012 to 2018, when between 220 and 280 individuals will reach retirement age each year.
- These projections represent the "best case scenario" and were based on the assumptions that all faculty would work until age 62 (average retirement age was 62.5 at the time) and that no additional faculty would leave teaching for personal or professional reasons. Keep in mind that faculty members teaching in 2001 who were 62 years and older could retire in most university systems at any time; and some younger faculty members are taking early retirement incentives because of institutional budget cuts, so the above projections are very conservative (Berlin & Sechrist, 2002a; 2002b).

10 Is there additional information about aging faculty?

The data are even more striking when the percentage of faculty over and under 50 years of age is plotted. In 1995 the percentage of doctoral faculty 50 and over and 50 and under was 55% and 45%, respectively. By 2005 the gap widened considerably, with almost 80% age 50 and over and 20% under 50 (Fig. 35–2). Master's faculty show an opposite pattern, with a wide gap in 1995 to a narrow gap in 2005 (Fig. 35–3).

11 What happened?

When considering doctoral faculty, the decline in those 36–45 years old was 14.2% (Fig. 35–4). For master's faculty, the same age category declined by 18.3%, going from 39.4% in 1995 to 21.1% in 2005 (Fig. 35–5). Some moved to the next age category, but younger teachers are leaving or not entering academia. This is a serious problem.

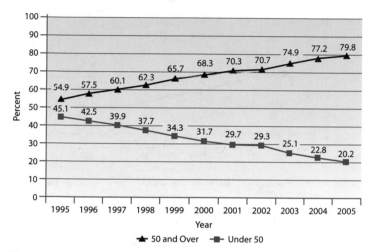

Figure 35–2. Percentage of doctoral faculty over and under the age of 50, 1995–2005 (AACN, 1995–2005a).

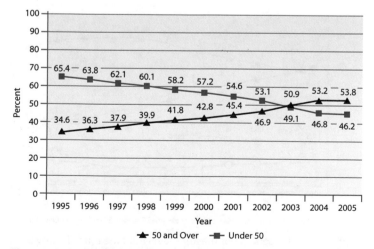

Figure 35–3. Percentage of master's-level faculty over and under the age of 50, 1993–2005 (AACN, 1995–2005a).

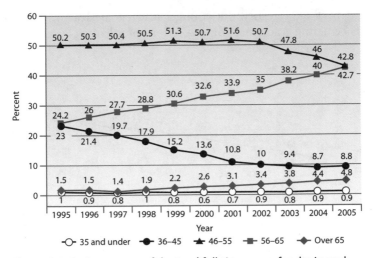

Figure 35–4. Percentage of doctoral full-time nurse faculty in each age category, 1995–2005 (AACN, 1995–2005a).

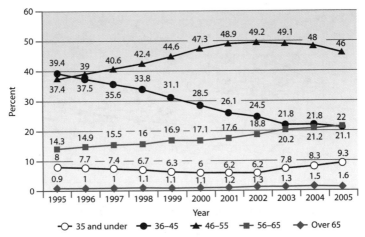

Figure 35–5. Percentage of master's-level full-time nurse faculty in each age category, 1995–2005 (AACN, 1995–2005a).

12 How do you know that younger faculty are leaving or not entering academia?

- Only 22.5% of individuals graduating from doctoral programs in nursing from 2003 to 2004 planned to work in settings other than schools (AACN, 2005a).
- Only 7% of the 12,099 nursing master's graduates from 2004 to 2005 majored in education (Fang, et al., 2006a).
- During academic year 2003–2004, data on faculty resignations of 36–45 years old indicated that, although 41% left to accept other school of nursing faculty positions, 36% left to assume nonacademic positions. The majority of these individuals held master's degrees (AACN, 2005b). Of graduates from nursing and nursing education doctoral programs during 2004–2005, 24% planned noneducation careers (National Opinion Research Center [NORC], 2007).
- Graduates planning teaching as a primary employment activity was 45%, a decline of almost 26% since 1980–1984 (NORC, 2001; 2007).

13 Is there a reason why younger faculty are not entering academia or are leaving?

One reason is noncompetitive salaries. In fall 2005, the median calendar year–based salary for instructional faculty at the rank of assistant professor was $59,572 and $71,092 for master's and doctoral faculty, respectively (Fang, et al., 2006b). Academic (9- or 10-month) salaries were converted to calendar year–based salaries so that they would be comparable to nonacademic salaries. A sample listing of nonacademic administrative and clinical nursing base salaries is presented in Table 35–1 and gives some idea about the competition (Salary.com, 2007). Although faculty salaries have increased somewhat over the past few years, there is still a considerable gap between academic and nonacademic compensation.

Table 35–1

Comparison of Nurse Faculty Salaries (School Year 2005–2006) and Selected Nonacademic Base Salaries (January 2007)

School of Nursing

Instructional Faculty Positions:	Median[1]
Assistant professor (Doctoral)	$71,092
Assistant professor (Master's)	$ 59,527
Clinical/Administrative Nonacademic Positions:	
Chief nurse executive (MSN)	$166,166
Nurse anesthetist (MSN)	$133,612
Nursing director (MSN)	$100,452
NP (specialty care)	$81,599
Certified nurse-midwife	$83,306
Head nurse, CCU (RN)	$84,054
Clinical nurse specialist (MSN)	$75,682
Nursing services instructor (RN)	$66,669
Staff nurse (RN)	$58,575

[1]The median is the same as the 50th percentile and is the salary midway between the lowest and highest value. Fang, et al., (2006b); Salary.com (January 2007).

14 Compensation is important, but job satisfaction could overcome this influence. Are there job satisfaction issues as well?

Yes, there are workplace issues related to overall job satisfaction, teaching workload demands, opportunities for advancement, effectiveness of leadership, and job security. In the National Study of Postsecondary Faculty, junior faculty (assistant professor, instructor, and lecturer) reported higher percentages of dissatisfaction than senior faculty (professor and associate professor) (U.S. Department of Education, 2001; Berlin & Sechrist, 2003).

15 Are there other factors that are influencing the number of faculty?

One factor relates to the past declines in the numbers of future teachers. These declines may be due, in part, to the increase in other career opportunities for women over the past few decades, thus diminishing the pool of people choosing nursing as a career.

16 How many doctoral programs are there, and how many people are graduating?

In fall 2005, there were 98 research-focused doctoral programs, with a total of 3,718 students, of whom 55% were part-time. Graduations from August 1, 2004, to July 31, 2005, totaled 431. Of these graduates, 65 were non-U.S. residents, so the pool of people available for faculty positions in the United States may be reduced further, assuming the majority of these graduates returned to their home countries. Graduates represented only 12% of enrollees, a reflection of the large number of part-time students. In addition, more individuals are pursuing postdoctoral study. There were 71 postdoctoral fellows in academic year 2005–2006 (Fang, et al., 2006a), almost 2.5 times as many as in 1995–1996 (Berlin, Bednash, & Scott, 1996). Postdoctoral study delays time-to-faculty status, but it is positive in terms of preparing increased numbers of nurse researchers.

17 Consequently, are there only approximately 300 people added to the faculty pool each year after accounting for non-U.S, residents and postdoctoral fellows?

Yes. However, there is another important consideration when talking about the faculty pool. Keep in mind that most new doctoral graduates were master's-level faculty prior to doctoral study. Therefore, the shift of master's-level faculty to doctoral student and ultimately to doctoral graduate does not bring that many new people into the faculty pool because most new doctoral graduates were already in the faculty pool as master's faculty.

18 Is there an upward trend in doctoral enrollees and graduates?

Yes. Enrollments have increased significantly over the past several years. However, over time there has not been a significant upward trend in graduations, which have been erratic and more or less static (Fig. 35–6). So, there are many students but too few graduates, a reflection of more part-time than full-time students. This is particularly disturbing given that the number of doctoral programs has increased from 62 in 1995 to 98 in 2005 (AACN, 1995–2005b).

19 What about the age characteristics of doctoral graduates?

Not only are there too few graduates, but most of them are older. The average age of graduates during academic year 2004–2005 was 45.6, which was 10 years older than doctoral graduates from all other research fields. The majority of graduates (almost 50%) were between the ages of 45 and 54 years, and 12% were 55 years and older (Fig. 35–7). Given that the mean age of retirement for doctoral faculty was 63 years in 2004, the number of productive teaching years is markedly curtailed (AACN, 2005b).

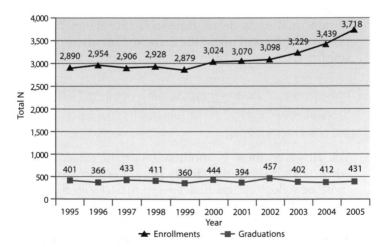

Figure 35–6. Enrollment and graduations in research-focused doctoral programs, 1995–2005 (AACN, 1995–2005b).

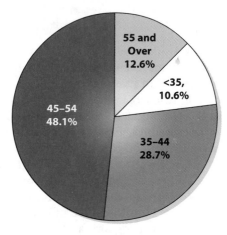

Mean=45.6   Median=46.8

Figure 35–7. Age distribution of graduates from doctoral programs in nursing and nursing education, 2004–2005 (valid N = 397) (NORC, 2007).

20 How long does it take these graduates to complete the doctoral programs compared with other disciplines?

The average number of years to completion of the doctorate after enrolling in the doctoral program was 7.5 years for nursing majors, compared with 6.6 years for all research doctoral majors. The median time from enrollment in a master's degree to achievement of the doctorate is 13.6 years, almost 5.5 years longer than for other disciplines (NORC, 2007).

21 What about the number of master's students and graduates?

In fall 2005, there were 439 schools with master's programs, and there are data on 89% of them. Master's enrollees totaled 46,444, and graduates from August 1, 2004, to July 31, 2005, totaled 12,099—almost four times more enrollees than graduates, a function of almost two (1.9) part-time students for every full-time student, which prolongs the time to graduation (Fang, et al., 2006a).

22 What about trends in master's graduates, and how do they influence the pipeline for future faculty?

A trend that did not receive much initial attention was the significant decline in master's enrollments that started in the late 1990s, reached a low point in 2001, and upturned dramatically beginning in 2002 (AACN, 1995–2005b). Graduations have not kept pace with enrollments because the high percentage of part-time students (65%) (Fang, et al., 2006a) has not translated into significant upward trend in the number of graduates. More master's graduates are critical. Not only are they the source of future doctoral students, but they comprise 75% of current full-time faculty in baccalaureate programs and approximately 22% in master's programs (AACN, 2007). In addition, the majority (83%) of full-time faculty in associate degree programs hold master's degrees (Kovner, Fairchild, & Jacobson, 2006) (Fig. 35–8).

23 Are there any positive signs for change ahead?

The situation with respect to the shortage of faculty is extremely serious but not hopeless. Building a viable pool

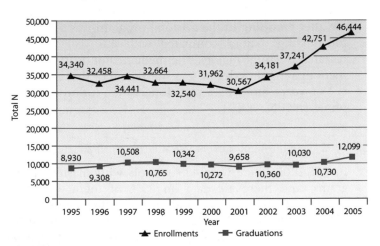

Figure 35–8. Enrollment and graduations in master's programs, 1995–2005 (AACN, 1995–2005b).

of faculty will not happen overnight. However, academic nursing is viewing the current situation as an opportunity to develop and implement a number of strategies that will ultimately overcome the shortage of current and future faculty. These include service and education partnerships to provide clinical education and address salary discrepancies; development of new graduate programs; increased numbers of students in current master's and doctoral programs; and role preparation for nurse educators as a component of graduate programs.

References

American Association of Colleges of Nursing. (1995–2005a). [Faculty age database]. Unpublished raw data.

American Association of Colleges of Nursing. (1995–2005b). [Enrollment and graduations database]. Unpublished raw data.

American Association of Colleges of Nursing. (2005a). [Employment plans of 2003–2004 doctoral graduates]. Unpublished raw data.

American Association of Colleges of Nursing. (2005b). [Faculty resignations and retirements from 2003-2004]. Unpublished raw data.

American Association of Colleges of Nursing (2006). [Special survey of AACN membership on vacant faculty positions for academic year 2006–2007]. Unpublished raw data.

American Association of Colleges of Nursing (2007). [Percent of master's prepared faculty teaching in baccalaureate and master's program for academic year 2005–2006]. Unpublished raw data.

Berlin, L.E., Bednash, G.D., & Scott, D.L. (1996). 1995–1996 enrollment and graduations in baccalaureate and graduate programs in nursing. Washington, DC: American Association of Colleges of Nursing.

Berlin, L.E., & Sechrist, K.R. (2002a). The shortage of doctorally prepared nursing faculty: a dire situation. Nursing Outlook, 50, 50–56.

Berlin, L.E., & Sechrist, K.R. (2002b). [Regression analysis of full-time master's prepared faculty in baccalaureate and graduate nursing programs]. Unpublished raw data.

Berlin, L.E., & Sechrist, K.R. (2003). [Analysis of selected variables pertaining to full-time nurse faculty from the 1999 national study of postsecondary faculty]. Unpublished raw data.

Berlin, L.E., Wilsey, S.J., & Bednash, G.D. (2005). 2004–2005 salaries of instructional and administrative nursing faculty in baccalaureate and graduate programs in nursing. Washington, DC: American Association of Colleges of Nursing.

Fang, D., Wilsey-Wisniewski, S.J., & Bednash, G.D. (2006a). 2005-2006 enrollment and graduations in baccalaureate and graduate programs in nursing. Washington, DC: American Association of Colleges of Nursing.

Fang, D., Wilsey-Wisniewski, S.J., & Bednash, G.D. (2006b) 2005–2006 salaries of instructional and administrative nursing faculty in baccalaureate and graduate programs in nursing. Washington, DC: American Association of Colleges of Nursing.

Kovner, C., Fairchild, S., & Jacobson, L. (2006). Nurse educators 2006: A report of the faculty census survey of RN programs and graduate programs. New York: National League for Nursing.

National League for Nursing (2006). NLN member update, July 31, 2006. New York: National League for Nursing. Available at http://www.nln.org/ newsletter/July 31 2006.htm

National Opinion Research Center, (2001). Survey of earned doctorates,1980–1984. Unpublished special report generated for the American Association of Colleges of Nursing. Chicago: NSF/NIH/USED/NEH/NASA.

National Opinion Research Center, (2007). Survey of earned doctorates, 2005. Unpublished special report generated for Dr. Linda Berlin. Chicago: NSF/NIH/USED/NEH/NASA.

Salary data (January 2007).[online salary information]. Available at http://www.salary.com

U.S. Department of Education. National Center for Education Statistics. (2001). National study of postsecondary faculty (NSOPF: 99). [Public use data analysis system (DAS)]. Washington, DC: NCES 2001–2003.

36

Beginning in the Faculty Role

Jackie McVey, PhD, RN

1 What are the main areas requiring mastery in the move from being a novice nurse educator to being more expert?

Nurse educators, along with all other higher education faculty, are evaluated in the categories of teaching, scholarship, and service.

- **Teaching:** Faculty members just beginning their nursing education careers spend the majority of their time in classroom and clinical teaching activities. Other responsibilities that support teaching include recruiting, advising, coaching, and evaluating students.
- **Scholarship:** In most institutions, experienced faculty members continue to teach, but they are also expected to do grant writing, research, and scholarly publication. In some institutions, even junior faculty are expected to engage in research as a significant part of their faculty role.
- **Service:** Committee and planning work for the nursing program and academic institution are forms of service, as are activities on behalf of the local community.

2 What similarities and differences are there between the nurse educator role and other nursing roles?

Expert nurse clinicians accomplish many teaching functions in a variety of professional contexts. Nurse clinicians are information sources for patients and families, role models for peers, leaders in developing clinical protocols, and facilitators of collaborative health team strategies. Nurse clinicians and nurse educators in academic settings share the common goal of promoting well-focused, efficient, and high-quality patient care. Part of effective teaching is for nursing faculty to be good role models in their areas of clinical expertise. The main difference between clinician and teaching roles is that nurse educators work more indirectly to influence patient care by teaching students about nursing judgment and competencies.

3 What makes teaching nursing students different from faculty roles in non-health academic majors?

All educators use specialty knowledge for planning, teaching, advising, and evaluating student learning. However, nursing is an applied discipline, legally and ethically bound to performance standards that ensure public safety. Students and faculty must therefore respond to these added challenges:

- Strict program entry and grading requirements
- Heavy laboratory and clinical load, with stringent evaluation standards
- Accelerated learning pace and increasing performance accountabilities
- Graduate requirement to pass a national standardized test to be eligible for licensure to practice

4 What attitudes and behaviors most contribute to success as a nursing teacher?

- **Teachable spirit:** Be open to learning and alert to program, faculty, and student strengths.
- **Willingness to participate:** Share your fresh ideas to make a contribution.

- **Patience in finding your place:** Fulfill varied teaching assignments until you find a good fit with your talents and interests.
- **Teamwork:** Give help generously, and receive help gratefully.
- **Self-care:** Remember to take time to maintain your own health, energy, and optimism.

---

5   What kind of mentors are needed, and how are they acquired?

Eventually, you will be assigned to an experienced faculty member who will orient you to faculty job expectations and available teaching resources. In addition, you will get advice and assistance from a number of short-term contacts from others in the nursing program and other departments. Only after months or even years on the job do genuine mentor relationships emerge, because they require the gradual discovery of compatible personal styles along with a willingness to commit to exploration of mutual interests and support. It is important to stay flexible and proactive in finding the type and amount of guidance needed at each stage of the nursing education role.

---

6   How can one best utilize one's experiences as a student nurse in teaching others?

Use your memories.

Remember the nest	Recall the ways you needed support and encouragement as you faced the academic, clinical, and personal pressures of nursing school. Develop ways to help your students feel a sense of belonging and hope for success.
Take the best	Identify specific individuals and experiences that helped you learn and adjust to the student nurse role. Use them as role models to develop your teaching style.
Leave the rest	The emphasis has moved from high-quantity teaching to high-quality learning. Devote yourself to helping students sort through health-care information by using creative teaching strategies such as mastery concepts and judgment-based learning exercises and tests.

7 How should my time be used most effectively in developing teaching plans?

Traditionally, almost all planning time for in-class teaching has centered on selecting and organizing lecture content. Little time was left for planning application exercises to teach nursing judgment. This trend has continued, even after increased patient acuities led nursing programs to evaluate learning with more judgment-based tests. Rather than follow the old content overload pattern, use a 50-50 rule of thumb so that only half your time is spent selecting material to support mastery concepts on nursing actions. In the remaining planning time, create active learning strategies to turn those concepts into judgment exercises that closely resemble real nursing situations.

8 How can I encourage students to take responsibility for their own learning in school and throughout their careers?

Accountability is a big part of all professional nursing roles. Teaching approaches based on active student learning contribute more to role ownership than more traditional methods based on the idea that teaching equals telling. Assignments including reflective clinical journals and group projects such as research posters often increase student competencies and confidence. Help students write and refine their personal philosophies of nursing and nursing education to include their responsibility for life-long learning. Career planning skills are developed through having them keep updated professional portfolios that reflect good use of print and Web resources on career decision making, résumés, job interviews, work performance, and continuing education options.

9 What are the stages of learning in nursing programs?

Most nursing programs have based their curriculum and teaching plans on the three categories of cognitive, psychomotor, and affective learning. Students are expected to progress through simple levels of knowledge and comprehension into more advanced levels of analysis, application, and evaluation. A recent trend is for faculty to emphasize planning, implementation, and evaluation steps of the nursing process as early as possible in the curriculum. Decisions and actions will form the core of course and lecture objectives and content, teaching approaches, and testing. Students must use steps of assessment and data analysis to apply good reasoning to nursing actions.

10 How can I encourage individual and creative learning styles without compromising standards necessary to guarantee safe and effective nursing care?

Become very knowledgeable about current standards for nursing and nursing education. Among others, these include national nursing licensure and practice regulations, accreditation criteria, and each program's conceptual framework, curriculum patterns, and evaluation plans. Also, find ways to stay updated with current nursing and health information. The secret to individualizing learning is to teach in ways that appeal to a variety of styles plus provide flexible ways for students to meet outcome goals. Collect material on learning strategies, and observe other teachers in order to build creativity into your teaching in ways that fit your own style.

11 What approaches can I use to help students integrate conceptual learning with clinical applications?

You can help students form judgment bridges between nursing concepts and nursing actions by emphasizing clinical reasoning. Your in-class learning exercises and examinations can be very practical and test clinical judgment. Clinical assignments should require students to provide rationales and evidence-based practice data to support nursing judgment. Without merging theory and clinical experiences through shared values, students may become brilliant thinkers and technically skilled practitioners, but they will not be professional nurses.

12 How do I grant more advanced students increased autonomy while providing the supervision necessary for safe patient care?

Do periodic assessments of how well each student is meeting clinical objectives to decide who is ready for more flexible assignments with less supervision. Consult with students on their own readiness for these experiences. You can build student autonomy and confidence while maintaining accountability in these ways:

- Plan group assignments with individual roles and responsibilities.
- Require all students to keep peers, faculty, and agency staff informed on plans and actions so that autonomy does not become independence.

13 How do I recognize and respond to the student who needs additional coaching or tutoring?

There are several resources for finding and helping students who need to improve their academic success and clinical performance:

- Material on methods to assess and promote study, testing, and clinical success
- Individual coaching and tutoring appointments
- Performance flow charts to identify problems
- Student academic records
- Current course test scores and clinical evaluations
- Standardized test scores used for program entry, progression, and graduation

Your aim in using these resources is to help students identify their learning styles, abilities, and problems in order to give appropriate guidance. A student may need help on how *not* to overplay a special strength such as decisiveness or conscientious analysis.

14 What are some secrets of time, energy, and stress management in the new faculty role?

- Know your own personal and professional strengths, and use them well.

- Stay hopeful and yet realistic in planning how to meet job expectations.
- Set timelines that benchmark role progress so successes are acknowledged.
- Become familiar with your job evaluation tool and keep records of your own performance.
- Take care of your whole self by staying healthy, taking breaks, and having fun.

---

15 How do I clarify my values, philosophy, and mission in nursing education?

- Explore the many self-assessment tools, and examine your scores for the ones you choose to utilize.
- Write your own philosophy of nursing and nursing education after studying those of other individuals.
- Get regular feedback from colleagues, mentors, and students on how they perceive your values and style.
- Do reflective exercises such as journaling, art, and interpretive movement.

---

16 What resources are available regarding career development and advancement in nursing education?

The many choices available to nurses create both the biggest opportunities and the most anxiety-producing challenges. One way to sort through this maze is to use a technique called "information interviewing." Ask for a few minutes to explore with other individuals how they have managed their careers and how happy they are in their current jobs. Also, books, seminars, and Web sites are available on career planning. Keep cumulative files of your explorations and decision-making exercises so that you can detect trends in your own career preferences.

---

17 To what extent are new teachers expected to conform to the norms of the faculty?

You want to find a teaching position in a nursing program that fits your own professional and personal style and plans. Informal networking can help you learn how much autonomy or direction you might have in a particular school. Most nursing programs provide many combinations of teamwork and individual projects. You can achieve a satisfactory balance of the two if you learn when and how to contribute your own creativity and ideas in ways that promote group goals.

---

18 What can be done to promote good outcomes when the teaching role creates a "sandwich" situation between students, faculty, agency nurses, and/or nursing program administrators?

Be sure all parties are in agreement regarding priorities and protocols. All individuals concerned with related questions or conflicts must be both pro-student and pro-program to the greatest extent possible. Faculty members can get caught in the middle because they are student advocates and student evaluators as well as representatives of program standards. Attempt to have the students, faculty, and administrators involved in the issue present together in major decision making meetings. This measure can prevent excessive second-hand information and facilitate problem solving.

---

19 How do I know if I am effective as an educator?

You will receive feedback from your course coordinators, program administrators, mentors, peers, and students on how well you are doing in the role. Utilize as many of the faculty development resources offered by your program as you can. Remember to keep your perspective and to deliberately seek ways to document evidence of your achievements. Ask trusted peers and mentors to help you keep on track with meeting job standards and to share in celebrating your successes.

Resources

Boyer, E.L. (1990). Scholarship reconsidered: Priorities of the professorate. Princeton: Carnegie Foundation.

Filene, P. (2005). The joy of teaching: A practical guide for new college instructors. Chapel Hill, N.C.: University of North Carolina Press.

Indiana University Programs in Teaching Nursing Online. Available at http://www.oncourse.iu.edu

Johns, C. (2002). Guided reflection: Advancing practice. Oxford, England: Blackwell Publishing.

Jones, L.B. (1996). The path. New York: Hyperion.

Kiersey Temperament Sorter. Available at http://www.humanmetrics.com

McVey, J. (2006). Critical thinking in novice nurse clinical learning. In M. Jackson, D.D. Ignatavicius, & B. Case (Eds.) Conversations in clinical judgment and critical thinking. Sudbury, Mass.: Jones & Bartlett.

Palmer, P. (1998). The courage to teach. San Francisco: Jossey-Bass.

Rayfield, S.W., & Manning, L. Pathways of teaching nursing: Keeping it real. Bossier City, La.: ICAN Publishing.

Smalley, G., & Trent, J. (1992). The two sides of love. Colorado Springs: Focus on the Family Press.

37

Nursing Within the College/University Environment

Carole Anderson, PhD, RN, FAAN

1 Where does nursing fit in the college/university?

The answer to this lies in knowing the *structure* of the college/university. Nursing can be a department, school, or college. It can be an independent organizational entity, or it can be part of a larger unit. The particular structure determines the amount of autonomy given to the head of the nursing unit. Knowing how nursing, a health profession, fits with the overall mission of the college/university provides the information as to the relative value of the nursing unit; the degree of *fit* is directly proportional to status.

2 Why is the amount of prestige important?

Prestige of any unit on campus is the extent to which the unit meets the overall mission and goals of the college/university. For example, in a research-intensive university, prestige is a function of the success of the research being done by nursing faculty. In a university where teaching is the primary mission, prestige is a function of student success, as measured by outcomes. In a liberal arts college, prestige will be measured by the success of the teaching and the extent to which the nursing program embraces and incorporates core liberal arts into the professional curriculum.

3 Who makes decisions about the nursing unit?

If the unit is an autonomous college, the dean of that autonomous college makes the decisions. If nursing is a department within a larger school or college, the nursing leader must consult the dean of the college. Ultimately, on major academic or budgetary decisions, the provost of the university/college has the final authority.

4 The word *quality* is often used in university/college publications. How is quality defined within the institution?

Typically, *quality* is used in referring to the student body or the faculty. The variables that are used to determine student quality are:

- Grade point and class standing
- Quality/reputation of institution previously attended
- Standardized test scores such as ACT, SAT, GRE
- Rigor of curriculum completed
- Engagement in extracurricular activities

When referring to faculty, the variables that are relevant are:

- Reputation of doctorate-granting institution
- Postdoctoral study
- Number and quality of scholarly works
- Relevance of scholarship to needs of the academic discipline
- Number of competitive research grants received (if applicable in the field)

5 How are the university and nursing funded?

University funding comes from multiple sources, including tuition, state support (if a public university), overhead from extramural grants, contracts, and endowment earnings. In recent years, tuition has become a larger percentage of the overall budgets for all universities. Nursing's funding comes from those same sources. Whether the nursing unit receives all of the income it generates from, for example, tuition, is a function of the budget model of the university.

---

6 How do the university/college and nursing mission statements influence what I should do?

The mission of the university/college is a statement of purpose or intent. This statement is usually followed by a statement of goals that are designed to fulfill the mission. For example, a research university's major mission is the generation of new knowledge through the conduct of research and the training of Ph.D. students. A college may have as its purpose the liberal education of undergraduates. If a college/university is state-funded, part of its purpose is the education of the state's residents. Some colleges/universities are affiliated with a religion; therefore, educating students within the precepts of that religion is part of the mission.

The nursing unit and its faculty must ensure that their program and practices are designed so as to conform to the mission. An example is a college/university whose mission is the education of high-ability students. In other words, it is highly selective. Nursing must gear its admission standards to be as selective as those of the university.

---

7 What is expected of faculty in the institution?

Faculty members are expected to teach, research, produce scholarship, and provide service to the institution and the profession. The amount of each depends on the mission of the institution. Faculty are judged on the quality of each by the use of metrics. Each institution should have guidelines that detail expectations in each of the core areas of teaching, scholarship, and service. Often, these are general statements, and teachers need to consult with senior faculty to learn specifics. For example, which journals are the most prestigious? What weight is given to student evaluations of teaching?

8 Are nursing instructors held to a standard different from that of other disciplines?

No. There was a period when nursing instructors were not held to research/scholarship standards because most were not research-trained, i.e., did not possess the Ph.D. However, that time has passed, and regular nursing faculty members are held to the same standard as other faculty in the college/university.

9 If I think the admission standards for the nursing program are too high compared with other disciplines, what can I do about it?

Admission standards are set by the faculty; concerns should be expressed at faculty meetings, making sure you have data to support your claim.

10 What are measures of good teaching?
- Student evaluation of teaching
- Peer evaluation of teaching
- Quality and organization of course materials
- Capacity to deliver material in an understandable manner
- Grading standards

11 Is the teaching of nursing perceived differently than teaching of other disciplines?

The main difference is that nursing faculty engage in clinical teaching that is time-intensive and difficult to evaluate. Often, the demands of this kind of teaching are not well understood by other disciplines, and the leader of the nursing unit needs to continuously educate others as to the nature of this type of teaching and the constraints placed by clinical agencies on the numbers of students that each faculty member can supervise at any one time.

12 How will I know I am a good teacher?

First, your students and your peers will let you know by their evaluations of your teaching. Another measure is student success on your portion of, for example, state boards or achievement tests. Feedback from faculty regarding students' knowledge of the subject matter you teach is another measure of your success. Your own continued enthusiasm for teaching and for the subject matter you teach is a clue that you are being successful.

13 How does scholarship/research in nursing compare with that in other disciplines?

It is difficult to do this comparison because the standards differ significantly for every discipline. In the humanities, for example, a major book is required. In the physical sciences, federal research funding and peer-reviewed, data-based articles in high quality journals are required.

Nursing is a developing profession in terms of research and scholarship; therefore, there is no long history or tradition. However, nursing does require research and scholarship to advance through the academic ranks. Differing types of institutions will have differing standards both in terms of quantity and type required.

14 Is federal funding required for research?

Federal research funding is the gold standard for research support. In a research-intensive university, there is no equal. At the same time, other national organizations, such as the American Heart Association, are also considered competitive, peer-reviewed funding agencies. The important concept is that research ideas undergo the test of peer review. The significance of extramural funding is linked to the ability to conduct research. Conducting research takes time and financial resources to be able to complete. That is why funding is so important; peer-reviewed funding is the most prestigious.

15 What does being a "good university citizen" mean?

It means becoming involved in university life by volunteering for various work groups or committees both within your unit and at the college/university level. This is the way faculty governance is put into practice. It is important for nursing faculty to participate with their colleagues from other units so as to learn different perspectives and also to allow others to learn from them. Join groups, volunteer for committees, eat at the faculty club or the local gathering place. Look for collaborators for your research/scholarship, attend research meetings in other units, and so on. The bottom line is to get out and involved across campus.

16 I am afraid to speak up at faculty meetings for fear I will say the wrong thing and will be punished for it later when I come up for promotion. Is this realistic?

Senior faculty members are expected to make promotion decisions based on objective evidence in the candidate's dossier, not on subjective feelings. This is at the heart of the promotion process, and violations are judged to be very serious infractions of faculty responsibility. Most institutions have appeal mechanisms to deal with unfair decisions or decisions not based on fact. Faculty who believe their work has not been objectively judged are urged to utilize this appeal process.

17 I like to work at home. Is that permitted?

A certain amount of working at home is acceptable in academic settings. However, you need to be alert as to whether you are spending sufficient time at work to become a contributing member of the intellectual community in your unit and to allow student interaction outside of the classroom. In the final analysis, what is important is what you produce.

18 Am I obliged to do university/college work during the summer, or can I use that time to work for extra money?

Summer is not considered vacation for faculty on 9-month academic appointments. Summer, the period without teaching responsibilities, is designed to allow faculty to concentrate on research/scholarship and to revise their courses. Although you may consider time spent in this manner working for the college/university, it is really working for yourself. In other words, you are concentrating on activities that ultimately will lead to *your* success and advancement.

19 How can I do everything?

Doing everything and doing it well require that the teaching assignments of faculty allow sufficient time to do it all. In nursing, that means that allowance is made for time-intensive clinical teaching. Each nursing unit must have assignments that allow faculty sufficient time to teach well, be scholarly, be productive, and provide service. The ability to meet expectations is a function of the quality of research training one has received, the interest in teaching, and good time management skills.

20 What is tenure?

Academic tenure is permanent employment and is achieved after serving a probationary period, most typically 6 years. Once tenure is achieved, service can be terminated only for extraordinary circumstances and financial exigencies.

21 Is there an unspoken limit on the number of faculty who can be tenured?

No. If an individual meets the standards for tenure, the institution is required to grant it. If tenure is not granted, the institution is liable for accusations of discrimination.

22 Does writing a textbook count for promotion and tenure?

Every college/university and nursing unit should have written standards for promotion and tenure. At some universities, authoring a textbook is considered to partially meet the criteria for teaching effectiveness, whereas at others it is considered to partially meet the scholarship criteria. Basically, writing a textbook does count, but count for what is the question that needs to be answered by reviewing the written standards for promotion and tenure.

23 If I do a presentation at a national/international meeting, does that mean I have a national/international reputation?

No. National/international reputations are built when a faculty members' work is known throughout the country/world. When that happens, the work is frequently cited in the literature, the person is invited to present his or her work at major meetings at sponsoring organizations' expense, and the person is sought for expert testimony by national organizations.

24 How can I combine having a family with promotion and tenure requirements?

This is a valid concern for women who choose academic careers. At last, the higher education community is recognizing the need to make accommodations so that women do not have to make a difficult choice of motherhood versus career. Specifically, many institutions are modifying their requirements such that additional years are added to the tenure clock to give women the opportunity to meet the standards for promotion and tenure.

25 Can I stop the tenure clock?

Yes. It depends on your institution's policies for promotion and tenure. Also, some institutions stop the tenure clock for such things as family caretaking responsibilities, illness, or circumstances beyond the faculty member's control (such as a delay in a faculty member's laboratory setup).

26 Are the standards for promotion and tenure always increasing?

The better senior faculty becomes, the higher the standards for junior faculty. Every college/university is increasing its standards for promotion and tenure in order to improve the quality of the faculty and hence improve their reputation rankings by the work done by well-qualified faculty. Faculty members must keep pace with these changing standards so as to have a promotion dossier that meets the standards at the time they are considered for promotion and tenure.

27 Why is it that senior faculty who are judging me today would not be able to meet the standards that they are using to judge me?

As standards continue to increase, faculty who were tenured at an earlier time may have difficulty meeting the current standards. However, active and productive faculty do keep up and know what standards need to prevail to continue to enhance the quality of the faculty and the academic unit. Make sure you are one of those active and productive faculty.

Resources

Boice, R. (2000). Advice for new faculty members. Needham Heights, Mass.: Allyn and Bacon.

Boss, J.M., & Eckert, S.H. (2006). Academic scientists at work: Navigating the biomedical research career, 2nd ed. New York: Springer.

Goldsmith, J., Komlos, J., & Gold, P.S. (2001). The Chicago guide to your academic career: A portable mentor for scholars from graduate school through tenure. Chicago: University of Chicago Press.

Lucas, C., & Murry, J.W. (2002). New faculty: A practical guide for academic beginners. New York: Palgrave Macmillan.

Schoenfeld, C., & Magnan, R. (1994). Mentor in a manual: Climbing the academic ladder to tenure, 2nd ed. Madison, Wis.: Atwood Publications.

38

Perspectives of the Nursing Dean at a Small Liberal Arts School

Judeen Schulte, PhD, RN

---

1 How is the smaller liberal arts school different from larger research-intensive schools and academic health centers?

There are a number of differences in focus:

- A smaller, liberal arts school usually has a primary allegiance to infusing a liberal arts perspective throughout the nursing undergraduate curriculum.
- A nursing faculty member in a liberal arts college often has a primary focus on teaching and scholarship, with research frequently assisting to improve pedagogy. As with other types of schools, the nursing faculty is expected to participate in institutional and community service.
- In liberal arts schools with nursing programs, the proportion of nursing faculty with a master's degree in nursing as the terminal degree is higher. If the smaller liberal arts school also has a graduate nursing program, however, there will usually be more doctoral faculty and a more diverse range of research involvements.

2 What is the role of the nursing dean or director? Does the role of the dean differ by program type or the individual's education?

Schools may call the chief nursing academic officer a dean, director, or chair, although the role is always to serve the learners and faculty and thus to contribute to the school's overall achievement of mission. Lofty as this may sound, day to day it means collaborating with others, both inside and outside the institution, to ensure that the resources—personnel, conceptual, emotional, physical, technological, clinical, financial—are available to facilitate the students' learning, faculty's teaching and scholarship, and staff's supporting the school's mission. The dean is also often the school's "public face" so, in many instances, the dean needs to have a doctorate in order to have the credibility to represent the discipline and to advocate internally for the resources and position and externally to advance the nursing program.

3 Does the organizational structure of the institution affect how the nursing unit operates as well as the role of the dean?

Definitely. If the nursing unit stands alone as a major institutional structure, i.e., a school or college, then the dean has more direct input into the overall functioning and decision making of the institution. If the nursing unit is one of several units that comprise a larger entity, for example, part of a school of allied health, the dean may function primarily as a program director. In most instances, the dean's influence in this situation is most directly within the nursing unit and with the immediate boss, the dean or director of the school of allied health. In an institution in which the faculty is unionized, additional rules apply for the faculty and the dean.

4 What are the typical issues that concern faculty? Do they differ by institutional type?

Across institutional types, the faculty is usually concerned with workload, scholarship opportunities, work environment, meeting the requirements for tenure or continuous appointment, salary, and opportunities to use personal talents in order to contribute to a larger goal such as the school's mission, the advancement of nursing, and the effective education of their students. People want to do a good job and they also want to be recognized for it. If the workload is manageable, opportunities exist to continue learning and deepening one's scholarship.

---

5   What are the typical issues that concern deans?

Deans are concerned about the same issues that faculty are: workload/responsibilities, scholarly productivity, work environment, meeting the requirements for tenure or continuous appointment, salary, opportunities to use personal talents to contribute to larger goals including achievement of the institution's mission, the advancement of nursing, and effective education of the institution's students. Deans are often required to take a broader, more system-oriented view than faculty, especially when competing for resources for nursing in relation to other schools or programs. Often, too, the dean needs to be concerned about ensuring that the school is contributing to the health of the local community as well as actively taking civic and political actions that will strengthen nursing's power base and increase its visibility and credibility. The dean is also responsible for facilitating faculty development and growth, and to engage in succession planning for leadership of the nursing academic unit.

---

6   Where do the resources that support the nursing unit come from, and what role does the dean have in securing resources?

Securing resources is a major responsibility. To fund the nursing academic unit, the dean competes within the university for internal resources, and also works to secure external funds, often in conjunction with grant writers and researchers. The mission, location (urban, rural), history and reputation, size and structure, program types and levels, student body, faculty, and administrative support all affect the institution's ability to secure and allocate resources. Within most institutions, resources come from institutional sources, such as tuition and fees, and external sources, such as grants and gifts. The budget of many institutions is highly dependent on tuition. Budgeting processes vary across institutions, but usually the nursing unit has a specific budget that is requested and negotiated each year, in relation to all other institutional units. In today's world of increased nursing students and the nursing shortage overall, many institutions are increasing nursing budgets and paying higher salaries to nursing faculty than are paid to faculty in other teaching units simply because of market demand.

7   As a faculty member, am I expected to have a role in helping the dean secure resources for the nursing program?

As a faculty member, your most critical role in helping the dean secure nursing program resources is doing your job well, even exceptionally. The reputation of every nursing unit accrues from the individual and collective work of the unit's members. In terms of human resources, many deans would also be delighted to have referrals of potential faculty members whom you believe have the needed credentials and experience to be a good match for the institution's needs.

8   How does a nursing unit maintain programs and/or grow new programs during periods of budget reductions?

In most institutions, programs are maintained based on outcomes produced by the responsible unit. In nursing, for instance, is the program graduating nurses who can pass the NCLEX-RN® or certification examinations? Does the practice of the graduates and alumni demonstrate the expected professional standards? Is the unit contributing effectively to the institution's mission and strategic goals? Are the costs of the nursing unit less than or about the same as the revenue it generates? Similarly, new programs are often approved, even in times of budget reduction, if the planning for the program sufficiently demonstrates need, matches with the institution's mission and resources, and has the long-range potential of enhancing the institution's mission, reputation, and revenues.

---

9   What external factors affect enrollment in nursing programs?

Historically, nursing has faced cycles of shortage and over-supply. Today, a number of factors are increasing the demand for nurses, including the increasing longevity among all people, advances in health care and technology, the need for new nurses to replace the current aging work-force, and the continued positive regard and respect for nurses and the profession. These and other factors suggest that high enrollment in nursing programs will continue well into the future. Having lived through times of dra-matic increases and declines in nursing enrollment, most institutions plan carefully so that faculty members are not terminated in times of enrollment decline. Rather, faculty attrition through retirement or choosing to move to a dif-ferent environment is often the way downsizing occurs.

---

10   How important is diversity to a unit in nursing?

Given the changing mix of cultures of persons who are seeking health care, it is increasingly important to demon-strate diversity within a nursing unit in terms of gender, race, culture, thought, lifestyle, educational background, and nursing practice. Therefore, it is a moral imperative for institutions to help educate increasingly diverse nurses. In this way, nursing units will contribute to more diverse staff in health-care organizations and create a pipeline for future faculty. Because the percentage of all nurses who are ethnically diverse is low (see the Department of Health and Human Service's nursing sample statistics or the American Association of Critical Care Nurses' Web site for specific information), institutions often pay higher salaries for ethnically diverse faculty.

11 What determines the mix of faculty and how they are assigned within nursing units?

The mix of faculty within a nursing unit depends on who is available and willing to work for the salary offered as well as who meets the requirements of the accrediting organization and/or the state's board of nursing. In Wisconsin, for example, to teach nursing, a master of science in nursing is required, even though the region's accrediting organization, the Higher Learning Commission of North Central, does not prescribe the academic credentials required. Faculty assignments are based on many factors, including unit history and patterns, needs, faculty expertise, and the potential to schedule the faculty member effectively. Faced with faculty shortages, institutions are being extremely creative in finding ways to facilitate student learning, often identifying ways to extend faculty, such as paying for teaching assistants in the classroom or in clinical. Regarding assigning faculty within their specialties, the dean knows that it is always to the advantage of the students, faculty, and the institution to have teachers work in their areas of expertise, even though that may not always be possible. It is therefore important for new faculty members to emphasize the range of areas that they can potentially address and to suggest areas in which they would be interested in developing expertise.

12 What is your biggest concern about how teachers teach? How can new faculty build competency in the faculty role?

Across educational and other environments, the trend is to identify and focus on outcomes as the product of the environment. In health-care environments, nurses are very familiar with the focus on outcomes but may think less about them in an educational context. Inexperienced faculty members may think more about how they want to prove their expertise instead of emphasizing what the students need to learn in order to function effectively as future nurses. Many nursing faculty primarily use a lecture mode rather than engage students in active learning. To build competency, read, ask questions, listen, try new approaches, and ask your dean if it would be possible to pair you with an experienced, effective teacher who can serve as your model and mentor.

13 What are some methods of maintaining a dynamic, responsive curriculum?

An active evaluation plan that is focused on using assessment results for improvement is highly recommended. Many institutions have identified specific processes for recommending curricular change that require faculty approval. In fact, most deans really understand that the faculty "own" the curriculum. If there are indicators that a total curriculum revision is needed, deans tend to work within the specific institutional structure to assign coordinating and leadership responsibilities for planning, implementing, and evaluating the change. Although the dean may contribute to the design processes, the dean's function at the time of curricular change is securing time, people, and/or financial resources so that faculty can execute the needed conceptualizing and planning. Because curricular change is complicated, the dean must also be an encourager, especially as the implementation begins and evolves semester after semester. The dean is responsible for knowing and facilitating institutional approval processes when total curricular change occurs. In addition, the dean is usually the liaison to the state board of nursing and/or accrediting agencies and is responsible for ensuring that the guidelines and regulations of such agencies are followed.

14 How do faculty habits and program traditions contribute to the capacity for change in a nursing program?

Each unit in institutions, as well as the institutions themselves, has history, habits, and traditions that tend to either support or dampen innovation and change. Knowing whether you are change-oriented or more inclined toward following what has been done is very important as you interview, so that you can match your preferences with the environment.

---

15 What is most critical for faculty development?

- Sufficient financial resources to support faculty participation in credit-bearing and noncredit-bearing educational opportunities that are high quality
- Sufficient time and faculty coverage to allow for faculty participation in development experiences

Keeping up with changes in health-care knowledge and best practices as well as changes in technology and educational best practices is not an option for faculty members if they are to fulfill their role as teacher.

---

16 How can I best prepare myself to assume the role of dean someday?

Start out by determining if becoming dean is truly your goal. If yes, start by becoming the best faculty member possible; deans of nursing are often appointed from within an institution. Pursue every opportunity to learn, within your unit and across the institution. If needed, take formal course work. Get to know people all across the institution. Volunteer when volunteers are requested. Attend campus activities to show your commitment and to be seen. Most important, focus your goals on learning and service— to your students, your peers, your profession, and your community.

The author acknowledges and thanks Dorothy Powell, EdD, RN, FAAN, Former Dean, College of Nursing and Health Sciences, Division of Nursing, Howard University, Washington, DC, who developed many of the questions used in this section.

39

Perspectives of the Nursing Dean at an Academic Health Center

Jeanette Lancaster, PhD, RN, FAAN

---

1 How is an academic health center (AHC) different from a small liberal arts school?

AHCs come in more than one type. The most prominent types are: (1) those that are part of a comprehensive university that has a variety of schools that have both health and other disciplines and (2) those that are only health related schools. AHCs also differ whether they own their own hospital, clinic, or other health-care site or if they partner with facilities with other ownerships. In the first type of AHC, the head of the nursing unit needs to be part of the leadership team of the university's academic division, which typically comprises all the schools including those devoted to the health professions. In the second type of AHC, the school of nursing may be the only one (or one of a limited number of schools) at the institution that educates undergraduates. Thus, the issues that the unit head must deal with will have some characteristics in common with those dealt with by unit heads in small liberal arts colleges.

2 How is the faculty role different in an AHC?

The mission and scope of responsibility for faculty in an
AHC is often different from that of faculty in liberal arts
schools. Specifically, faculty on tenure-earning lines in
AHCs are expected to be engaged in research, and this is
often translated into having funded research. Teaching and
service remain a part of their role, but these two areas may
be less significant than the research mission. There is also
a greater expectation that the faculty in AHCs will be
skilled in interdisciplinary work. This aspect is expected to
grow in regard to research with the shift in funding priorities at the National Institutes of Health. Major funding will
be based on what is called translational research, i.e., the
transfer of knowledge from the bench scientist to the recip-
ient of care. It is also expected that funding will depend on
the quality and scope of the interdisciplinary work, that it
will include researchers from across the university, and that
it will not be limited to those in health care.

3 What is the role of the nursing dean or director?

The nursing dean is primarily responsible for leading and
providing vision for the academic unit. This includes
recruitment of faculty, overseeing the school's planning,
developing and implementing the budget, lobbying for
institutional funds for the nursing unit, overseeing the evaluation process, and representing and advocating for the
nursing unit both within and outside the university. The
dean sets priorities and leverages resources. Consistently,
there are more needs and desires than there are resources to
satisfy them. To garner resources, the nursing dean must
also be active in securing private resources and, if the dean
is at a public institution, state resources when approval to
do so is permitted by the institution. The dean fosters collaboration among internal and external stakeholders to
move the school forward. In many ways, the dean is the
chief advocate for the unit, seeking support for its mission,
goals, and priorities from a range of entities.

4 To what extent is the dean involved in planning?

Planning is a key feature of most institutions of higher learning. At the unit level, the leadership for planning is typically the dean's responsibility. The dean often involves key faculty and administrative stakeholders in this process. Many times the planning process includes a much wider range of constituents, such as students, alumni, practice partners, and others, who have an investment and interest in the direction the unit takes. A part of planning is fiscal management and priority setting. Adhering to the established priorities is basic to the dean's role. This is not always easy, because faculty and other constituents often call attention to new opportunities that seem hard to decline; deviating from set priorities should be done with care. Deans must have a clear view of the aspirations and priorities of the nursing unit as well as those of the parent institution. Specifically, nursing program development must be consistent with the overall mission of nursing and the institution.

5 How does the dean engage in the selection and retention of faculty?

The dean has a sizable role in selection, retention, promotion, and adequate compensation of faculty and staff. For example, once the search committee completes its work and makes recommendations to the dean, the dean is responsible for recruiting the most highly ranked candidates to the school. This includes clarifying salary, benefits, teaching responsibilities, and other expectations in the areas of service and scholarship. The relative weight attributed to each component of the faculty role will vary by institution. The dean also works over time to help sustain a culture and climate that is attractive and supportive of faculty and staff. If the persons hired are capable and contribute to the mission and work of the unit, then it is important to retain them and help them grow in their careers. Unfortunately, there are times when hiring decisions do not prove beneficial to either the unit or the employee. Once that becomes apparent, it is best for all involved to move quickly, fairly, and with professional respect for the person. Neither the unit nor the employee benefits when a person is retained in a situation that suggests a poor fit.

---

6 Does the organizational structure of the institution affect how the nursing unit operates and the role of the dean?

Yes. For example, organizations differ in regard to the person to whom the dean reports. The dean should help the chief academic officer understand and value the profession of nursing. The dean may report to a health professional, or to a provost who does not come from a health discipline. However, one cannot assume that individuals from health-care professions truly understand the scope of nursing education any better than individuals from other disciplines. Thus, inviting the provost to join a clinical group or spend time in a simulation laboratory with students can provide valuable information about the discipline of nursing. Regardless of the reporting relationship, it is important that the dean participate in institutional decision making consistent with that of the other deans. This may mean that the nursing dean needs to participate both within the university decision-making structure as well as that of the health system.

The keys for successful reporting relationships are presenting the case for support and having the persons making the decisions understand the need to appreciate the value of growing and supporting the nursing unit. Regardless of the reporting structure, it is important to be accurate, honest, forthright, and well prepared with data when making requests.

---

7 Who develops the nursing school budget?

Typically in an AHC, the dean of the school develops the budget, with input from others within the school's administrative team. Budgets must be balanced, and this can be difficult given the ebb and flow of grant funds. It is important not to make long-term financial commitments with funds that are not guaranteed. Be careful about hiring faculty on tenure lines unless the base budget exists to support their salaries and benefits. The key to effective budgeting is effective decision making. What are the priorities? What is essential? What can the nursing unit afford? Where can more funds come from?

---

8   Where do the resources come from to support the nursing unit?

They come from a variety of sources, depending on institutional type. For example, in some private schools the nursing unit may receive funds from tuition, fees, and other sources such as private donors including foundations and corporations. The unit then pays an overhead charge to the college or university. In other models, schools receive a direct subsidy from the state. This mechanism varies, with some schools receiving state funds via the institution based on precise enrollment numbers; other schools receive the same funds, but the formula is not tied directly to enrollment.

In all instances, there are opportunities for policies and politics to affect the allocation of resources to nursing. It is important for deans to understand how their funds are allocated and what options are available to them for influencing the decision making regarding funds. If your school has an opportunity to request additional funds that are added to the base budget, think carefully about which of the school's needs and priorities most closely align with those of the persons who control the budget. Deans can benefit by asking two important questions when considering essential new resources and where to secure them: If the school receives the requested resources, what is the benefit, and who will benefit? For example, if you are seeking funds for a new building in order to increase enrollment, who benefits from more nursing graduates? Most likely the answer will include practice partners. Therefore, you need to ask what have practice partners contributed, or what could they contribute to the proposed building?

9 How similar are concerns of the dean and those of the faculty?

Deans and faculty share many concerns. Both want the nursing unit and their contributions to be appreciated and valued at the institution. They also want to recruit, retain, and matriculate capable students who are likely to contribute to nursing. Both want students to succeed, and each knows that when students do not succeed, actions must be taken. At times, students may need extra tutoring or remediation. At other times, it is in the best interests of the student and the school for the student to separate from the institution. When this situation arises, faculty and other administrative persons such as program directors or associate deans need to be supported by one another and by the dean.

Deans and faculty seek to understand what is expected of faculty in order to be retained, promoted, and equitably rewarded. For example, in most AHCs, there is an expectation that faculty will be good teachers; contribute to the service mission of the school, university, and profession; and be productive in scholarship. The latter may be directly translated into being a funded researcher.

There are some concerns that faculty and deans do not share. Teachers often focus on their area of expertise rather than the global concerns of the nursing unit. They must succeed in their roles in order to be retained, promoted, and tenured. They want others in the organization to support them when possible, and this is a reasonable expectation.

Deans, unlike faculty, must take a more holistic view and balance the vision of the nursing unit and individual needs of faculty with the external demands and strategic plans of the institution including the education of students. A dean's perspective is ideally "other-focused."

10 What are the typical issues that concern deans?

Deans at an AHC are concerned about ensuring shared governance and in developing faculty to take an active role in such activities as recruiting faculty colleagues and making policy recommendations. Many of the concerns deans face center on resources, whether they be human, fiscal, or facilities. Deans are often most concerned about recruiting the best possible faculty to accomplish the goals of the institution. A challenge is retaining those who show the most promise to contribute significantly to teaching and, if appropriate, to the research mission. A closely related challenge is securing the resources to hire adequate numbers of high-quality faculty and staff. Fiscal concerns are also linked to providing physical space and furnishings, including information technology, to meet the teaching and research missions. Effective deans educate key internal and external stakeholders about the complex scientific and caring aspects of nursing. As well, deans help to resolve conflicts that interfere with mission accomplishment.

---

11 **What external factors affect enrollment in nursing programs, and how do fluctuations in institutional enrollment affect the nursing unit?**

Historically, enrollment in schools of nursing has fluctuated within a 5- to 7-year cycle that correlates with federal reimbursement for health care. For example, reductions in Medicare payments to hospitals led to less revenue for hospitals. Consequently, some administrators chose to lay off nurses and others announced a hiring freeze. Applicants to schools began to question the viability of nursing as a career. Applications decreased, and enrollment dropped. During the period 1995–2000, enrollments in nursing schools decreased by over 25%; there were subsequent declines in faculty. Fluctuations in enrollments are problematic to schools as are census fluctuations in health care. When enrollments decline, budgets are cut, and there are fewer teachers. Schools have difficulty rapidly increasing enrollment because students must have an adequate number of well-qualified faculty.

As the interest in nursing increased in 2000, schools were limited in their ability to respond readily to this renewed interest. It took time to recoup the budget decreases that occurred when enrollments declined as well as to recruit faculty. A variety of factors have influenced the heightened interest in nursing. Examples include multiple disasters in the country, which have rekindled a commitment to service; the publicity related to nursing as a career with many options; and the creation of consumer-sensitive designs of programs.

12 How does a nursing unit maintain programs or develop new programs during periods of budget reduction?

During periods of budget reduction, the importance of setting priorities is acute. Then, it is essential to determine if increasing enrollments will lead to more funds for faculty. In order to increase enrollment by a certain number of students per year, you will need a specific amount of money to support faculty, staff, and such resources as computers, use of telephones, and other support. This is also the time to look at programs with low enrollment. Should they be eliminated? Should you admit every other year in order to have a student cohort in each class that equates to the formula you use for workload allocation? Should you look at new delivery mechanisms? For example, if the program is RN-to-BSN, and you have been offering it in a face-to-face format with classes once per week, you could consider following a more executive format with condensed classes on consecutive days, or you could use a Web-based format with or without condensed classes. A first step is to conduct a needs assessment to determine what the population you hope to serve prefers. You can also develop new alliances with practice partners. For example, if you conduct a certain amount of your clinical instruction in the facility, can the facility support faculty positions, or can advanced practice nurses serve as your faculty?

13 How important is diversity to a nursing unit, and what are the implications of diversity for a nursing program?

Diversity within the faculty and the student population is essential. As the demographics of the country change, the need to emphasize diversity and teach students to be culturally competent has grown. In general, the diversity within nursing has not paralleled the population. The place to start is to increase the diversity of faculty so that students who represent minority groups are taught by faculty members who are positive role models, represent their ethnic background, and value the richness of an eclectic faculty and student body. There are several aspects to diversity: first, ideally the population within the school would be diverse. Secondly, it is key to have either a course related to cultural competence or have this content threaded throughout courses so students learn to appreciate working with people whose culture differs from their own.

---

14 **What are the challenges to maintaining dynamic curriculum and program offerings?**

In this time of rapid change in health care, it is crucial that faculty maintain a dynamic curriculum. This takes time and energy. Thus, it is important to inspire and reward creativity and innovation. For example, for many years at my school, we have had an Innovative Teaching Award program. Faculty can apply for a grant to try out an innovation in teaching. This enables instructors to use their creativity. Students benefit from new learning methods or additional content. The goal is to spark the creative spirit in faculty and nourish it. Faculty members need to attend conferences to learn about other programs and ways of doing things. Both when they present and attend solely as listeners there are opportunities to learn, grow, and develop networks

---

15 **How important is succession planning?**

Increasingly in nursing and throughout higher education, succession planning is important. Part of effective succession planning is identifying talent and providing opportunities for the person to grow and develop in order to be part of the next generation of leaders. Deans need to be vigilant in identifying opportunities to nominate and support their faculty and staff in programs, courses, or other learning arenas that will develop new skills. Deans serve as role models for faculty and students just as faculty serve as role models for one another and for students. People watch one another to see if they want to aspire to that role or position. Deans, as are many others in the organization, should be leaders, and strong leadership is built on service to others.

---

16 How can I best prepare to assume the role of dean someday?

There are a number of beneficial ways to prepare oneself to be a dean or director. First, there are development programs offered by organizations such as the American Association of Colleges of Nursing that are designed to provide skill development in academic administration. These programs offer content, networking, and mentoring. Many universities offer programs that are designed for leadership development. There is a growing awareness in academia of the importance of investing in leadership development. Read what you can on the subject in nursing and related literature; take advantage of appropriate programs, workshops, and institutes; and find a mentor who will provide guidance and support.

The author acknowledges and thanks Dorothy Powell, EdD, RN, FAAN, Former Dean, College of Nursing and Health Sciences, Division of Nursing, Howard University, Washington, DC, who developed many of the questions used in this section.

40

Faculty Roles and Expectations

Jane Marie Kirschling, DNS, RN

---

1 What are the different types of faculty positions?

The types of available faculty positions will depend on the institution for which you are interested in working. Key aspects of a faculty position include whether it is a tenure track versus non-tenure track and expectation of performance in a single or multiple missions (e.g., teaching, research/scholarship, service).

All institutions of higher education recognize the importance of the teaching mission, and this is commonly an expectation of all faculty. What varies is the amount of time dedicated to teaching and whether a faculty member can be granted tenure solely on the basis of his or her contributions to the teaching mission. Research-intensive universities often have the option of offering a research-focused faculty appointment, which typically carries an expectation that a significant portion, if not all, of the individual's time is funded through external sources. Certain institutions (especially academic health centers) may offer the opportunity for a practice-focused faculty appointment, which carries expectations for clinical practice as well as teaching, service, and clinical scholarship.

2 What key questions should I ask during my interview?

- Is the position tenure-track? If yes, and if you have a master's degree, do you need to obtain your doctoral degree in order to be tenured? What is the time frame for review of tenure, and what happens if tenure is not granted? If the position is not tenure-track, what is the duration of your contract (e.g., 1 year, 2 years), and are there any limitations on renewal? How will your performance be evaluated and at what time intervals?

3 If I am interested in an academic-year versus fiscal-year position, what implications does this have for benefits and vacation?

Typically, faculty in academic year (9- or 10-month) and fiscal year (11- or 12-month) positions have the same health-care benefits and the same retirement benefits proportional to their salary. Academic-year faculty typically do not accrue vacation but are off on holidays recognized by their institutions. Some universities close during extended holidays. Fiscal-year faculty usually accrue vacation; it is important to understand how many hours you can carry forward from one year to the next. Sick time is handled differently across institutions; it is important to understand what you are eligible for at the time of hire.

4 What is included in my faculty workload?

The Southern Regional Educational Board Council on Collegiate Education for Nursing (2002) defined the nurse educator role to include the teacher role, scholar role, and collaborator role. However, institutions vary in their expectations on how faculty will contribute to this traditional tripartite role. It is essential that you understand how workload is determined. Establishing a solid teaching foundation, including reflecting on student and peer feedback, is important, particularly during the initial years of your faculty appointment. Explore whether you will have the opportunity for some stability in your teaching assignment from semester to semester or year to year. Discuss what the expectations are in relation to research/scholarship productivity. Finally, understand how service to the nursing program, university, community, and profession is valued. The tendency of new faculty is to overcommit to the service mission, often at the expense of research or scholarship. Before accepting a new committee responsibility, remember that "working smart requires transforming existing commitments and resources into opportunities for creating scholarly products that are shared with the broader nursing community" (Witt & Heinrich, 2000, p. 71).

5   Am I expected to teach across levels of nursing students (e.g., undergraduate, master's, doctoral)?

Although some faculty will be presented with the opportunity to teach across the continuum of nursing educational programs, most will teach within one or two levels of nursing. Each level of nursing student presents unique teaching opportunities and challenges. Consequently, teaching all levels in any given academic year can place considerable demands on the faculty member's time and expertise. Undergraduate nursing students are learning about the complexities of the human body and are truly novices as they enter health care. The development of critical thinking skills is foremost on faculty members' minds as they engage undergraduate students in learning how to become a nurse. The majority of master's students bring health-care experience with them into the classroom. Faculty must encourage these students to draw from their past experiences while educating them as specialists. Key is optimizing graduate students' ability to lead, initiate change, and use evidence to inform decision making. Doctoral students, often novices in research, require considerable support to develop their technical writing skills, to maintain their research focus, and to actively engage in research.

6 How much time will I need to develop and revise courses and prepare for class?

The first time you offer a course or clinical, you will find that considerable preparation time will be needed. Preparation of a 3-hour class, for example, may require 9–12 hours the first time it is offered. However, after the first offering, the preparation time should decrease to 1–3 hours, depending on how stable the course content is and the extent of revisions you may want to make. Often, faculty members will share their lecture notes, course assignments, and test banks. Simply giving someone else's lecture may save you time, but the richness of the learning opportunity may be lost. Although you can spend more time preparing, it is important to find a balance that also allows you to engage in research/scholarship and service.

7 If scholarship is expected in my faculty role, what criteria are used to evaluate my work?

Having a clear understanding of the criteria that will be used to evaluate your scholarship is essential. For example, you need to find out whether you will be expected to have peer-reviewed publications, secure grant funding, serve as a primary investigator, and/or present in national venues. If you are in a tenure-track appointment, carefully review promotion and tenure criteria not only within your academic unit but also within the larger university. Often the criteria will include the concept of "sustained productivity." In essence, once tenure is granted, the institution has made a lifetime commitment. Consequently, the institution wants to see a consistent pattern of high-level productivity that is likely to continue in future years. As well, discover whether your institution expects you to have a regional, national, and/or international reputation in your area of expertise. The higher the expectation, the more important it is to have a highly focused plan for your scholarship.

Prior to 1990, scholarship was synonymous with research, and nursing faculty members were expected to generate new knowledge. In his 1990 book *Scholarship*

Reconsidered: Priorities of the Professoriate, Ernest Boyer challenged higher education to expand scholarship to include four components: discovery (research), application (practice), integration, and teaching. Since then, nursing and other disciplines have embraced the broader conceptualization, especially at non–research-intensive universities (Bartels, 2007). If you are in an institution that has adopted Boyer's conceptualization, it would be useful to read his original work. Also, read Lee Shulman's work on scholarship of teaching and learning (Alferink, 2006; Glassick, 2000). In addition, the nursing literature includes models that have been adopted at specific institutions (e.g., Sherwen, 1998; Shoffner, Davis, & Bowen, 1994; Stull & Lantz, 2005), and institutions such as Pennsylvania State University have done considerable work amplifying the broader definition of scholarship (Hyman, et al., 2000).

---

8 What resources are available to support my scholarship?

Faculty in research-intensive environments often have access to internal funding for pilot research, editorial support for grant writing and manuscript preparation, ready access to statisticians, and financial support to present in peer-reviewed venues. Faculty in non–research-intensive environments may also have access to pilot funding on a smaller scale, some travel support, and access to statistical or editorial consultation on a case-by-case basis.

---

9 What is expected of me in terms of writing grants for external funding?

Writing and securing grant funding will depend on the type of institution and type of faculty position. Tenure-track and research-track nursing faculty in research-intensive institutions are expected to support their program of research and a portion of their salaries through external funding. To be competitive for external funding, pilot work and release time for scholarship are essential, in addition to having access to colleagues in other disciplines with complementary research interests who can serve as primary investigators and co-investigators.

10 How do I prioritize opportunities to be active in my academic unit and the university?

Some schools of nursing have explicit guidelines for the amount of service that is expected within the academic unit; for example, every faculty member is expected to serve on one school committee and one department committee. If there are no explicit guidelines, talk with the person to whom you report in order to find out the "norm" for new faculty. It is important to find a balance that includes actively participating in the work of your academic unit but not at the expense of the other missions. University service, although important, should not be pursued during your initial years on faculty. In many institutions, it is not uncommon to protect junior faculty from heavy service commitments within the university and to reserve these opportunities for tenured and/or senior faculty.

11 How much and in what types of community service should I be engaged?

Community service involves activities outside of the university and can include a range of opportunities. Examples include serving on boards or committees of community organizations (e.g., American Cancer Society), engaging in community fund-raising for a health-related cause (e.g., American Heart Association Heart Walk), and doing health screening of children attending a summer camp. As you consider community service, ask how the opportunity enhances your areas of expertise. If there is not a direct link to your area of expertise, then it makes sense to pass on the opportunity. Examples of a good fit include agreeing to serve on a local hospice quality committee (if your teaching and scholarship focus on end-of-life care) and agreeing to serve on a governor's council on health and fitness (if you teach pediatric nursing and your research focuses on obesity in children). Community service is important for institutions that are actively engaged in their city, region, and state; however, be strategic in your community service activities, because doing more is not necessarily better, especially if you are pursuing tenure.

---

12 What type, and how much, professional service should I pursue?

Professional service provides an excellent opportunity to engage with colleagues in your specialty area and in your state, region, and nation. Be selective when volunteering; it is typical that new members in professional nursing organizations have to work their way up the organization. A good first step is to determine how the organization selects individuals to serve on committees or the board of directors. Then volunteer, knowing that your offer to become involved may not be immediately acted on. The key in professional service is to balance it with your other commitments and not to do it in place of the contributions you are expected to make in the other missions.

---

13 What is the faculty member's role in advising students?

Expectations for advising vary across institutions and degree programs. As a new faculty member, talk with senior advisors, whether staff or faculty, to learn about the resources that are available to support you as an advisor (Light, 2001). When working with traditional students, there is often a need to provide structure and to make sure they understand how to navigate within the institution. If the student is shy, you may find that you initially do most of the talking. The key over time is to support the student. Adult learners, whether they are in second degree, master's, or doctoral programs, are likely to need support that "more closely resembles a trustworthy peer relationship than a mentorship" (Marques & Luna, 2005, p. 5). Whatever the level of student, it is essential that the faculty advisor serve as a student advocate and understand the degree requirements and sequencing of course offerings to ensure students have practical advice.

14 How available should I be to students?

Many schools of nursing require that faculty have posted office hours during the academic year, and you should be prepared to spend some time after class or clinical to answer student questions. In addition, determine your preference in terms of students reaching you during the work week, whether through your office phone number, e-mail, home phone, or cell phone. It is normally not expected that you allow contact during non–work hours; if you do so, put limits on when students can call you (e.g., before 9 p.m.). Consequently, access your voice mails and e-mails on a regular basis, ideally daily, so that you can respond to student inquiries in a timely manner.

15 How do I prioritize my time to accomplish all that is expected of me?

Know your daily schedule in terms of time management: when do you do your best work, need for blocks of time to engage in scholarly writing, requirements for class preparation, and what strategies you have to be most effective in organizing your work to meet deadlines. It is important that you recognize the amount of time that will be needed to complete a specific project and be realistic in how much time you actually have available to accomplish what is necessary. Develop a strategy for managing the volume of daily communication. Finally, make sure you have downtime from work. Given the volume and nature of the work, there is a tendency to have it spill over into weekends and vacations. It is important to find balance in your life to sustain quality work over time.

16 What resources are available to support my professional development, including development as a teacher?

Universities often have teaching support centers that assist faculty in enhancing classroom instruction through workshops and consultation. Some institutions also offer graduate course work in teaching. Inquire whether there is a mentorship program for new faculty (Brown, 1999). For nursing faculty who have clinical assignments, it is likely that you will need to look inside the nursing program for support and seek advice of seasoned clinical instructors. When you receive your student evaluations, meet with the person who is responsible for your evaluation to review the feedback and to get a sense of how the feedback compares with that of others. Develop a plan for addressing any concerns, especially if there is a consistent pattern in the feedback (e.g., grading criteria were not clear). Depending on your comfort level, you may want to be explicit with students about any major changes you have made in the course based on their feedback. This sends a strong message that you value student feedback. Finally, determine whether there are funds to support your attendance at regional or national nursing meetings that will support your development as a teacher or researcher.

---

17 How can I best compete for faculty development funds for attending state, national, or international meetings?

First, learn from your unit and institution about what funds are available and what is involved in the application process. Your rationale for wanting to attend a particular meeting should include a clear statement as to what you hope to gain from the experience and how it will contribute to your ability to meet the expectations of your faculty position. Being clear about how you will disseminate what you have learned at the meeting will also enhance your application. It is important to note that future requests for development funding may be evaluated within the context of the positive outcomes from past investments.

---

18 I am very interested in maintaining a faculty practice. Is this possible with a full-time faculty position?

Schools of nursing vary in how they handle faculty practice, whether as a registered nurse or advanced practice registered nurse. Some schools have faculty practice plans that serve as sources for revenue generation. The faculty practice plan will specify whether faculty members are eligible for compensation in addition to their faculty salary. Other schools of nursing may, within the policies of the home institution, allow faculty to practice for additional compensation up to 1 day a week. Given this variability, it is important to understand how faculty practice is managed within your school.

Typically, it is expected that faculty involved in clinical instruction of undergraduate students will maintain practice expertise. In some cases, this may include personal experience in caring for individuals, families, communities, or populations. In other cases, providing clinical supervision within the undergraduate program is allowed instead. Discuss faculty practice expectations as part of the interview.

Nursing faculty members who are advanced practice registered nurses must maintain a clinical practice to remain certified. The time involved in actual practice will vary depending on the needs of the nursing program, faculty member interest, and availability of a practice site. Whether you are teaching in an undergraduate program and/or a graduate program, it is important to acknowledge the actual time involved in your faculty practice and to strategize how to orient the practice opportunity in support of your work across missions.

---

19 In addition to my teaching position, can I work elsewhere?

Discuss the ability to be employed elsewhere with the person to whom you report. As previously stated, many institutions allow faculty to spend up to a day a week in outside activities (e.g., consulting) as long as this work does not interfere with university responsibilities.

---

20 What strategies should I use to get to know my nursing colleagues?

It is important that you participate in faculty, committee, and course meetings as a way of connecting with your colleagues. In addition, find out whether faculty gather in a common area for lunch, and join in as time allows. Some new faculty have also found it helpful to form a group with other new members as a means of support (e.g., Jacelon, et al., 2003; Lewallen, et al., 2003).

---

21 What computer and other skills are important for my success as a faculty member?

With the commitment that every faculty member has a computer on his or her desk comes the expectation that you will be proficient with word processing; presentation software; e-mail; online course management systems (e.g., Blackboard); and other software that is unique to your teaching assignment or research interests, e.g., using handheld computers or personal digital computers in clinical instruction (George & Davidson, 2005) and statistical software for analyzing research data. Instructors who teach online courses are expected to become proficient with the technology for online instruction (Barker, 2003).

As with other work environments, faculty members need to have proficient verbal and writing communication skills, be committed to creating an environment that is characterized by civility, be willing to work in groups to accomplish common goals, and be responsive to deadlines. Within the academy, the concept of collegiality is often discussed. Balsmeyer, Haubrich, and Quinn (1996) describe collegiality through four broad statements: "willingness to serve on committees and perform work necessary to departmental operations, willingness to provide guidance and help colleagues in their professional duties, respect for the ideas of others, and conduct of one's professional life without prejudice toward others" (p. 264).

---

22 If the faculty at my institution is unionized, what does this mean to me?

If you work in a unionized institution, read the union contract to see what is included in relation to salary, workload, and so on; determine how active the nursing faculty is in the union; and ask whether the faculty has gone on strike or limited work within the university (e.g., suspended involvement in university committee work) in response to contract negotiations.

23 Whom should I turn to if I have questions or concerns?

Although you might solicit informal advice from your faculty colleagues, it is important that you establish a solid working relationship with the person to whom you report. This individual is the best person for answering your questions or advising you with whom you should talk.

24 How are faculty members evaluated?

Newly hired faculty are typically evaluated annually according to the university's format for evaluation. The evaluation process typically involves review with at least one administrator and often a peer review committee. The evaluation should include the opportunity to address the missions that are a part of your faculty position.

Ask colleagues if they are willing to share their evaluation materials with you as examples. This will facilitate your understanding of the level of detail that you should provide as part of your evaluation. Early on, you should become familiar with the promotion and tenure criteria for your academic unit, and be prepared to demonstrate how your work is meeting or exceeding the criteria.

25 How is student feedback obtained on my teaching, and who sees student evaluations?

Once grades have been posted, teachers have the opportunity to review their student and course evaluations. Someone in administration, for example an associate dean, reviews all student feedback on teaching effectiveness to identify areas of concern that require follow-up. Once you review your student evaluations, do not hesitate to ask for a meeting with your supervisor to discuss the feedback. Course evaluations are reviewed by administration as well as by the appropriate program committee.

26 Should I invite faculty peers to observe my classroom and/or clinical teaching?

Determine whether your academic unit requires some form of classroom or clinical observation; if so, find out how the feedback will be used in your evaluation. If you do not agree with the feedback, share your concerns with the observer, and prepare a written response as part of the evaluation materials. If you choose to invite peer observation, provide the individual with specific information on what you would like him or her to evaluate. For example, if you have recently revised the class to include small group assignments, ask the observer for feedback on how engaged the students appeared to be in the assignment. Encourage the observer to be honest with recommendations for improvement.

27 What documents should I save for reappointment, promotion, and tenure?

Early on in your faculty appointment, ask what types of documents you should retain; when in doubt, keep the document. Some institutions encourage faculty to save thank-you letters for guest lecturers, unsolicited feedback from students, and conference brochures that list your presentation or poster title. Others are less stringent. Having a central repository is key, whether it is a file drawer or a box. Every 6–12 months, you should review and organize the materials that you have saved and update your curriculum vitae.

28 What attributes are likely to foster my success in the faculty role?

Key attributes that will foster your success in the faculty role include collegiality with faculty and staff, good follow-through, sound communication skills, a willingness to say, "I don't know the answer but will find out," and a commitment to continuous improvement, whether in the classroom, in your research or scholarship, or in your service activities. Hard work is a given, so being able to follow your passion is important.

References

Alferink, L.A. (2006). Making teaching public. PsychCRITIQUES, 51(50).

Balsmeyer, B., Haubrich, K., & Quinn, C. (1996). Defining collegiality within the academic setting. Journal of Nursing Education 35, 264–267.

Barker, A. (2003). Faculty development for teaching online: Educational and technological issues. Journal of Continuing Education in Nursing 34, 273–278.

Bartels, J.E. (2007). Preparing nursing faculty for Baccalaureate-level and graduate-level nursing programs: Role preparation for the academy. Journal of Nursing Education, 46, 154–158.

Boyer, E.L. (1990). Scholarship reconsidered: Priorities of the professoriate. Princeton: The Carnegie Foundation for the Advancement of Teaching.

Brown, H.N. (1999). Mentoring new faculty. Nurse Educator 24(1), 48–51.

George, L.E., & Davidson, L.J. (2005). PDA use in nursing education: Prepared for today, poised for tomorrow. On-Line Journal of Nursing Informatics 9(2).

Glassick, C.E. (2000). Boyer's expanded definitions of scholarship, the standards for assessing scholarship, and the elusiveness of the scholarship of teaching. Academic Medicine 75, 877–880.

Hyman, D., et al. (2000). UniSCOPE 2000: A multidimensional model of scholarship for the 21st century. University Park, Pa.: The UniSCOPE Learning Community.

Jacelon, C.S., et al. (2003). Peer mentoring for tenure-track faculty. Journal of Professional Nursing 19, 335–338.

Lewallen, L.P., et al. (2003). An innovative strategy to enhance new faculty success. Nursing Education Perspectives 24, 257–260.

Light, R.J. (2001). The power of good advice for students. The Chronicle of Higher Education 47(25), B811.

Marques, J.F., & Luna, R. (2005). Advising adult learners: The practice of peer partisanship. Recruitment and Retention in Higher Education 19(6), 5–6.

Sherwen, L.N. (1998). When the mission is teaching: Does nursing faculty practice fit? Journal of Professional Nursing 14(3), 137–143.

Shoffner, D.H., Davis, M.W., & Bowen, S.M. (1994). A model for clinical teaching as a scholarly endeavor. Image: Journal of Nursing Scholarship 26(3), 181–184.

Southern Regional Education Board Council on Collegiate
    Education for Nursing. (2002). Nurse educator competencies.
    Atlanta, GA: Author.
Stull, A., & Lantz, C. (2005). An innovative model for nursing
    scholarship. The Journal of Nursing Education 44, 493–497.
Witt, B.S., & Heinrich. K.T. (2000). Working smart: Turning every-
    day commitments into scholarly outcomes. Journal of
    Continuing Education in Nursing 31(2), 71–75.

41

Anticipating an Academic Career

Katharyn A. May, DNSc, RN, FAAN

1 Are there particular personal traits or characteristics that are especially important for nurse educators?

- All of the personal characteristics associated with professional practice are essential in nursing education. These include:
- High standards in regard to knowledge, skill, judgment, and practice of the profession
- A strong sense of responsibility and accountability
- Excellent interpersonal skills and the ability to establish and maintain rapport with individuals who may not be at their best

2 Are there other traits that are particularly important because of the unique culture and working life of the educator?

- First, one must be willing to work hard to achieve results that may not be evident today or tomorrow. While the nurse in practice can usually identify benchmarks or changes in patients that result from professional nursing care, nurse educators usually must wait longer to see the results of their work. Nurse educators are creating the future of nursing by preparing nurses—clinicians, leaders, scientists—most of whom will go on to practice well beyond the view of faculty. Change in nursing education, while brisk, is not as rapid as change in the practice world, if for no other reason than academic programs change gradually, i.e., usually only from one academic year to the next and no faster than the rate of graduating classes.

Nurse educators should also respect the fact that they work surrounded by others who may have very different perspectives on time and work. Consider the daily life of students—their fears and concerns, the pace of classes and clinical practice, their personal life—and contrast that with the faculty member's very different time schedule—judging performance over weeks and months, planning and completing projects over months or years, or completing a research program over a decade. Nurse educators work for the future rather than the more immediate present. Although all nurse educators become frustrated with the pace of change sometimes, if this lengthened time perspective that is part of the world of the educator seems too slow, that may be an indication that full-time engagement in an academic career may not be the best choice for you.

LIFE OF THE MIND

- Nurse educators must have an appetite for "the life of the mind," meaning that the world of ideas must be as compelling as the world of practice. Usually, individuals who are drawn to a career in education already know they love to learn and to teach. However, that is not, in and of itself, sufficient. One must also enjoy intellectual discourse, that is, the process of testing knowledge and ideas through systematic thought, discussion, and debate. In many ways, nurse faculty members are paid to think, and the products of their work are ideas, new approaches, critiques of old practices, and creation of new knowledge, either by transmitting it (i.e., teaching) or by creating it (i.e., scholarship and research). In order to be successful as a nurse scholar or scientist, one must be able to focus on problems and build expertise and experience in a delimited area, just as clinicians focus within a specialty.

COMMUNICATION

- Educators must communicate their knowledge, not only through teaching students, but also through publishing, presenting to peers and allowing critique of their work in order to refine and improve it. An old nursing adage in practice stated, "If it wasn't charted, it wasn't done." In the academic world, if new knowledge is not published (or communicated and accessible to critique by a wider audience), it has not really been "learned" or "taught."

---

3   Is the culture of nursing education really so different from the culture of practice?

Yes. Professional nursing prides itself on a strong foundation in liberal arts education and a commitment to *education* rather than *training* for practice. This requires nursing education to stand a bit apart from nursing practice and to use that distance to ask questions and search for new knowledge. That distance permits a broader range of thinking and exploration and often results in educators having a perspective slightly different from that of practice leaders regarding where the profession is and where it should go. While too wide a gap between education and practice is unhealthy, some slight separation of thought is in keeping with the historic function of universities, and its importance must not be underestimated.

As a result, the culture of nursing education has values that emanate from the profession and the academy. Success in the practice world, therefore, does not necessarily predict success in the education world. It is important for those considering a faculty career to think about how the unique elements of academic culture may enhance or inhibit their ability to be successful and to understand that academic cultures vary a great deal by type of institution and by style of institutional and school or department leadership. It is also important to recognize that nursing education is struggling to become evidence-based, as is nursing practice. Much of what is done in education derives from the fact that teachers have a tendency to teach as they were taught. Unless faculty members examine assumptions, traditions, and norms in academic life, unproductive and sometimes even destructive patterns are perpetuated (Hall, 2004).

Some elements of nursing education culture parallel the practice world. Nursing education has very strong values associated with excellence in performance; often, nursing instructors are widely regarded as among the best teachers and the strongest and most effective academic citizens on a university campus. However, nursing education also tends to be a bit insular and self-absorbed, allowing faculty to become too removed from the realities of professional practice and to cling to faulty frames of reference. Furthermore, teachers may communicate that graduate education and engagement in research are more important than undergraduate clinical teaching and professional service, despite compelling evidence to the contrary.

---

4 How can new faculty maximize success in the educational institution?

Faculty must become students of the culture in their own institution in order to understand its value structure and how that fits with their individual aspirations as well as the aspirations of the profession. Typically, one can learn a great deal by reading statements of philosophy, mission and purpose, progression and promotion guidelines, and strategic plans. Beyond that, senior faculty colleagues, department chairs, and deans have some responsibility to help those beginning their academic careers to be successful, so conversations with those individuals are also important. In the end, a successful academic career is always a product of "fit": a faculty member whose passion for professional work fits well with the culture and the mission of the institution.

---

5 How are faculty members recognized and evaluated?

The reward structure for faculty varies according to the type of institution and school or department. Expectations and standards should be published and widely available, and academic administrators (i.e., deans, directors, department chairs) are generally responsible for interpreting evaluation standards and processes. Recognition and reward for faculty performance typically occurs in three ways: promotion through ranks; formal awards given by students, peers, or academic administrators to acknowledge achievement; and special allocation of resources useful to the individual faculty member.

---

6   What does promotion mean in an academic sense?

Promotion is usually the most formalized process of recognition and is closely tied to the overall institutional mission. For example, teaching-intensive institutions expect evidence of excellence in teaching with some productivity in scholarship, and promotions are based largely on teaching performance. Research-intensive institutions expect excellence both in teaching and research but will likely value research productivity more heavily in considering promotion. Commonly, academic rank progresses through lecturer, instructor, assistant professor, associate professor, and professor. In addition, the exceptionally qualified full professor can be designated as distinguished professor, university professor, or a named chair. There are also promotions into administrative positions, such as director of the undergraduate program, chair of the acute care nursing department, or associate dean. Usually, these competitive positions go to teachers who are particularly well-suited to the role and who meet exacting criteria.

---

7   Is tenure the ultimate indicator of faculty success?

In institutions where tenure is conferred, the promotion to tenure is usually the most significant step in the process, as conferral of security of position is based not only on evaluation of past performance but also on the potential for future sustained contributions. Many nursing programs have separate promotion guidelines and criteria for tenure-track and clinical-track faculty. This differentiation usually reflects the expectation for research and scholarship for the tenure track and for clinical expertise and leadership for the clinical track. However, tenure is not necessarily the "gold standard" in all institutions or for all faculty within the same institution. Faculty members who are appointed in non-tenure tracks will have other rewards for performance, such as longer employment contracts, salary increases, and perhaps more desirable teaching and service assignments.

8   What are some other rewards?

Conferral of awards for achievement, either by students, peers, or academic leaders, is a less formalized but still meaningful process of reward and recognition. Awards for exemplary teaching, research and scholarship, and community, public, or professional service are relatively common in academic nursing and in higher education in general. Such awards may be only honorary or may include a cash prize and may be given at the department, school, or university level. Performance may also be rewarded by allocating useful resources to high-performing faculty, in the form of funding for certain activities (travel or scholarship expenses) or in a reduction in teaching or service responsibilities.

9   How often are faculty members evaluated?

Timing of faculty performance appraisals should be specified in policies and procedures. Typically, faculty performance is reviewed annually, and these reviews may be tied to merit pay or progression through steps within a particular title. Reviews for promotion to higher rank (with or without tenure) are usually on a longer cycle. Some institutions have rigid cycles (i.e., tenure must be achieved within 5–6 years or employment is terminated), whereas others are flexible. Faculty in non-tenure track may be evaluated only when employment contracts are under review or may be reviewed at set intervals when promotion may also be considered.

10 How is faculty salary determined?

Compensation is usually linked to the institution's formal evaluation structure. Many public institutions have campus-wide grids that link salary to rank and step within rank; in these systems, salaries increase primarily through promotion. Some systems also allow for salary increments based on merit, separate from promotion review.

11 What information is typically important in evaluating faculty?

Again, this depends on the institution's overall mission and is specified in faculty evaluation and promotion guidelines. Evidence of strong teaching performance is always important, and usually evidence of productive service to school/department, university, and the profession or the public is also a factor. In research universities, evidence of a sustained program of scholarship and research productivity is essential. Accomplishments and achievements are recorded in the curriculum vitae, but more direct forms of evidence, such as student and peer evaluations of teaching, letters testifying to the impact of service activities, and external appraisals of publications and scholarly presentations are typically found in promotion dossiers. Usually, faculty members are responsible for writing statements about their approach to their work (i.e., teaching philosophy, overall plan of research/scholarship) as well as an appraisal of their own performance. Often, faculty members are asked to state goals for their work and identify resources needed to achieve those goals. The curriculum vitae is always a critical part of information used in faculty evaluation; it is important to keep copies of publications and records of honors, awards, and invitations to speak and consult and to use these materials to update the curriculum vitae at least annually.

12 How are faculty evaluated in terms of teaching?

Regardless of the type of institution, teaching evaluation is based on student as well as peer appraisal, demonstrable learning outcomes, objective measures (e.g., test scores, progression and pass rates), evaluation of course materials by peers or external reviewers, and awards or recognitions for teaching. Many nursing programs use teaching portfolios to document faculty teaching and to communicate activities focused on the scholarship of teaching (Reece, et al., 2001). Most institutions expect progressive improvement and increasing sophistication and effectiveness in teaching over time. Other forms of teaching, such as invited presentations and lectures, consulting, and use of new technologies, may be important, and evidence of effectiveness of these activities may be required by the institution. Written products, such as manuals and textbooks and publications related to teaching, are also considered.

---

13 Are student and peer evaluations of teaching really important?

Yes, even in research-intensive institutions where research productivity is highly valued. Teaching records do not necessarily need to be perfect; in fact, evidence that a faculty member has changed and ultimately improved teaching based on constructive feedback is usually viewed quite positively. The critical point here is faculty members must take their teaching responsibilities seriously and use feedback about their performance to improve, regardless of how productive they may be in other aspects of their academic role.

---

14 How are faculty members evaluated in regard to research and scholarship?

In research-intensive institutions, faculty performance is judged against performance of others working in comparable institutions in the same field. This is done through external appraisals of the faculty member's impact on a particular field, judged through peer-reviewed publications and grant proposals, and expert reviewers' opinions of the quality and significance of the work. In teaching-intensive institutions, faculty performance in research and scholarship is likely to be judged by systematic and effective efforts to improve teaching and learning as well as evidence of dissemination of scholarship through publications, presentations, and other forms of teaching. Many nursing programs have a number of different faculty roles or tracks, usually designated with a different title series (i.e., tenure-track, clinical or scientist track). Because expectations for time and effort spent in research and scholarship in these roles are different, criteria for evaluation will be different. Nevertheless, expectations should be published and readily available, and those teachers responsible for guiding and mentoring new faculty should be clearly identified and accessible (Foley, et al., 2003; Jones & Van Ort, 2001).

---

15 How true is "publish or perish" in nursing education?

Faculty members are primarily responsible for developing and disseminating knowledge, and publishing is the primary means of dissemination. In research-intensive institutions, faculty members are expected to publish original research as well as synthesis/analysis papers in peer-reviewed nursing and interdisciplinary journals. Typically, there is no special number of publications expected, as quality is more important than quantity. However, a sustained and progressive pattern of dissemination is expected over time, and the impact of the work will be evaluated, evidenced by the numbers of times papers are cited by others, invitations for lectures and keynote speeches, and invitations to serve on scientific committees and expert panels. In teaching-intensive institutions, publications are also likely to be required for progression and promotion. However, there may be less emphasis on original research and scholarship (i.e., developing new knowledge in nursing) and more emphasis on scholarship related to teaching, professional issues in the field, or on clinical publications.

---

16 How are faculty members evaluated for service to their department or school, institution, and the profession?

Research-intensive institutions may expect most service to be in the realm of scientific service (i.e., reviewing and editing journals, membership on funding agencies or scientific panels), whereas teaching-intensive institutions are more likely to emphasize school and campus service related to the teaching mission. Because nursing is a practice discipline, faculty members are also expected to be engaged in professional or public service. Again, specific expectations will depend on campus norms, the specific type of faculty appointment, and the stage of faculty career development. Often, junior faculty members are advised not to overdo service commitments as they are building their own program of teaching and research/scholarship, especially if meeting expectations for tenure is a consideration. In many institutions, extensive and highly effective service may balance out less robust performance in research and scholarship. However, it rarely compensates for persistent and unresolved problems in teaching performance or absence of progress in research/scholarship.

---

17 How do schools ensure that standards for appraising faculty performance are applied fairly and consistently?

Academic institutions generally have well-established procedures to ensure fair and consistent reviews, and academic administrators are responsible for ensuring procedures result in an impartial appraisal. Periodic review of processes and criteria by faculty and administrators is necessary so that a common understanding and consistent interpretation of standards are maintained. However, even though published guidelines may not change, expectations for performance are a product of social interaction and are therefore dynamic. As institutions evolve, so do definitions of success; for this reason, faculty members should rely on guidance and mentorship as much as on published review criteria (Byrne & Keefe, 2002; Wills & Kaiser, 2002).

---

18 Who is promoted to the executive-level academic leadership positions?

Not long ago, there were essentially two models of success in academic nursing: the tenured full professor and the dean, director, or department chair. Both models were primarily defined by the norms of the academy, and individuals who attained these positions typically did so near the end of their careers, after years in professional practice. Typically, full professors and chief academic nursing officers stepped from these positions into retirement.

New patterns are emerging, with nurses moving earlier and more frequently between positions in education and practice into roles in nursing education that did not exist just a decade ago. This dynamic is driven by growing concerns about the aging of the nursing professoriate and by pressures on nursing education to increase faculty productivity across all three critical mission areas, education, research, and academic nursing practice. It is likely that benchmarks for success in nursing education will shift in response to these trends, just as many believe that tenure will diminish in importance as higher education evolves to meet the demands of the information age.

19 What does a successful career in academic nursing look like?

The primary responsibility for developing, testing, and transmitting new knowledge is that of the nursing faculty. The professional lives of faculty members are increasingly as complex and demanding as those of colleagues in the practice world. Just as in practice, educators move through a predictable progression over time. They move from focusing largely on their own students and their own program of teaching and scholarship to a larger responsibility for mentoring advanced students and less experienced faculty and for revising curricula and helping to build new academic programs.

Eventually, success in the faculty role means that one's circle of influence extends beyond school and department to the wider university and professional community. Leadership in academic nursing is expected through sustained and progressive programs of research and scholarship that have a genuine impact on practice, through focused engagement that influences the direction of nursing and nursing education for the future, and through academic administrative leadership that builds the nursing education infrastructure to ensure continued progress.

Resources

American Association of Colleges of Nursing. (2005). Academic leadership in nursing: Making the journey. Washington, DC: Author.

Byrne, M., & Keefe, M. (2002). Building research competence in nursing through mentoring. Journal of Nursing Scholarship 34(4), 391–396.

Foley, B., et al. (2003). Determining faculty development needs. Nursing Outlook 51, 227–232.

Glanville, I., and Houde, S. (2004). The scholarship of teaching: Implications for nursing faculty. Journal of Professional Nursing 20(1), 7–14.

Hall, J. (2004). Dispelling desperation in nursing education. Nursing Outlook 52, 147–154.

Heinrich, K. (2005). Halfway between giving and receiving: A relational analysis of doctorate-prepared nurse scholars' first five years after graduation. Journal of Professional Nursing 21(5), 303–313.

Jones, E., & Van Ort, S. (2001). Facilitating scholarship among clinical faculty. Journal of Professional Nursing 17(3), 141–146.

Reece, S., et al. (2001). The faculty portfolio: Documenting the scholarship of teaching. Journal of Professional Nursing 17(4), 180–186.

Wills, C., & Kaiser, L. (2002). Navigating the course of scholarly productivity: The protégé's role in mentoring. Nursing Outlook 50, 61–66.

Index

A

Abilities
development of
into learning situations, example of, 111
program outcomes related to, 112
vs. developing competence, in learning process, 109
leveling of, in ensuring appropriate learning, 110–111
for success in nursing practice environment, 110
Absences, clinical, management of, 207
Abuse, substance, student with, handling of, 204
Academic career
anticipation of, 531–542
being active in, prioritizing opportunities for, 520
successful, described, 541–542
Academic difficulties, maintaining academic standards and empathy in students experiencing, 407–408
Academic health center (AHC)
faculty role in, 506
nursing dean or director's role in, 506–508
organizational structure of institution, effects on nursing unit operation, 508
perspectives of nursing dean at, 505–514
maintaining programs on nursing unit during periods of budget reduction, 512
organizational structure of institution, 508
succession planning, 513–514

vs. concerns of faculty, 510
types of, 505
vs. small liberal arts school, 505
Academic institutions, distance education at, reasons for, 163–164
Academic misconduct, types of, 418–419
Academic standards, in students experiencing academic difficulties, maintaining of, 407–408
Academic year positions, vs. fiscal year positions, benefits and vacations, 516
Accelerated bachelor's degree, 45
Accommodations, in dealing with conflict, 442
Accountability, 427
Accreditation, achievement tests supporting, 334–335
Accreditation guidelines
curriculum effects of, 156
following of, procedures for, 156
Achievement awards, for faculty, 536
Achievement tests
content-specific, selection of, factors in, 328–329
standardized, 327–337. *See also* Standardized achievement tests
Achievement test business, surge in, 327–328
Achievement test companies, 337
Active involvement, in adult learning, 7
Activism, 423–433
activities reflecting, promoting student involvement, 430
clinical proficiency and, 429
communication in, 431–432
competencies reflecting, 427–428
described, 423
electronic media in, 431–432

543